Recent Advances in
OPHTHALMOLOGY–13

Recent Advances in Ophthalmology–13

Editors

HV Nema MS
Former Professor and Head
Department of Ophthalmology
Institute of Medical Sciences, Banaras Hindu University
Varanasi, Uttar Pradesh, India

Nitin Nema MS DNB
Professor
Department of Ophthalmology
Sri Aurobindo Institute of Medical Sciences
Indore, Madhya Pradesh, India

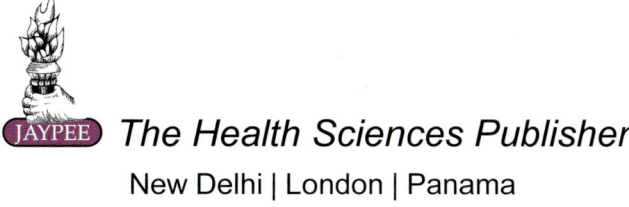

JAYPEE *The Health Sciences Publisher*
New Delhi | London | Panama

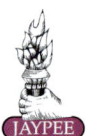
Jaypee Brothers Medical Publishers (P) Ltd

Headquarters
Jaypee Brothers Medical Publishers (P) Ltd
4838/24, Ansari Road, Daryaganj
New Delhi 110 002, India
Phone: +91-11-43574357
Fax: +91-11-43574314
Email: jaypee@jaypeebrothers.com

Overseas Offices

J.P. Medical Ltd
83 Victoria Street, London
SW1H 0HW (UK)
Phone: +44 20 3170 8910
Fax: +44 (0)20 3008 6180
Email: info@jpmedpub.com

Jaypee-Highlights Medical Publishers Inc
City of Knowledge, Bld. 235, 2nd floor, Clayton
Panama City, Panama
Phone: +1 507-301-0496
Fax: +1 507-301-0499
Email: cservice@jphmedical.com

Jaypee Brothers Medical Publishers (P) Ltd
17/1-B Babar Road, Block-B, Shaymali
Mohammadpur, Dhaka-1207
Bangladesh
Phone: +08801912003485
Email: jaypeedhaka@gmail.com

Jaypee Brothers Medical Publishers (P) Ltd
Bhotahity, Kathmandu, Nepal
Phone: +977-9741283608
Email: kathmandu@jaypeebrothers.com

Website: www.jaypeebrothers.com
Website: www.jaypeedigital.com

© 2017, Jaypee Brothers Medical Publishers

The views and opinions expressed in this book are solely those of the original contributor(s)/author(s) and do not necessarily represent those of editor(s) of the book.

All rights reserved. No part of this publication may be reproduced, stored or transmitted in any form or by any means, electronic, mechanical, photocopying, recording or otherwise, without the prior permission in writing of the publishers.

All brand names and product names used in this book are trade names, service marks, trademarks or registered trademarks of their respective owners. The publisher is not associated with any product or vendor mentioned in this book.

Medical knowledge and practice change constantly. This book is designed to provide accurate, authoritative information about the subject matter in question. However, readers are advised to check the most current information available on procedures included and check information from the manufacturer of each product to be administered, to verify the recommended dose, formula, method and duration of administration, adverse effects and contraindications. It is the responsibility of the practitioner to take all appropriate safety precautions. Neither the publisher nor the author(s)/editor(s) assume any liability for any injury and/or damage to persons or property arising from or related to use of material in this book.

This book is sold on the understanding that the publisher is not engaged in providing professional medical services. If such advice or services are required, the services of a competent medical professional should be sought.

Every effort has been made where necessary to contact holders of copyright to obtain permission to reproduce copyright material. If any have been inadvertently overlooked, the publisher will be pleased to make the necessary arrangements at the first opportunity.

Inquiries for bulk sales may be solicited at: jaypee@jaypeebrothers.com

Recent Advances in Ophthalmology–13

First Edition: 2017

ISBN: 978-93-86322-78-4

Printed at: Samrat Offset Pvt. Ltd.

Dedicated to

Loving memory of Pratibha

Editorial Board

Devindra Sood MD
Director
Glaucoma Imaging Centre
New Delhi, India

Frank Goes MD
Director
Oagchirurgie-Oagheelkunde
Antwerp, Belgium

Jorge L Aliö MD PhD
Director
Vissum Instituite of Ophthalmology
Universidad Miguel Hernández
Alicante, Spain

Jyotirmay Biswas MS FMRF FNAMS FIC (Path) FAICO
Director
Department of Uveitis and Ocular Pathology
Sankara Nethralaya
Chennai, Tamil Nadu, India

Lingam Gopal MS FRCS
Associate Professor and Consultant
Department of Ophthalmology
National University Health System
Singapore
Department of Vitreoretinal Services
Sankara Nethralaya
Chennai, Tamil Nadu, India

Suresh R Chandra MD
Professor
Department of Ophthalmology and Visual Sciences
University of Wisconsin School of Medicine and Public Health
Madison, Wisconsin, USA

Contributors

Amol D Kulkarni MD
Retina Specialist
SSM Health Davis Duehr Dean Eye Care
Adjunct Assistant Clinical Professor
Department of Ophthalmology and Visual Sciences
University of Wisconsin
Madison, Wisconsin, USA

Arindam Chakravarti MS DNB
Consultant Vitreoretinal Surgeon
Department of Ophthalmology
Centre for Sight
New Delhi, India

Arshee Ahmed DO DNB
Associate Consultant
Department of Uvea
Sankara Nethralaya
Chennai, Tamil Nadu, India

Arshi Misbah MS
Senior Resident
Department of Ophthalmology
Maharani Laxmibai Medical College
Allahabad, Uttar Pradesh, India

Arun Gupta MD (Radiodiagnosis), PDCC (Vascular and Interventional Radiology)
Department of Neuroimaging and Interventional Radiology
National Institute of Mental Health and Neurosciences
Bengaluru, Karnataka, India

B Sowkath Ali MS Fellow
Department of Uvea
Sankara Nethralaya
Chennai, Tamil Nadu, India

Charmaine Chai MBBS MMed (Ophth)
Associate Consultant
National University Hospital
Singapore

Chetan Videkar MS Retina Fellow
LV Prasad Eye Institute
Hyderabad, Telangana, India

Dhananjay Shukla MS MAMS
Senior Consultant and Director
Retina-Vitreous Service
Ratan Jyoti Netralaya
Gwalior, Madhya Pradesh, India

Eliza Anthony DNB Fellow
Department of Uvea
Sankara Nethralaya
Chennai, Tamil Nadu, India

Fairooz P Manjandavida MS
Department of Ocular Oncology
Narayana Nethralaya
Bengaluru, Karnataka, India

Govinda Jha B Optom
Center for Ocular Regeneration
Srujana Center for Innovation
LV Prasad Eye Institute
Hyderabad, Telangana, India

Hima Pendharkar DMRD DNB (Radiodiagnosis) DM (Diagnosis and Interventional Neuroradiology)
Associate Professor
Department of Neuroimaging and Interventional Radiology
National Institute of Mental Health and Neurosciences
Bengaluru, Karnataka, India

Jayesh Vazirani MS
Cornea and Ocular Surface Service
Maheshwari Eye Care Hospital
Rajkot, Gujarat, India

Jorge L Aliö MD PhD
Director
Vissum Instituite of Ophthalmology
Universidad Miguel Hernández
Alicante, Spain

Jyotirmay Biswas MS FMRF FNAMS
FIC (Path) FAICO
Director
Department of Uveitis and Ocular Pathology
Sankara Nethralaya
Chennai, Tamil Nadu, India

Kamaljeet Singh MS
Professor and Head
Department of Ophthalmology
MLB Medical College
Allahabad, Uttar Pradesh, India
Secretary
UP State Ophthalmological Society
Past-President
Intraocular Implant and Refractive
Society, India

Krushna Gopal Panda MS Fellow
LV Prasad Eye Institute
Kallam Anji Reddy Campus
Hyderabad, Telangana, India

Lalit Verma MD DNB
Director
Centre for Sight
New Delhi, India

Lingam Gopal MS FRCS
Associate Profession and Consultant
Department of Ophthalmology
National University Health System
Singapore
Department of Vitreoretinal Services
Sankara Nethralaya
Chennai, Tamil Nadu, India

Malarchelvi Palani DO DNB FICO(UK) FTERF
Consultant
Department of Glaucoma
MN Eye Hospital
Chennai, Tamil Nadu, India

Manotosh Ray MD FRCSEd
Senior Consultant
National University Hospital
Assistant Professor
Yong Loo Lin School of Medicine
National University of Singapore
Singapore

Mayuri Bhargava MS
Senior Resident Physician
Department of Ophthalmology
National University Hospital
Singapore

Mihir Kothari MS DNB FPOS FAICO
Diploma in Pediatric Ophthalmology and
Strabismus (USA)
Director
Jyotirmay Eye Clinic
Jyotirmay's Ocular Motility and Binocular
Vision Lab and Pediatric Low Vision Center
Mumbai, Maharashtra, India

Mohamed El Bahrawy MD
Consultant
Vissum Institute of Ophthalmology
Alicante, Spain

Murali Ariga MS DNB FAICO
Head
Department of Glaucoma Services
MN Eye Hospital
Director
Swamy Eye Clinic
Chennai, Tamil Nadu, India

Neha Mohan MS
Consultant
Drishticone Eye Care
New Delhi, India

Contributors

Nivean Madhivanan MS FMRF
Consultant- Vitreo-retina
MN Eye Hospital
Chennai, Tamil Nadu, India

Parthopratim Dutta Majumder MS
Associate Consultant
Department of Uveitis and Ocular Pathology
Sankara Nethralaya
Chennai, Tamil Nadu, India

Ronnie Jacob George MS
Senior Glaucoma Consultant
Department of Glaucoma
Sankara Nethralaya
Chennai, Tamil Nadu, India

Sangeetha Rajagopal DO DNB
Consultant-Retina
MN Eye Hospital
Chennai, Tamil Nadu, India

Santosh G Honavar MD FACS
Director
Department of Ocular Oncology
Centre for Sight
Hyderabad, Telangana, India

Shefali Vyas MD FAAP
Associate Director
Children's Kidney Center
RWJ Barnabas Health
West Orange, New Jersey, USA

Su Xinyi MMed PhD
Consultant
Department of Ophthalmology
National University Hospital
Singapore

Suresh R Chandra MD
Professor
Department of Ophthalmology and Visual Sciences
University of Wisconsin School of Medicine and Public Health
Madison, Wisconsin, USA

TP Das MS
Vice-Chairman
LV Prasad Eye Institute
Kallam Anji Reddy Campus
Hyderabad, Telangana, India

Umesh C Behera MS Fellow
LV Prasad Eye Institute
Suddhananda School of Management and Computer Science Campus
Bhubaneswar, Odisha, India

Upender Wali MS
Senior Specialist and Consultant
Department of Ophthalmology
College of Medical and Health Sciences
Sultan Qaboos University Hospital
Muscat, Oman

Vaibhavi Subhedar MSc (Microbiology)
Consultant Microbiologist and Infection Control Incharge
Bombay Hospital
Indore, Madhya Pradesh, India

Virender Sangwan MS
Dr Paul Dubord Chair in Cornea
Director, Center for Ocular Regeneration
Director, Srujana-Center for Innovation
LV Prasad Eye Institute
Kallam Anji Reddy Campus
Hyderabad, Telangana, India

Preface

The year 2017 marks the 25th year of publication of *Recent Advances in Ophthalmology* (RAO). The main objective of the publication of RAO is to keep abreast the postgraduate students and practicing busy ophthalmologists of South East Asia with the recent development in ophthalmology. It is a tremendous task in which a galaxy of national and international ophthalmologists has been supporting us right from the inception of the book. We received thumbing response from readers and reviewers.

Like its predecessors, the 13th volume of RAO contains selected topics on cornea, uvea, glaucoma, retina and systemic diseases. Editorials on imaging in glaucoma and intravascular interventions in ophthalmic disorders are included to highlight the diagnostic treatment aspect of these diseases respectively.

Refractive lenticule extraction (ReLEx), small incision lenticule extraction (SMILE) is a bladeless and flapless procedure wherein a corneal lenticule is removed by femtoseconed laser. It is less invasive and does not cause dryness and is free of corneal flap complications. However, it is in an evaluation stage. SMILE has several limitations such as, it cannot treat hyperopia and takes longer time for visual recovery. On the other hand, laser-assisted in situ keratomileusis (LASIK) is an established technology which can provide good visual acuity in a short time. It has a versatile ablation profile and can correct all types of ametropia. Aliö and coworker have presented a critical account of both types of refractive surgery.

Many patients with ocular tuberculosis may not present any evidence of primary tuberculosis. It is reported that only 1.4% of patients with primary tuberculosis develop ocular manifestations. Ocular tuberculosis is unilateral and asymmetrical. It may result from hematogenous spread. It may cause a wide spectrum of lesions ranging from ocular surface to optic nerve. Biswas and associates have described the ocular lesions of tuberculosis and summarized the ongoing research and development in the diagnosis and treatment.

Some cases of uveitis pose a challenge to the treating ophthalmologists because they are chronic, recalcitrant and sight threatening. They remain refractory to systemic corticosteroid and immunosuppressant therapy. Both these drugs cause unacceptable side effects; therefore, intravitreal administration of biologicals is considered relatively safer and effective. Majumder and Biswas described the importance of intravitreal therapy.

We know that diabetic macular edema (DME) is the leading cause of blindness in patients with diabetic retinopathy. A poor glycemic control, impaired blood retinal barrier integrity, release of vasoreactive substances and altered vitreoretinal interface play their complex role in the pathogenesis of DME. The control of metabolic factors, laser photocoagulation therapy, and vitrectomy are effective, sight-saving interventions. Das and associates have discussed DME in some details with the help of nice illustrations.

Classical case studies of postoperative endophthalmitis are presented by Verma and Chakravarti in the chapter on endophthalmitis. The pictorial case studies reveal not only the mode of presentations but also their response to the given treatment. Management of endophthalmitis mainly comprises intravitreal antibiotics and pars plana vitrectomy. Authors have described prophylaxis, availability of newer intravitreal antibiotics, cluster infection and legal issues related to endophthalmitis also.

Toxic anterior segment syndrome (TASS) may be confused with blinding endophthalmitis. Hence, it is also included in the volume. The differentiating points between these two conditions are detailed.

Prevention of postoperative endophthalmitis is a joint responsibility of operating surgeons, staff of the theater and paramedical staff. Viewpoints of an experienced microbiologist are projected in the chapter on control of infection in ocular surgery.

Oxidative stress, chronic inflammation and genetic and environmental factors largely contribute to the occurrence of age-related macular degeneration (AMD). Chandra and Kulkarni have reviewed the role of anti-oxidative stress therapies, anti-inflammatory therapies, visual cycle modifying agents, choroidal blood flow enhancing agents and regenerative stem cell therapies in the prophylaxis of AMD and concluded that these therapies lack definitive evidence of benefit. Therefore, Age-related Eye Disease Study (AREDS) formulation remains the mainstay of prophylaxis. Anti-VEGF agents have a definite place in the treatment of wet AMD, but they need repeated intravitreal injections, and develop drug resistance and tissue atrophy from chronic use.

Idiopathic polypoidal choroidal vasculopathy (IPCV) is an ill-understood clinical entity that has some common features of AMD. Whether AMD and PCV represent two different and distinct entities or are variants of the same disease? Gopal and coauthors have tried to answer these queries. Presence of orange nodules, large hemorrhages, absence of drusen and typical indocyanine green (ICG) angiography picture helps to differentiate the two different disease entities.

Chapters on ocular sarcoidosis, retinoblastoma, ocular surface disorder, macular phototoxicity, herpes, nystagmus, Behçet's disease, and cystinosis have also been included in this volume.

Recent developments in ophthalmology have significantly revolutionized the treatment of eye diseases and improved the quality of patient's life. It is hoped that readers especially postgraduates, and residents and general practitioners will find the book useful in the examination and day-to-day care of their patients, respectively.

HV Nema
Nitin Nema

Acknowledgments

We express our sincere thanks and appreciation to all authors of *Recent Advances in Ophthalmology-13* for their very informative contributions. Dr Ronnie George and Dr Arun Gupta deserve our grateful thanks for writing the editorials on a short notice.

We are thankful to Shri Jitendar P Vij (Group Chairman), Mr Ankit Vij (Group President) of M/s Jaypee Brothers Medical Publishers (P) Ltd, New Delhi, India, and staff for their continued interest in the publication of the *Recent Advances in Ophthalmology Series*.

Contents

1. **SMILE vs LASIK** — 1
   Jorge L Aliö, Mohamed El Bahrawy
   - Recent Evolution of Laser Refractive Surgery of the Cornea 1

2. **Herpetic Eye Disease** — 11
   Charmaine Chai, Manotosh Ray
   - Epidemiology 11
   - Etiology 12
   - Clinical Presentation 12
   - Risk Factors 14
   - Complications 16
   - Management 16

3. **Recent Advances in Management of Ocular Surface Disorders** — 24
   Jayesh Vazirani, Virender Sangwan, Govinda Jha

4. **Intraocular Tuberculosis** — 32
   Arshee Ahmed, B Sowkath Ali, Jyotirmay Biswas
   - Epidemiology 32
   - Pathogenesis 32
   - Management 42

5. **Ocular Sarcoidosis** — 45
   Eliza Anthony, Parthopratim Dutta Majumder, Jyotirmay Biswas
   - Epidemiology 45
   - Etiology 45
   - Clinical Features 46
   - Diagnosis 49
   - Treatment 53

6. **Advances in Intravitreal Therapeutics in Uveitis** — 56
   Parthopratim Dutta Majumder, Jyotirmay Biswas

7. **Current Role of Imaging in Glaucoma Management** — 65
   Malarchelvi Palani, Sangeetha Rajagopal,
   Nivean Madhivanan, Murali Ariga
   - Scanning Laser Polarimetry 65
   - Confocal Scanning Laser Ophthalmoscope 69

- Heidelberg Retinal Tomography III *72*
- Optical Coherence Tomography *73*
- Scanning Laser Polarimetry *81*
- Confocal Scanning Laser Ophthalmoscope *82*
- Optical Coherence Tomography *85*
- Future Developments in Glaucoma Imaging *93*

8. Postoperative Endophthalmitis 99
Lalit Verma, Arindam Chakravarti

- Bacterial Endophthalmitis *100*
- Fungal Endophthalmitis *108*
- Chronic Endophthalmitis *109*
- Prevention and Prophylaxis *112*
- Newer Intravitreal Antibiotics *113*
- What to Do, in Case of Infection? *114*
- What to Do in Cluster Infections or Outbreak? *114*
- Legal Issues Related to Endophthalmitis *115*

9. Toxic Anterior Segment Syndrome 117
Kamaljeet Singh, Arshi Misbah

- Epidemiology *117*
- Etiology *118*
- Clinical Features *119*
- Prevention *122*
- Treatment *122*
- Clinical Outcome and Prognosis *122*

10. Control of Infection in Ocular Surgery 125
Vaibhavi Subhedar

- Progress in Intraocular Cataract Surgery *125*
- Epidemiology of Postoperative Endophthalmitis *126*
- Risk Factors for Endophthalmitis *127*
- Pathogens *128*
- Prophylaxis *129*
- Policy *133*

11. Diabetic Macular Edema 139
Neha Mohan, Chetan Videkar, Umesh C Behera, Krushna Gopal Panda, TP Das

- Risk Factors *139*
- Pathogenesis *139*
- Classification *141*
- Symptoms and Signs *145*
- Treatment *146*
- Surgery: Vitrectomy *155*

12. New Frontiers in the Treatment of AMD 160
Suresh R Chandra, Amol D Kulkarni

- Emerging Therapeutic Options in Dry AMD *161*
- Emerging Therapeutic Options in Wet AMD *165*

13. Polypoidal Choroidal Vasculopathy 170
Lingam Gopal, Mayuri Bhargava, Su Xinyi

- Demographics *170*
- Clinical Presentation *170*
- Management *174*

14. Macular Phototoxicity 185
Dhananjay Shukla

15. Retinoblastoma 193
Fairooz P Manjandavida, Santosh G Honavar

- Genetics *193*
- Classification and Staging *194*
- Clinical Features *195*
- Diagnosis *196*
- Management *197*

16. Endovascular Interventions in Ophthalmic Disorders 206
Hima Pendharkar

- Case 1: Idiopathic Intracranial Hypertension *208*
- Case 2: Intracranial Dural Arteriovenous Fistula *212*
- Case 3: Cavernous Internal Carotid Artery Aneurysms *215*
- Case 4: Carotid Cavernous Fistula *218*
- Case 5: Posterior Communicating Artery Aneurysm *223*
- Case 6: Occipital Arteriovenous Malformation *224*

17. Nystagmus 230
Mihir Kothari

- Management *244*

18. Cystinosis 255
Shefali Vyas

- Clinical Manifestations *256*
- Extrarenal Manifestations *256*
- Pathogenesis *257*
- Diagnosis and Management *258*
- Treatment *259*

19. Behçet's Disease 261
Upender Wali

- Historical Aspect *261*

- Nonocular Manifestations *264*
- Ocular Manifestations of Behçet's Disease *267*
- Behçet's Disease in Children *273*
- Behçet's Disease in Pregnancy *274*
- Ancillary Tests *277*
- Differential Diagnosis in Behçet's Disease *278*
- Treatment *279*
- Prognosis for Vision in Behçet's Disease *282*

Index *289*

Editorial 1

Evolution of Imaging Technology in Glaucoma

Ronnie George

The past two decades have seen the availability of commercially available instruments that could image the optic head and nerve fiber layer. This was an exciting development as various reports had suggested that more than 20% nerve fiber layer loss occurred before the then available functional tests could detect visual field damage.[1] Development of these techniques—the Heidelberg Retinal Tomograph (HRT) and GDx Nerve Fiber Analyzer gave rise to the possibility that it was now possible to image and detect the optic disc damage early. However, early studies demonstrated sensitivities and specificities in the mid-eighties—not really consistent with a paradigm shift in our ability to diagnose glaucoma in everyone earlier than would be possible with conventional perimetry.[2]

This poor diagnostic performance is primarily a function of the huge inter-individual variability seen in optic disc morphology. Since, optic disc size itself shows an almost 600% variation. It is unlikely that any device would accurately classify optic discs as normal or glaucomatous with very high accuracies.[3] This led to the realization that the true potential of imaging would be in the field of progression and reports demonstrated that imaging had the potential to detect change before it occurred on visual fields.

The advent of the GDx gave us the ability to actually measure the nerve fiber layer parameters and was a new clinical parameter entirely. It demonstrated extremely good diagnostic capability in the initial reports, subsequent reports however put its diagnostic ability on par with the other imaging devices. The GDx also had the misfortune of having three significant hardware changes during its lifetime. These were carried out as a way to minimize the effect that other birefringent structures had on the nerve fiber layer measurements. While this resulted in improved testing accuracy this came at the cost of no backward compatibility with earlier versions of the device. This effectively limited its utility in assessing progression since few patients had long-term follow-up on a single device. The advent of the spectral domain optical coherence tomography (OCT) effectively sounded the death knell for the GDx since you now had a device which could measure nerve fiber layer (NFL) at higher resolutions in addition to having retinal applications too.

While, the OCT revolutionized macular imaging, its impact on glaucoma was less dramatic with time domain technology. While, it was as effective as the HRT and GDx in detecting the disease there were concerns about the follow-up scans not being obtained from the same locations as the baseline scans because of poor image registration. This limited its utility in assessing progression as compared to the HRT where good image registration was available.

The resolution of the OCT was further enhanced with the spectral domain OCT. This was made possible by the improved hardware and the improved computation power available. However, these generational changes were also backward incompatible rendering a lot of follow-up data useless. The HRT was in this respect an excellent tool because the hardware changes still permitted backward compatibility with earlier scans. The longest optic disc follow-ups for glaucomatous eyes is possibly available on the HRT because of the backward compatibility making it possible to use patient data from earlier devices for comparison. However, the HRT III will no longer be manufactured while support will be provided for existing devices. This has effectively limited the future utility of the HRT since most newly detected glaucoma patients would be imaged on the OCT.

The spectral domain OCT promised superlative resolutions. However, these resolutions are rarely seen in clinical practice partly because of issues with eye movements and scan artefacts. In spite of this, the level of detail available and measurement accuracies mean that it is better at detecting progression than earlier devices. However, the large number of device manufacturers is an issue since measurements between various devices are not the same and patients would have to be imaged on the same device for meaningful data on progression.

While the devices are helpful in classifying disease one must always remember that "abnormal" values on imaging are statistical abnormal and in the absence of corroborating clinical data should not be taken at face value as evidence of disease. The over diagnosis of glaucoma because of the so called "red disease" is very common and results in unnecessary medications and hardship to the patient. It is also worth keeping in mind that most normative databases include only eyes with "normal" optic disc morphology. There are very few macrodiscs or microdiscs. Tilted and otherwise anomalous discs are also not included. Using any imaging tool on such eyes will invariably result in abnormal results which do not necessarily indicate glaucomatous damage. It is also important to keep in mind that the imaging techniques perform better at detecting glaucoma progression early in the disease. In more advanced disease, perimetry is still more sensitive in detecting progression.

The adaptive optics devices promise almost cellular resolutions. They are currently limited by very small image windows which limit their utility in glaucoma detection.

Further improved resolutions and testing algorithms on the OCT will make it possible to perhaps detect progression earlier. This would require a rethink of our clinical strategies. Unfortunately, too rapid changes in technology are sometimes detrimental in glaucoma since in a slowly progressive disease our patients need to be tested for years before we can detect slow rates of progression. While highlighting the importance of imaging keep in mind its limitations and the need for clinical judgment before any major diagnostic or therapeutic decisions are made.

■ REFERENCES

1. Kerrigan-Baumrind LA, Quigley HA, Pease ME, Kerrigan DF, Mitchell RS. Number of ganglion cells in glaucoma eyes compared with threshold visual field tests in the same persons. Invest Ophthalmol Vis Sci. 2000;41(3):741-8.
2. Garway-Heath DF. Early diagnosis in glaucoma. Prog Brain Res. 2008;173(08):47-57.
3. Jonas JB, Mardin CY, Gründler AE. Comparison of measurements of neuroretinal rim area between confocal laser scanning tomography and planimetry of photographs. Br J Ophthalmol. 1998;82(4):362-6.

Editorial 2

Endovascular Interventions in Ophthalmic Disorders
Arun Gupta

Common orbital vascular lesions include cavernous hemangioma, lymphangioma, varix, arteriovenous malformation and vascular fistulas.[1-3] A correct diagnosis is important because natural history and proper management are often dramatically different among no-flow, slow-flow, and higher-flow lesions.

Most of orbital lesions clinically present with proptosis, conjunctival congestion, chemosis, conjunctival bleeding, hemorrhage, pain, dropping of eyelids and restriction in eye movements. Due to these symptoms, patients come to the hospital early to seek the treatment.

For the patients with orbital lesions, a complete evaluation is essential to plan further diagnostic and treatment strategy. A complete high-resolution imaging with computed tomography (CT) or magnetic resonance imaging (MRI) has become most important investigations. Digital subtraction angiography has been considered the gold standard for vascular lesions including orbital lesions. Angiography can provide information about arterial blood supply, venous drainage, vessel caliber, collateral circulation, flow velocity, arteriovenous shunting, and presence of flow-related aneurysms which is essential for planning the interventions. CT and CT-angiography can provide excellent visualization of large and medium-sized blood vessels with dynamic information about blood flow to a vascular orbital lesion.

The various ophthalmic pathologies which can be diagnosed accurately and few of them can be treated using interventional radiological techniques are:
- Orbital vascular lesions
    - Arterial and arteriovenous lesions
        - Arteriovenous malformations
        - Arteriovenous fistulas: Congenital, spontaneous, post-traumatic
        - Ophthalmic artery aneurysms
- Arteriovenous fistulas
    - Carotid-cavernous fistula (CCF): Direct and indirect
        Type A: Direct CCF—cavernous internal carotid artery (ICA) to cavernous sinus
        Type B: Feeders from dural branches of internal carotid artery
        Type C: Feeders from dural branches of external carotid artery
        Type D: Feeders from dural branches of both internal and external carotid arteries.
    - A complex venous anomaly: Deep orbital varix
    - Highly vascular lesions and vascular tumors

- Miscellaneous: Coats disease
- Thrombolysis for central retinal artery
- Venous lymphatic malformations—capillary, cavernous, and cystic lymphatic malformations.

Surgery for these lesions is difficult due to high-risk of bleeding. The highest degree of success has been found when vascular malformations are treated by a multidisciplinary team. Image-guided therapy has proved highly effective with good to excellent results possible in 75–90% of patients.[4] Interventional radiologists have taken a central role in the multidisciplinary team.

To treat vascular lesions of the orbit various routes had been tried with mixed results which are:
- Percutaneous
- Arterial
- Venous
- A combination of above.

Percutaneous Treatment

Various slow flow orbital vascular malformations can be treated via percutaneous route. Most of the malformations can be successfully punctured by needle under guidance of X-ray fluoroscopy, CT, duplex sonography, or MRI. The next step is sclerotherapy of the lesion with the volume estimation of sclerosing agent.[4-7]

The necessary steps for safe performance of sclerotherapy include precise preprocedural lesion visualization and characterization, accurate needle placement, determination of the correct volume of sclerosing agent for injection, and real time monitoring of venous egress during the injection procedure.

Arterial Route

- **Carotid-cavernous fistula (CCF):** Interventional radiology has changed the management of all types of CCFs. The direct CCFs are treated using balloons, coils, stent-assisted coiling or by covered stents with complete cure. The Onyx injection with coils also has been tried with good result.[8]
  The other types of CCF are in reality dural AV fistulas and are treated either by arterial route or via venous route or a combination of it using the same materials. However, venous route using coils and Onyx gives good result and is popular among interventional radiologists.
- **Orbital arteriovenous malformation:** Orbital arteriovenous malformations are rare vascular lesions of the orbit. Endovascular treatment of these lesions is challenging and has to be planned in stages mainly via transarterial route embolization.[9] Onyx and/or n-butyl cyanoacrylate (n-BCA) along with Lipiodol (Guerbet, Villepinte, France) is the choice of the embolic agent. However, there is a small-risk of embolization of the central retinal artery.
- **Arteriovenous fistula other than CCF:** These are rare lesions. Identification of site of fistula and embolization at the site of fistula cures the lesion.
- **Ophthalmic artery aneurysms:** Proper ophthalmic artery aneurysms are extremely rare. The carotid-ophthalmic artery aneurysms are more common but account for a small percentage of cerebral aneurysms. They arise at the origin of the ophthalmic artery from the supraclinoid internal carotid artery. Small aneurysms are asymptomatic but large ones can cause compression of the optic nerve and produce visual symptoms. They may rupture causing intracranial subarachnoid hemorrhage. Depending on the size, they are

treated either only by coils, or stent-assisted coiling or by flow diverters with good result.
- **Thrombolysis for central retinal artery:** Acute sudden vision loss may be due to occlusion of central artery of retina. It is treated as a case of local stroke. If patient reports in time, the thrombolysis can prevent the vision loss.

Venous Route

It is mainly used when lesion cannot be approached through arterial route.

For success of endovascular interventions of orbital lesion, detail knowledge of vascular anatomy, various materials used for procedure, embolic agents is very essential. Predicting the complications and their management is important to obtain good long-term results.

■ REFERENCES

1. Wisnicki JL. Hemangiomas and vascular malformations. Ann Plast Surg.1984;12: 41-59.
2. Wright JE, Sullivan TJ, Garner A, et al. Orbital venous anomalies. Ophthalmology. 1997;104:905-13.
3. Greene AK, Burrows PE, Smith L, Mulliken JB. Periorbital lymphatic malformations: clinical course and management in 42 patients. Plast Reconstr Surg. 2005;115(1):22-30.
4. Burrows PE, Mason KP. Percutaneous treatment of low flow vascular malformations. J Vasc Interv Radiol. 2004;15:431-45.
5. Baker LL, Dillon WP, Hieshima GB, Dowd CF, Frieden IJ. Hemangiomas and vascular malformation of the head and neck: MR characterization. AJNR Am J Neuroradiol. 1993;14:307-14.
6. Goyal M, Causer PA, Armstrong D. Venous vascular malformations in pediatric patients: comparison of results of alcohol sclerotherapy with proposed MR imaging classification. Radiology. 2002;223:639-44.
7. Lewin JS, Merkle E, Duerk JL, Tarr RW. Low-flow vascular malformations in the head and neck: safety and feasibility of MR imaging-guided percutaneous sclerotherapy–preliminary experience with 14 procedures in three patients. Radiology. 1999;211: 566-70.
8. Hayashi N, Masumoto T, Okubo T, et al. Hemangiomas in the face and extremities: MR-guided sclerotherapy—optimization with monitoring of signal intensity changes in vivo. Radiology. 2003;226:567-72.
9. Gupta AK, Purkayastha S, Krishnamoorthy T, Bodhey NK, et al. Endovascular treatment of direct carotid cavernous fistulae: a pictorial review. Neuroradiology. 2006;48(11):831-9.

Chapter 1

SMILE vs LASIK

Jorge L Alio, Mohamed El Bahrawy

RECENT EVOLUTION OF LASER REFRACTIVE SURGERY OF THE CORNEA

The concepts of modern refractive surgery witnessed its breakthrough when Professor Jose I Barraquer described in 1949 his coined technique of keratomileusis, setting the foundation for all following innovation in this field. The name excimer laser came as an abbreviation of "excited dimer", introduced by the Russian, Nikolay Basov, in 1970 using a xenon dimer gas. Few years later, the argon-fluoride excimer laser was developed and was first tried on an organic tissue by IBM scientists. The introduction of excimer laser to be used in the human eye was done by Stephen Trokel as a precise and safe tool of corneal shaping, these concepts later defined the refractive techniques widely used now, when Marguerite McDonald under the supervision of Steve Kaufmann, performed the most commonly used epithelium removal technique photorefractive keratectomy (PRK). Peyman, presented the first patency of using excimer laser as a corneal refractive tool, and it was accepted in June 1989 (personal correspondence Gholam Peyman). Following Ioannis Pallikaris, among others, introduced the most widely used and commonly accepted technique of laser in situ keratomileusis (LASIK) in 1990.[1] Laser refractive surgery has been performed for decades, and there have been tremendous advancements in terms of technique and technology, making it increasingly precise and highly predictable.[2] LASIK is currently the most common laser refractive procedure for the treatment of myopia—its advantages include early postoperative improvement in visual acuity and minimal postoperative patient discomfort. Although LASIK patients report 95% satisfaction, a spectrum of complicated side effects can negatively impact results.[3]

Femtosecond laser technology was first developed by Dr Kurtz at the University of Michigan in the early 1990s,[4] and was rapidly adopted in the surgical field of ophthalmology. Femtosecond lasers emit light pulses of short duration (10–15s) at 1053 nm wavelength that cause photodisruption of the tissue with minimum collateral damage.[5] The femtosecond laser has revolutionized corneal and refractive surgery with respect to its increased safety, precision, and predictability over traditional microkeratomes. Advantages of bladeless femtosecond assisted LASIK (FS-LASIK) over conventional microkeratome assisted LASIK (MK-LASIK) include reduced dry eye symptomatology, reduced risk of flap button hole or free cap formation.[6,7]

Ever since femtosecond lasers were first introduced into refractive surgery, the ultimate goal has been to create an intrastromal lenticule that can then be manually removed as a single piece thereby circumventing the need for incremental photoablation by an excimer laser. A precursor to modern refractive lenticule extraction (ReLEx) was first described in 1996 using a picosecond laser to generate an intrastromal lenticule that was removed manually after lifting the flap,[8,9] however, significant manual dissection was required leading to an irregular surface. The switch to femtosecond improved the precision[10] and studies were performed in rabbit eyes in 1998[11] and in partially sighted eyes in 2003[12] but these initial studies were not followed up with further clinical trials. Following the introduction of the VisuMax femtosecond laser (Carl Zeiss Meditec, Jena, Germany) in 2007,[13] the intrastromal lenticule method was reintroduced in a procedure called femtosecond lenticule extraction (FLEx). The 6-month results of the first 10 fully seeing eyes treated were published in 2008[14] and results of a larger population have since been reported.[15,16] The refractive results were similar to those observed in LASIK, but visual recovery time was longer due to the lack of optimization in energy parameters and scan modes; further refinements have led to much improved visual recovery times.[17] Following the successful implementation of FLEx, a new procedure called *small incision lenticule extraction (SMILE)* was developed. This procedure involves passing a dissector through a small 2–3 mm incision to separate the lenticular interfaces and allow the lenticule to be removed, thus eliminating the need to create a flap. The SMILE procedure is now gaining popularity following the results of the first prospective trials.[18-29]

Small Incision Lenticule Extraction (SMILE) Outcome

Since, the development of the SMILE technique, the exciting new concept of the flapless nature of the technology, namely the *3rd generation laser refractive surgery*, has driven many authors to approach it and report the results of SMILE outcomes alone or in comparison with LASIK.

In a study we conducted, we compared the outcomes of a matched case of SMILE versus 6th generation excimer laser LASIK patient, where the cases were matched by age, gender and spherical equivalent. In the SMILE group; 50% females, 34 years (23:49), –4.59 diopters (–2.125:–8.37), the LASIK group; matching SMILE/FLEx cases: of same gender, age (±1 year), spherical equivalent (±0.5 D). The study included 16 eyes in each group, and we reported both SMILE and LASIK had comparable results in terms of safety, efficacy and predictability, in follow up of 6 months duration (Table 1.1).

TABLE 1.1: Refractive outcome of comparative study between SMILE and LASIK

Comparison		SMILE	FS-LASIK
Efficacy	20/20 or more	93.75%	92.18%
	20/25 or more	100%	96.87%
	20/40 or more	100%	100%
	No loss of lines	96.87%	93.43%
	Lost more than 2 lines	0%	0%
	Gained lines	18.75% (1 line)	18.64% (1–3 lines)
Predictability	% of cases ± 0.5 D	84.43%	86.25%
	% of cases ± 1.0 D	100%	100%

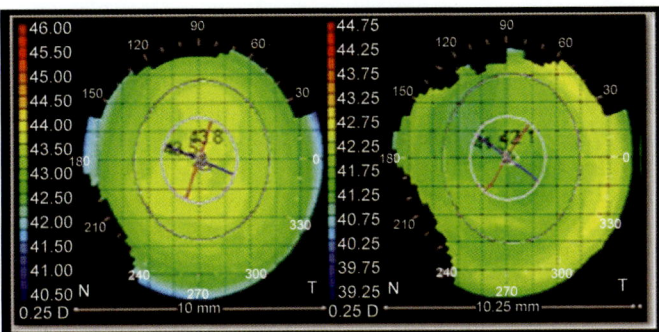

A −2.25D: (Left) Preoperative; (Right) After SMILE correction

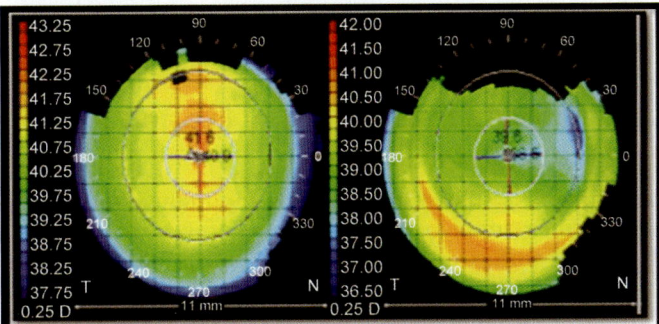

B −2.00D: (Left) Preoperative; (Right) After LASIK correction

Figs 1.1A and B: Topographical changes in moderate myopia

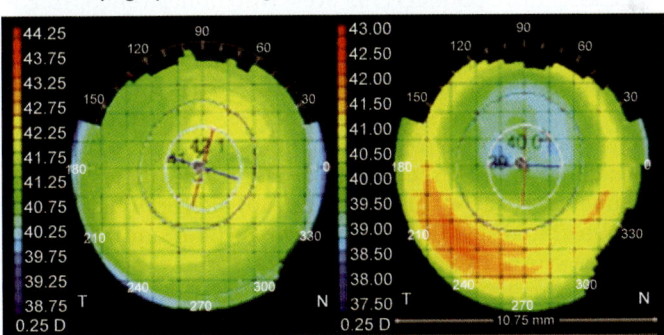

A −8.00D: (Left) Preoperative; (Right) After SMILE correction

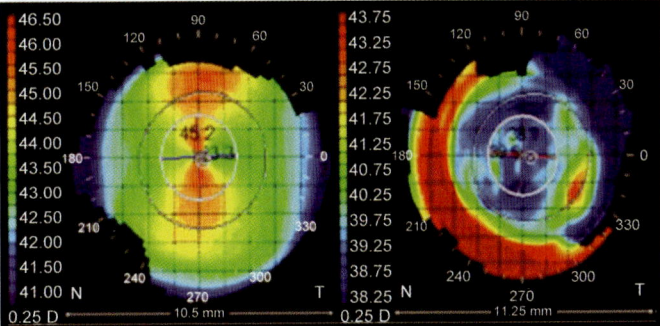

B −9.25D: (Left) Preoperative; (Right) After FLEx correction

Figs 1.2A and B: Topographical changes in high myopia

Many other authors reported similar outcomes, still with a disadvantage of slower refractive recovery in SMILE patients, which is currently witnessing significant improvements due to the development of different energy and spot spacing setting.[17,21] Kim et al. reported that age may be a predictor that influenced visual outcome, as outcomes were better in younger patients of his study sample but its effect appeared clinically insignificant.[22] SMILE surgery was effective and safe in correcting low to moderate astigmatism, and stable refractive outcomes were observed at the long-term follow-up. The preoperative cylinder ranged from –2.75 D to –0.25 D (average of –0.90 ± 0.68 D), and the mean postoperative cylinder values were –0.24 ± 0.29 D, –0.24 ± 0.29 D, and –0.20 ± 0.27 D at 1 month, 6 months, and 12 months, respectively.[23]

On the other side topographic changes and barometric changes were significantly lower in SMILE patients compared with LASIK patients whether in mild to moderate myopia or high myopia as reported by results of our study (Figs 1.1 and 1.2).

Advantages of SMILE in Cases of Dry Eye and Ocular Surface Disease

The flapless nature of SMILE will preserve the important anterior corneal phase, this will preserve the natural integrity of corneal nerves, which will significantly influence the ocular surface and tear film stability (Fig. 1.3).

Central corneal sensitivity exhibited a small decrease and a faster recovery after the SMILE procedure compared to FS-LASIK during the first three postoperative months. Corneal sensitivity after SMILE and FS-LASIK was similar at 6 months after surgery.[24] Qiu et al. in a longitudinal retrospective study studied ninety-seven consecutive patients (193 eyes) who underwent SMILE for myopia. Parameters evaluated included: subjective dry eye symptoms (dryness, foreign body sensation and photophobia), tear film breakup time (TBUT), Schirmer's test without anesthesia, tear meniscus height (TMH) and corneal fluorescein staining. Each parameter was evaluated before, and subsequently at 1 day, 1 week, 1 month and 3 month after surgery. The results showed that compared with preoperative data, dryness was noted to be significantly increased at 1 week and 1 month postoperatively ($P < 0.01$). Symptoms of photophobia and foreign body sensation demonstrated significant differences at 1 day and 1 week as compared with preoperative scores respectively ($P < 0.01$). These values were decreased at 1 and 3 month postsurgery ($P > 0.05$). Conversely the corneal staining scores were higher than the preoperative data at 1 day, 1 week and 1 month ($P < 0.01$), but were close to the preoperative level at 3 months postoperatively. There was a significant decrease in TMH at 1 week and 1 month ($P < 0.01$), but the value

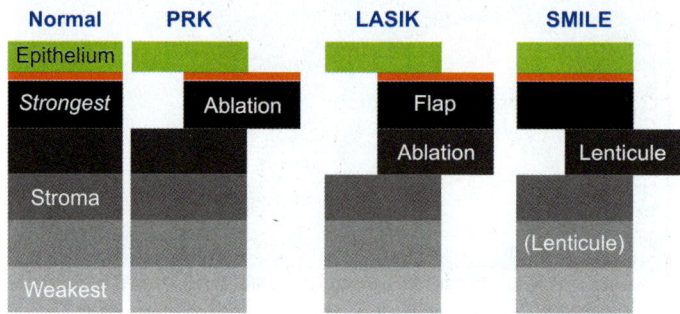

Fig. 1.3: Effect of different refractive procedures on the anterior corneal surface

was close to the preoperative level at 3 months postoperatively (P = 0.16). The examination outcomes of ST were significantly increased at 1 day then reduced at 1 week after surgery (P <0.01). Each value subsequently returned to the baseline value at 1 and 3 months (P >0.05). TBUT was significantly decreased at all postoperative time points (P < 0.01). It is reported that SMILE resulted in mild dry eye symptoms, tear film instability and ocular surface damages; however, these complications can recover in a short period of time.[25] This was confirmed when compared with FS assisted LASIK by Li et al. as he reported that SMILE surgeries resulted in a short-term increase in dry eye symptoms, tear film instability, and loss of corneal sensitivity. Furthermore, SMILE surgeries have superiority over femto-LASIK in lower risk of postoperative corneal staining and less reduction of corneal sensation.[26]

Tear Inflammatory Mediators in SMILE

In a study by Gao et al. Tears were collected and analyzed for interleukin-6 (IL-6), tumor necrosis factor alpha (TNF-α), nerve growth factor (NGF) and intercellular adhesion molecule-1 (ICAM-1) levels using multiplex magnetic beads. All measurements were preformed preoperatively and 1 day, 1 week, 1 month and 3 months postoperatively. They reported that In the early postoperative period, ReLEx SMILE results in milder ocular surface changes than FS-LASIK. Furthermore, the tear inflammatory mediators IL-6 and NGF may play a crucial role in the ocular surface healing process following ReLEx smile and FS-LASIK.[27] SMILE induces less keratocyte apoptosis, proliferation and inflammation compared with femtosecond laser LASIK.[28]

Biomechanical Properties of the Cornea in SMILE

Randleman et al. suggested that the cohesive tensile strength of the stroma is based on how the stromal lamellae are held together, which decreases from anterior to posterior within the central corneal region. Reinstein et al. used a mathematical model to predict that the postoperative tensile strength would be higher after SMILE than both LASIK and PRK, given the fact that the strongest anterior lamellar layer remains intact, enabling it to correct higher levels of myopia with a better safety profile. In our investigation, we studied biomechanical corneal properties by comparing targeted vs obtained radius of curvature (Fig. 1.4).

The mean values and standard deviation of the curvature change coefficient are: [*(Paired T-test) SMILE: –1.77 ± 1.72 (%), FS-LASIK: –1.82 ± 3.76 (%)*]. A good

---

Coefficient of Biomechanical Response:

$$C = \frac{R_{post} - R_S}{R_S} \times 100$$

R_{post}: Postsurgical corneal radius (1 month after)

R_s: Surgical radius sculpted on corneal stroma by laser ablation (calculated)

- C characterizes the change in corneal curvature due to biomechanical response of the corneal surface after the flap cut and relocation (LASIK) or lenticule cut and extraction (SMILE and FLEX)
- **Meaning:** $C>0$ $R_{post} > R_S$ *Flattening (overcorrection)*
  $C<0$ $R_{post} < R_S$ *Steepening (undercorrection)*

Fig. 1.4: Mathematical model for calculation of corneal tensile properties

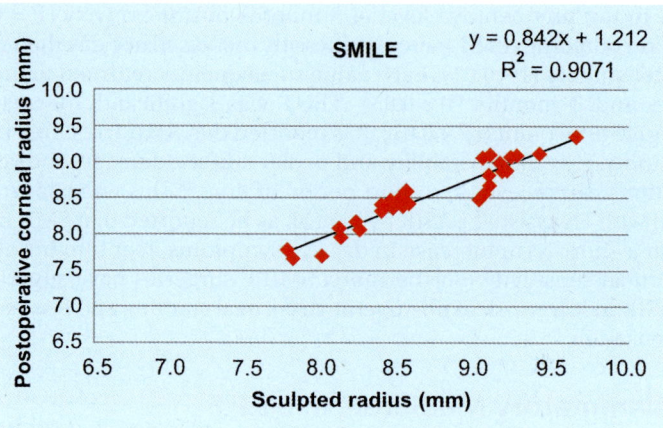

Fig. 1.5: Results of biomechanical tensile changes in SMILE and FS-LASIK

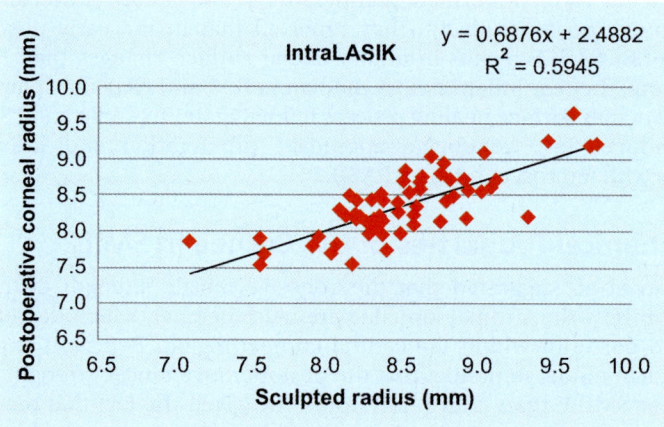

Fig. 1.6: Results of biomechanical tensile changes in SMILE and FS-LASIK

correlation for the linear fit: *(Pearson Correlation) R = 0.95 for SMILE group R = 0.85 for FLEX group.* There are not statistically significant differences (P>0.1) between two groups. However, the low standard deviation of the SMILE group demonstrates a better predictability for this technique (Figs 1.5 and 1.6).

Other study used Scheimpflug-based noncontact tonometer, concluded that no significant modifications in biomechanical properties were observed after SMILE so this procedure could induce only minimal transient alterations of corneal biomechanics.[29] When correlating corneal biomechanical properties with the induced high-order aberrations. The preoperative CRF was significantly correlated with the induced 3rd–6th order HOAs and spherical aberration of the anterior surface and the total cornea after SMILE and FS-LASIK surgeries (P<0.05), postoperatively. The CRF was significantly correlated with the induced vertical coma of the anterior and posterior surfaces and the total cornea after SMILE surgery (P<0.05). There was a significant correlation between the CRF and the induced posterior corneal horizontal coma after FS-LASIK surgery (P = 0.013). This indicates that corneal biomechanics affect the surgically induced corneal

HOAs after SMILE and FS-LASIK surgery, which may be meaningful for screening the patients preoperatively and optimizing the visual qualities postoperatively.[30] On the other hand in high myopic patients, FS-LASIK demonstrated a greater increase in posterior corneal elevation than SMILE only at 12 months as well as a greater reduction of CRF than SMILE, but there were no significant difference between the two groups over time.[31]

Confocal Microscopy in SMILE

In confocal microscopy study, the mean backscattered light intensity (LI) at all measured depths and the maximum backscattered LI were higher in the SMILE group than the femto-LASIK group at all postoperative visits. LI differences at 1 week and 1 month and 3-month visits were statistically significant ($P< 0,05$). LI differences at 6 months were not statistically significant. There was no difference in the number of refractive particles at the flap interface between the groups at any visit. It may be concluded that SMILE results in increased backscattered LI in the anterior stroma when compared with femto-LASIK.[32] The decrease in sub-basal nerve fiber density was less severe in the SMILE group than the FS-LASIK group in the first 3 months following the surgery. The sub-basal nerve density was correlated with central corneal sensitivity.[33]

Corneal Cap Precision in SMILE

There is a significant change in corneal deformation parameters following SMILE procedure. The changes may be caused predominantly by stromal lenticule extraction, while lenticule creation with femtosecond laser may not have an obvious effect on corneal deformation properties.[34] A study conducted investigating the morphology of SMILE cap using anterior segment optical coherence tomography reported that corneal caps of SMILE are predictable with good reproducibility, regularity and uniformity. Cap morphology might have a mild effect on refractive outcomes in the early stage.[35] and the predictability of cap thickness in SMILE surgery does not differ from the femto-LASIK flaps created using the same femtosecond laser platform.[36]

Enhancements after SMILE Surgery

One of the most important challenges facing SMILE technology is the enhancement methodology in postoperative refractive residuals. In a study enrolled 28 eyes 27 underwent the VisuMax® Circle pattern procedure for refractive enhancement, and 1 for residual lenticule extraction. In 100% of cases (28 eyes) the lifting of the flap was possible, as planned. In all cases of refractive enhancement (27 eyes) by LASIK, the exposure of the stromal bed was sufficient for the necessary excimer laser ablation. No eyes lost two or more Snellen lines of corrected distance visual acuity (CDVA) and no procedure or flap related complications or serious adverse events occurred. This initial case series demonstrates that VisuMax® Circle pattern is efficacious and a suitable method to create a corneal flap for enhancement, following small incision lenticule extraction.[37]

Innovative Indications of Laser Lenticular Extraction

1. *The technique of cryopreservation of corneal lenticules extracted after small incision refractive lenticule extraction (ReLEx SMILE) and initial results of*

femtosecond laser intrastromal lenticular implantation for hyperopia: The technique seems to be a safe method of long-term storage of refractive lenticules extracted after ReLEx SMILE for use in allogeneic human subjects. It may potentially be a safe and effective alternative to excimer laser ablation for hyperopia because of the low risks of regression, haze, flap-related complications, postoperative dry eye, and higher-order aberrations.[38]
2. *ReLEx SMILE Xtra, small-incision lenticule extraction with accelerated cross-linking; in patients with thin corneas and borderline topography:* Based on the initial clinical outcome it appears that SMILE Xtra may be a safe and feasible modality to prevent corneal ectasia in susceptible individuals.[39] Also this has been investigated in *forme fruste* keratoconus and irregular corneas, combined small-incision lenticule extraction and intrastromal corneal collagen cross-linking are a promising treatment option for patients for whom conventional laser refractive surgery is contraindicated.[40]
3. Finally, A feasibility study reported that LASIK can be performed following lenticule re-implantation to create presbyopic monovision. The tissue responses elicited after performing LASIK on corneas that have undergone SMILE and subsequent lenticule re-implantation are similar to primary procedure.[41]

REFERENCES

1. El Bahrawy M, Alió JL. Excimer laser 6th generation: state of the art and refractive surgical outcomes. Eye Vis (Lond). 2015;2:6.
2. Alio J. Refractive surgery today: is there innovation or stagnation? Eye Vis (Lond). 2014;1:4.
3. Alio JL, Muftuoglu O, Ortiz D, Pérez-Santonja JJ, Artola A, Ayala MJ, et al. Ten-year follow-up of laser in situ keratomileusis for high myopia. Am J Ophthalmol. 2008;145:46-54.
4. Soong HK, Malta JB. Femtosecond lasers in ophthalmology. Am J Ophthalmol. 2009;147:189-97.
5. Ratkay-Traub I, Ferincz IE, Juhasz T, Kurtz RM, Krueger RR. First clinical results with the femtosecond neodymium-glass laser in refractive surgery. J Refract Surg. 2003; 19:94-103.
6. Salomao MQ, Wilson SE. Femtosecond laser in laser in situ keratomileusis. J Cataract Refract Surg. 2010;36:1024-32.
7. Morshirfar M, Gardiner JP, Schliesser JA, Espandar L, Feiz V, Mifflin MD, et al. Laser in situ keratomileusis flap complications using mechanical microkeratome versus femtosecond laser: retrospective comparison. J Cataract Refract Surg. 2010;36: 1925-33.
8. Krueger RR, Juhasz T, Gualano A, Marchi V. The picosecond laser for nonmechanical laser in situ keratomileusis. J Refract Surg. 1998;14:467-69.
9. Ito M, Quantock AJ, Malhan S, Schanzlin DJ, Krueger RR. Picosecond laser in situ keratomileusis with a 1053-nm Nd:YLF laser. J Refract Surg. 1996;12:721-28.
10. Kurtz RM, Horvath C, Liu HH, Krueger RR, Juhasz T. Lamellar refractive surgery with scanned intrastromal picosecond and femtosecond laser pulses in animal eyes. J Refract Surg. 1998;14:541-8.
11. Heisterkamp A, Mamom T, Kermani O, Drommer W, Welling H, Ertmer W, et al. Intrastromal refractive surgery with ultrashort laser pulses: in vivo study on the rabbit eye. Graefes Arch Clin Exp Ophthalmol. 2003;241:511-7.
12. Ratkay-Traub I, Ferincz IE, Juhasz T, Kurtz RM, Krueger RR. First clinical results with the femtosecond neodynium-glass laser in refractive surgery. J Refract Surg. 2003;19:94-103.

13. Reinstein DZ, Archer TJ, Gobbe M, Johnson N. Accuracy and reproducibility of Artemis central flap thickness and visual outcomes of LASIK with the Carl zeiss meditec VisuMax femtosecond laser and MEL 80 excimer laser platforms. J Refract Surg. 2010;26:107-19.
14. Sekundo W, Kunert K, Russmann C, Gille A, Bissmann W, Stobrawa G, et al. First efficacy and safety study of femtosecond lenticule extraction for the correction of myopia: six-month results. J Cataract Refract Surg. 2008;34:1513-20.
15. Blum M, Kunert KS, Engelbrecht C, Dawczynski J, Sekundo W. Femtosecond lenticule extraction (FLEx)—results after 12 months in myopic astigmatism. Klin Monbl Augenheilkd. 2010;227:961-5.
16. Vestergaard A, Ivarsen A, Asp S, Hjortdal JØ. Femtosecond (FS) laser vision correction procedure for moderate to high myopia: a prospective study of ReLEx(®) flex and comparison with a retrospective study of FS-laser in situ keratomileusis. Acta Ophthalmol. 2013;91(4):355-62.
17. Shah R, Shah S. Effect of scanning patterns on the results of femtosecond laser lenticule extraction refractive surgery. J Cataract Refract Surg. 2011;37:1636-47.
18. Sekundo W, Kunert KS, Blum M. Small incision corneal refractive surgery using the small incision lenticule extraction (SMILE) procedure for the correction of myopia and myopic astigmatism: results of a 6 month prospective study. Br J Ophthalmol. 2011;95:335-9.
19. Shah R, Shah S, Sengupta S. Results of small incision lenticule extraction: All-in-one femtosecond laser refractive surgery. J Cataract Refract Surg. 2011;37:127-37.
20. Reinstein DZ, Archer TJ, Gobbe M, et al. Small incision lenticule extraction (SMILE) history, fundamentals of a new refractive surgery technique and clinical outcomes. Eye Vis (Lond). 2014;1:3.
21. Vestergaard A, Ivarsen AR, Asp S, Hjortdal JO. Small-incision lenticule extraction for moderate to high myopia: predictability, safety, and patient satisfaction. J Cataract Refract Surg. 2012;38:2003-10.
22. Kim JR, Hwang HB, Mun SJ, Chung YT, Kim HS, et al. Efficacy, predictability, and safety of small incision lenticule extraction: 6-months prospective cohort study. BMC Ophthalmol. 2014;14:117.
23. Zhang J, Wang Y, Wu W, Xu L, Li X, Dou R, et al. Vector analysis of low to moderate astigmatism with small incision lenticule extraction (SMILE): results of a 1-year follow-up. BMC Ophthalmol. 2015;15:8.
24. He M, Huang W, Zhong X, et al. Central corneal sensitivity after small incision lenticule extraction versus femtosecond laser-assisted LASIK for myopia: a meta-analysis of comparative studies. BMC Ophthalmol. 2015;15:141.
25. Qiu PJ, Yang YB. Early changes to dry eye and ocular surface after small-incision lenticule extraction for myopia. Int J Ophthalmol. 2016;9(4):575-9.
26. Li M, Zhao J, Shen Y, Li T, He L, et al. Comparison of dry eye and corneal sensitivity between small incision lenticule extraction and femtosecond LASIK for myopia. PLoS ONE. 2013;8:10.
27. Gao S, Li S, Liu L, Wang Y, Ding H, et al. Early Changes in Ocular Surface and Tear Inflammatory Mediators after Small-Incision Lenticule Extraction and Femtosecond Laser-Assisted Laser In Situ Keratomileusis. PLoS ONE. 2014;9:9.
28. Dong Z, Zhou X, Wu J, et al. Small incision lenticule extraction (SMILE) and femtosecond laser LASIK: comparison of corneal wound healing and inflammation. Br J Ophthalmol. 2014;98:263-9.
29. Mastropasqua L, Calienno R, Lanzini M, et al. Evaluation of corneal biomechanical properties modification after small incision lenticule extraction using Scheimpflug-based noncontact tonometer. Biomed Res Int. 2014;2014:290619.

30. Wang Y, Wu W. The Correlation Analysis between Corneal Biomechanical Properties and the Surgically Induced Corneal High-Order Aberrations after Small Incision Lenticule Extraction and Femtosecond Laser In Situ Keratomileusis. J Ophthalmol. 2015;2015:758196.
31. Wang B, Zhang Z, Naidu RK, et al. Comparison of the change in posterior corneal elevation and corneal biomechanical parameters after small incision lenticule extraction and femtosecond laser-assisted LASIK for high myopia correction. Cont Lens Anterior Eye. 2016;39(3):191-6.
32. Agca A, Ozgurhan EB, Yildirim Y, et al. Corneal backscatter analysis by in vivo confocal microscopy: fellow eye comparison of small incision lenticule extraction and femtosecond laser assisted LASIK. J Ophthalmol. 2014;2014:265012.
33. Li M, Niu L, Qin B, et al. Confocal comparison of corneal reinnervation after small incision lenticule extraction (SMILE) and femtosecond laser in situ keratomileusis (FS-LASIK). PLoS One. 2013;8(12).
34. Shen Y, Zhao J, Yao P, et al. Changes in corneal deformation parameters after lenticule creation and extraction during small incision lenticule extraction (SMILE) procedure. PLoS One. 2014;9(8):e103893.
35. Zhao J, Yao P, Li M, et al. The morphology of corneal cap and its relation to refractive outcomes in femtosecond laser small incisionlenticule extraction (SMILE) with anterior segment optical coherence tomography observation. PLoS One. 2013;8(8).
36. Ozgurhan EB, Agca A, Bozkurt E, et al. Accuracy and precision of cap thickness in small incision lenticule extraction. Clin Ophthalmol. 2013;7:923-6.
37. Chansue E, Tanehsakdi M, Swasdibutra S, et al. Safety and efficacy of VisuMax® circle patterns for flap creation and enhancement following small incision lenticule extraction. Eye Vis (Lond). 2015;2:21.
38. Ganesh S, Brar S, Rao PA. Cryopreservation of extracted corneal lenticules after small incision lenticule extraction for potential use in human subjects. Cornea. 2014;33(12):1355-62.
39. Ganesh S, Brar S. Clinical outcomes of small incision lenticule extraction with accelerated cross-linking (ReLEx SMILE Xtra) in patients with thin corneas and borderline topography. J Ophthalmol. 2015;2015:263412.
40. Graue-Hernandez EO, Pagano GL, Garcia-De la Rosa G, et al. Combined small-incision lenticule extraction and intrastromal corneal collagen crosslinking to treat mild keratoconus: Long-term follow-up. J Cataract Refract Surg. 2015;41(11):2524-32.
41. Lim CH, Riau AK, Lwin NC, et al. LASIK following small incision lenticule extraction (SMILE) lenticule re-implantation: a feasibility study of anovel method for treatment of presbyopia. PLoS One. 2013;8(12):e83046.

Chapter 2

Herpetic Eye Disease

Charmaine Chai, Manotosh Ray

INTRODUCTION

Herpetic keratitis is an infection of the cornea caused by the herpes simplex virus (HSV) type 1 or 2. Like many viruses, the herpes simplex viruses are present in most adults. The viruses in the herpes family usually live around the nerve fibers in humans without ever causing any problem. Occasionally, the viruses will start to multiply, or they will move from one area of the body to another, and that is when herpetic disease breaks out. This often happens when some other disease process significantly weakens the immune system of the body. It can manifest in various forms depending on the level of the corneal involvement. The pathogenesis and management differs between an epithelial keratitis, stromal keratitis or endotheliitis along with iridocyclitis. Early diagnosis is necessary in order to initiate the appropriate treatment.

This chapter describes the common manifestations of herpetic keratitis and their management based on our experience.

EPIDEMIOLOGY

Herpes simplex virus keratitis can affect all ages. Herpes simplex virus is endemic throughout the world and humans are the only known natural reservoir. Studies suggest that nearly 90% of world population is infected by latent HSV1 infection by the time they are 60 years old. HSV1 is primarily transmitted through direct contacts. The rate of infection is affected by the amount of exposure to potential sources of infection. Socioeconomic status of the patient plays a significant role. Children with lower socioeconomic status have higher rate of seroconversion than with middle class and above. The reported incidence of new cases of ocular HSV is about 8.4 to 13.2 cases per 100,000 per year.[1-3] HSV1 has been found to be the main causative virus in herpetic eye disease, accounting for about 95% of ocular HSV. HSV 2 is less commonly isolated, and more commonly associated with genital herpes.

Herpes simplex virus is a common cause of corneal infection and one of the leading infectious causes of corneal blindness worldwide. Ocular herpes is typically unilateral. However, bilateral herpetic manifestations have been observed in children[4] and atopic individuals.[5,6] The Herpetic Eye Disease Study (HEDS), a multi-arm placebo controlled trial was designed to determine best treatments and prophylaxis for HSV keratitis as well as to investigate the risk factors of the disease. Herpes simplex virus epithelial keratitis and stromal keratitis accounted for 47% and 16% of ocular HSV infection respectively in the

HEDS trial.[7] The study focussed on use of oral acyclovir to prevent the epithelial and stromal keratitis and thus provided valuable epidemiological data, especially in regards to the recurrence rates of the disease. HEDS found an ocular HSV recurrence rate of 32% over 1 year.[7] A history of previous episode of HSV stromal keratitis and a high number of previous episodes were associated with a higher risk of subsequent attacks. The reported risk of recurrence after the first episode is about 9.6% in the first year, and 22.9% at 2 years. The cumulative risk of recurrence was about 50% at 10 years.[1] The number of recurrences was strongly associated with past episodes. Therefore, a history of HSV stromal keratitis and a high number of previous episodes increase the risk of future recurrence. The study also suggested that short interval between attacks tend to be associated with shorter intervals between future attacks.[7]

Ocular HSV infection is responsible for visual disability in approximately 1,000,000 people each year world-wide. It is also estimated that there are 1,000,000 new cases and 900,000 recurrent infections each year globally. The average time from onset of symptoms to resolution of an active herpetic eye infection varies between 17 and 28 days. Therefore, the number of global man-hour loss from HSV eye infection is alarmingly significant.

ETIOLOGY

Herpes simplex virus keratitis is caused by the HSV I and HSV II, that are part of the human herpes virus family. These are double-stranded DNA viruses made up of a core DNA surrounded by icosahedral-shaped capsid. HSV I and HSV II are typically differentiated by virus specific antigens. HSV I primarily affects the oropharynx region while HSV II typically involves the genital area, although there are exceptions of the rule. Transmission of the disease occurs by direct contact with infected secretions or lesions.

After primary infection, the HSV virus can remain dormant within the trigeminal nerve or manifest with frequent reactivation. Primary infection can be asymptomatic or present as a benign form of blepharoconjunctivitis. Ocular manifestations are the result of ocular inflammation and viral activity. This is more often secondary to viral reactivation as compared to primary infection. Active viral replication has been demonstrated in tear samples collected from patients with active epithelial and stromal disease.[8] The viral load detected in the tears was found to be higher in epithelial compared to stromal keratitis.[9] Periodic shedding of HSV into the tears can occur even in asymptomatic individuals. Hence, virus transmission can also occur through asymptomatic individuals.

CLINICAL PRESENTATION

Herpes simplex virus (HSV) keratitis has multiple manifestations. The nature of these manifestations is distinctive and can readily be distinguished by careful examination of individual layers of the cornea. HSV keratitis involving different layers of cornea has functionally distinct pathogenesis. HSV epithelial keratitis is believed to be a result of direct infection of epithelial cells, while immune mechanisms are involved in HSV stromal keratitis. Therefore, epithelial keratitis typically requires anti-viral therapy, while stromal keratitis would require topical steroids in addition to anti-viral therapy.

Primary ocular herpes may manifest as blepharitis, conjunctivitis or HSV keratitis. Typically these patients present with unilateral red eye, vesicles on the

TABLE 2.1: Classification of herpes simplex keratitis

Type of HSV keratitis	Clinical manifestation

• Epithelial
  – Dendritic
  – Geographic
	Dendritic ulcer with terminal bulb that stains with fluorescein

• Stromal keratitis
  – Necrotizing
  – Non-necrotizing, immune stromal keratitis
	Stromal infiltrates with or without ulceration
	Deep stromal vascularization
	Immune ring

• Endothelial keratitis
  – Disciform keratitis
  – Diffuse keratitis
  – Linear keratitis
	Corneal edema with keratic precipitates

lids and occasionally with punctate epithelial keratitis. Recurrent disease can manifest as corneal or adnexal infections. HSV keratitis is classified according to the level of involvement of the corneal layers (Table 2.1). The pathogenesis differs depending on the type of manifestation.

Herpes simplex virus epithelial keratitis manifests as a dendritic or geographic ulcer. Dendritic ulcers are the most common presentations of HSV keratitis. Classical features of the ulcer are linear branching pattern with terminal bulbs and swollen epithelial borders. Untreated, dendritic ulcers progress to form geographic ulcers characterized by swollen epithelium and scalloped or geographic borders. This occurs as a result of direct virus infection of the corneal epithelial cells. Hence, antiviral therapy is the mainstay of treatment. Neurotrophic keratopathy may present with punctate epithelial erosion or irregular corneal surface. Eventually, these lesions may progress to a persistent epithelial defect. Typically, these are interpalpebral oval lesions with smooth borders. Stromal ulceration is not uncommon in advanced stage.

Herpes simplex virus stromal keratitis may be the primary manifestation of herpetic keratitis or it may be secondary to other form of keratitis, e.g. epithelial, neurotrophic or even endothelial form of HSV keratitis. Nearly one quarter of epithelial keratitis patients develop stromal keratitis. HSV stromal keratitis may manifest as necrotizing or non-necrotizing forms. Their manifestation is primarily attributed to immune related mechanisms. Hence, topical steroids are necessary on top of topical antiviral therapy. Necrotizing stromal keratitis is believed to result from active viral replication in stromal keratocytes and thereby producing a severe host inflammatory response. Clinical lesion is characterized by dense stromal infiltrate, ulceration and necrosis and often difficult to differentiate from other forms of microbial keratitis. Non-necrotizing stromal keratitis is less severe focal or multifocal stromal infiltrates associated with immune ring and deep corneal neovascularization. Multiple recurrences are common.

Though disciform keratitis can present with stromal involvement, it is more accurately a form of endothelial keratitis presenting with a focal area of corneal edema, associated keratic precipitates, anterior chamber reaction associated with accompanying corneal hypoesthesia.

Herpes simplex virus endotheliitis can manifest either as disciform, diffuse or linear endotheliitis based on the area of corneal involvement. Herpetic endotheliitis is characterized by keratic precipitates, stromal and epithelial edema in absence of any stromal vascularization. Corneal edema is due to endothelial decompensation.

RISK FACTORS

Various factors may increase the virus reactivation. Compromised cell mediated immunity has been suggested to increase the risk of HSV disease and recurrences (Table 2.2). Both systemic and local factors that alter the host immunity can increase the risk of HSV keratitis.

Higher incidence of reactivation have also been reported in HIV,[10-12] atopic and diabetic patients. However, the incidence of HSV keratitis was found to be similar in HIV positive patients compared to those who were tested negative for HIV.[11] Atopic individuals were found to have a higher risk of HSV keratitis, and this risk was greater in patients with severe atopy.[13] Various factors have been postulated to contribute to this. These patients have altered cell mediated immunity with relative imbalance between the T-helper 1 and T-helper 2 (Th-1 and Th-2) response, with a reduction in Th1 response allowing virus reactivation.[14] In addition, many of these patients remain on chronic immunosuppression treatment for their atopic condition. A patient with severe eczema was treated with a course of oral prednisolone and long-term topical steroids. She presented with conjunctival injection and blurring of vision shortly after starting the oral prednisolone. On examination, a geographic ulcer was seen (Figs 2.1A and B). The patient was given topical acyclovir and the oral steroid was stopped. The lesion responded well to treatment and healed within 2 weeks.

Herpes simplex virus keratitis can present more aggressively in children, with more exaggerated inflammatory response and frequent recurrences leading

TABLE 2.2: Risk factors for HSV keratitis

Systemic risk factors	Local risk factors

• Pre-existing conditions that reduce host immunity:
  – HIV infection[11 12]
  – Organ transplant recipients
  – Diabetes mellitus
  – Measles infection
 	
• Altered immunity:
  – Children
  – Atopy
  – Prolonged use of systemic immunosuppression
  – Immune stressors
	• Chronic use of topical medications
	  – Corticosteroids
	  – Prostaglandin analogs[60]
	
	• Surgical procedures
	  – Laser procedures
	  – LASIK
	  – Collagen Cross-linking
	  – Cataract surgery
	  – Corneal transplant

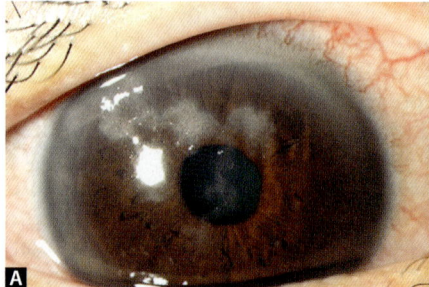
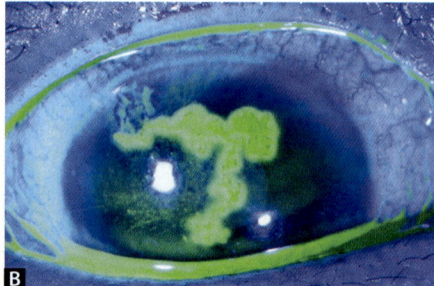

Figs 2.1A and B: Anterior segment photographs of a patient with severe eczema who presents with epithelial keratitis after starting oral steroids

to increased corneal scarring. This is especially detrimental since children are susceptible to amblyopia secondary to corneal opacity and the induced astigmatism.[15] Bilateral disease is also seen more frequently as compared to adults.

Herpes simplex virus reactivation has also been reported to occur as a result of local trauma. Several case reports have been published reporting incidences of HSV keratitis after YAG laser,[16,17] photodynamic therapy,[18] Argon laser trabeculoplasty[19] and laser in situ keratomileusis (LASIK).[20] Recurrences have also been reported after collagen cross-linking.[21-23]

Surgical trauma is a risk factor for recurrences, which is further augmented by the use of postoperative topical steroids. Antiviral prophylaxis can be considered in a select group of patients with a history of HSV keratitis. Few case reports of HSV Keratitis during the first few postoperative weeks after cataract surgery have been reported.[24,25] A patient who presented with left eye irritation and redness 1 week after an uneventful phacoemulsification was on tobramycin and dexamethasone eye drops (Figs 2.2A and B). He responded well to acyclovir therapy and his vision remained good (6/7.5).

The reported incidence of newly acquired herpetic keratitis post penetrating keratoplasty is 1.2 per 1000 person-years and usually occurs in the first 2 postoperative years.[26] Herpetic keratitis can occur as a new onset post-transplant or as a reactivation.[27,28] Recurrence of herpetic keratitis is the main reason for graft failure in patients who undergo keratoplasty for HSV keratitis.[29] Thirty three percent of donor corneas with primary graft failure were found to be positive for HSV1 DNA.[30] Recurrence may be related to regeneration of corneal innervation or due to virus shedding into the tear film. Oral antiviral prophylaxis is recommended in patients with a history of herpetic keratitis and may be continued while the patient is maintained on topical steroids or for the first one to two years post-transplant.[31,32] This has been found to reduce the recurrence rate and graft failure in this group of patients.[33,34] Although there is no clear regime or guideline, studies suggest a maintenance dose of 400 mg oral acyclovir twice a day. Topical acyclovir prophylaxis, on the other hand, is not routinely used as it may lead to epithelial toxicity and is possibly not as effective in preventing recurrence.[35]

A patient who underwent an endothelial keratoplasty about 2.5 years back and was maintained on long-term topical prednisolone acetate eye drops, as part of his postoperative regime, presented with a dendritic ulcer in the right eye (Figs 2.3A and B). His ulcer resolved upon treatment with topical acyclovir but he subsequently developed a metaherpetic ulcer with an overlying epithelial defect and corneal thinning. The epithelial defect healed after 3 weeks with treatment but the residual stromal thinning remained. His vision was 'counting fingers,'

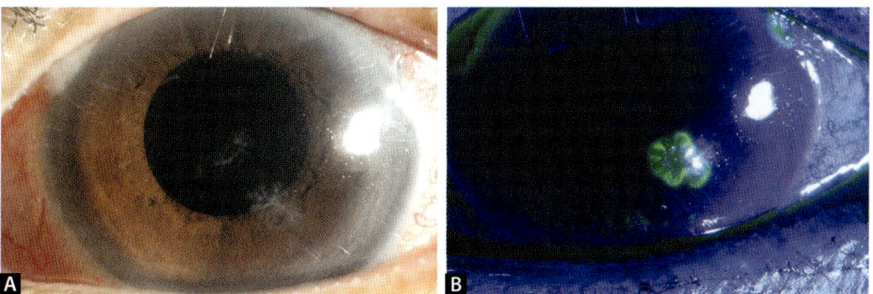

Figs 2.2A and B: Anterior segment photographs of a patient who presents with a herpetic dendritic ulcer 1 week after cataract surgery

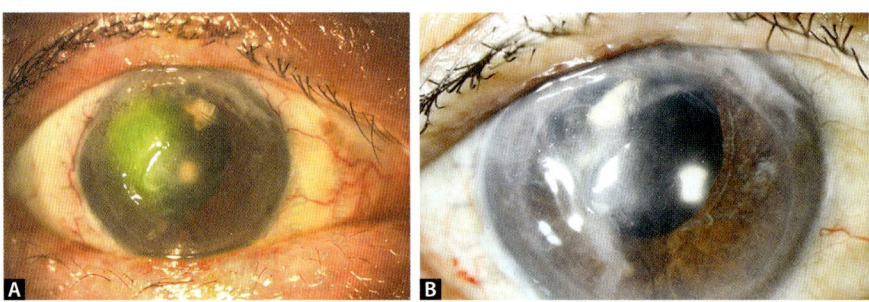

Figs 2.3A and B: Anterior segment photograph at presentation and upon resolution of a patient with metaherpetic ulcer after endothelial keratoplasty

which was contributed by his advanced glaucoma which was being treated with topical anti-glaucoma therapy.

COMPLICATIONS

Corneal Scar

Recurrent keratitis can lead to visual loss from scarring and induced astigmatism. A visible corneal scar was seen in 18% of primary presentation and 28% of recurrent disease. About 73–90% still maintained a visual acuity of 6/12 or better for at least 5 years. Significant scarring and astigmatism may require subsequent keratoplasty.

Neurotrophic Keratopathy

Herpetic keratitis can result in corneal neurotrophy and persistent corneal defect. Metaherpetic ulcers can occur following dendritic or geographic ulcers due to the inability of the epithelium to heal. It occurs in the absence of any live virus. The edges of the ulcer may be rolled up and do not stain with rose Bengal, while the base of the ulcer will stain, exhibiting a 'reverse staining pattern'. Without adequate treatment, this can progress to corneal thinning and perforation.

Bullous Keratopathy

Endothelial decompensation can result from chronic endotheliitis. The reported incidence of endothelial dysfunction is about 0.01% from recurrent ocular HSV.[1]

Corneal Perforation

Destructive intra-stromal inflammation in necrotizing stromal keratitis may lead to devastating complications including severe corneal thinning and corneal perforation. The complication may occur within a short span of time in spite of adequate treatment.

MANAGEMENT

Epithelial Keratitis

Epithelial keratitis is the most common ocular presentation of HSV, accounting for 50 to 80% of ocular herpes. It can occur due to actively replicating virus. It

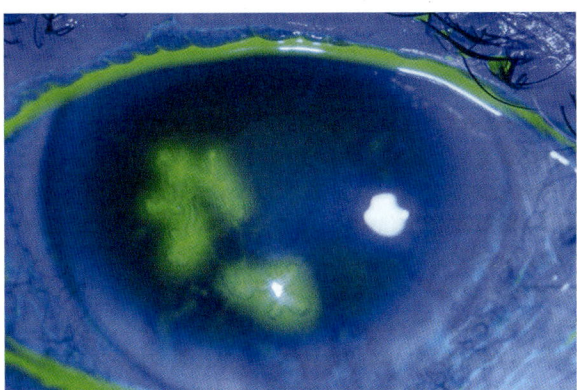

Fig. 2.4: Anterior segment photograph demonstrating a dendritic ulcer, which stains with fluorescein

classically presents as a dendritic ulcer (Fig. 2.4) with branching pattern or a geographic ulcer. This pattern stains with fluorescein or Rose Bengal, highlighting the branching lesions with terminal bulbs. Management of epithelial keratitis is primarily with antivirals. The use of steroids is contraindicated in the presence of epithelial involvement.

Antiviral agents stop viral replication by interfering with viral DNA synthesis during transcription of the viral genome. Various topical antiviral therapies have been investigated. A Cochrane systemic review compared the relative effectiveness of antivirals agents, interferon and corneal debridement in the treatment of HSV epithelial keratitis.[36] The review found that trifluridine and acyclovir are more effective than idoxuridine or vidarabine. Ganciclovir was also found to be at least as effective as acyclovir. Oral acyclovir alone or a combination of oral acyclovir and a topical antiviral appeared as effective as a topical antiviral monotherapy. The review found that there is no strong evidence supporting the efficacy of combining antiviral treatment with either Interferon or corneal surface debridement. Corneal debridement was thought to physically remove or destroy the virus infected cells. However, debridement alone is not an effective form of treatment.

Oral acyclovir may be an alternative to a topical antiviral agent. Oral acyclovir 400 mg 5 times a day is at least as efficacious as topical acyclovir ointment.[37,38] Despite the widespread use of acyclovir, HSV resistance still appears low.[39] The efficacy of valacyclovir and famciclovir in the treatment of herpetic epithelial keratitis is not known.

Stromal Keratitis

There are 2 main forms of stromal keratitis. Non-necrotizing keratitis accounts for about 88% and necrotizing stromal keratitis accounts for about 7%. The remaining 5% is a mix of both. Disciform keratitis has frequently been considered as a form of stromal keratitis, though it is primarily an endothelitis with secondary stromal edema.[40] 20–60% of recurrent herpetic keratitis presents as stromal keratitis. This can lead to significant visual impairment as a result of stromal inflammation and scarring.

Necrotizing keratitis is often characterized by necrosis and ulceration and can progress to corneal perforation without treatment. This is due to combination of immunological and viral related mechanisms. Non-necrotizing stromal keratitis is marked by stromal inflammation. This is likely due to recruitment of T-lymphocytes causing an immunopathologic response.[41,42] The host response contributes to scarring and corneal vascularization. The role of viral antigen in the pathogenesis of non-necrotizing stromal keratitis is not clear.

Management strategies of stromal keratitis have been largely drawn from evidence from the Herpetic Eye Disease Study (HEDS).[43] HEDS comprises of 2 randomised, double-masked, placebo-controlled multicentre studies that were performed to look at the role of topical steroids in stromal keratitis, and the role of oral acyclovir when used together with topical antiviral (1% trifluridine) and topical steroids (1% prednisolone phosphate). The study established the efficacy of using topical steroids in controlling the host immune response in stromal keratitis, but did not find a benefit of adding oral acyclovir for patients already on treatment with a topical antiviral and topical steroid. The study methodology treated these patients with 10 weeks of tapered topical steroids and antivirals. However the optimal duration of taper of topical steroids remains unanswered and is often based on clinical response. Hence, topical steroids and antivirals remain the mainstay of treatment in stromal keratitis to reduce inflammation and halt viral replication.

Topical acyclovir penetrates the corneal wall in the presence of an intact epithelium,[44] and is preferred over topical trifluridine or ganciclovir. Topical trifluridine and topical gancyclovir do not penetrate the cornea well in the presence of an intact epithelium. Also, long-term use of topical trifluridine is associated with epitheliopathy. Where topical acyclovir is unavailable, oral acyclovir can be used instead together with topical steroids. In patients with stromal keratitis and epithelial disease, topical steroids should be withheld or used judiciously until the epithelial disease has resolved.

Other forms of treatment that have been reported include:
1. Cyclosporin A (CsA)
   Several small studies suggest a benefit of CsA in the treatment of stromal keratitis, even after failing treatment with topical steroids.[45-47] These studies found a resolution of inflammation in about 83% of non-necrotizing disease, and about 50% in necrotizing disease.[48] However, these studies lack a control group. CsA serves as a steroid-sparing agent and is particularly useful in patients with exaggerated adverse response to steroids or in those that require prolong treatment with topical steroids.
2. Amniotic membrane transplant
   Amniotic membrane transplant (AMT) has been investigated in the treatment of necrotizing stromal keratitis.[49,50] Amniotic membrane may help reduce the stromal inflammation and stabilize the ocular surface. It is a possible treatment option in patients with severe and persistent corneal inflammation. However, these have been limited to small retrospective series and further randomized controlled trials are necessary to establish their role.

Herpetic Endotheliitis

Herpetic disciform keratitis is a form of endotheliitis. It presents with a focal, discrete area of corneal edema with associated keratic precipitates and anterior chamber activity. The treatment is similar to stromal keratitis, with the use of topical antivirals together with topical steroids.[51,52] Oral acyclovir appeared to be as effective as topical acyclovir ointment.[53] Oral acyclovir may be preferred in the absence of topical acyclovir, since topical trifluridine and ganciclovir do not achieve adequate corneal penetration.

A woman presented with a first episode of eye redness and blurring of vision for one month before seeking consultation. On examination, there was a focal area of cornea edema seen inferiorly with associated keratic precipitates, posterior synechiae and mild cellular activity (Fig. 2.5A). Her best corrected visual acuity was 6/12 and her intraocular pressure was elevated at 28 mm Hg. Antiviral treatment together with topical prednisolone eye drops was started and slowly tapered over few months with good response. Other patient with disciform keratitis presented with recurrent episodes of keratouveitis (Fig. 2.5B). She was previously treated elsewhere and had about 7–8 episodes of recurrence over 13 years. She responded well to oral acyclovir with topical steroids and was subsequently started on long-term prophylactic acyclovir at 400 mg twice a day. Treatment guideline for HSV keratitis is shown in Table 2.3.

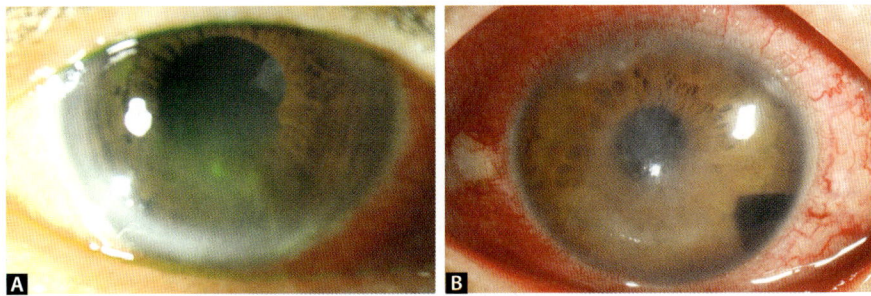

Figs 2.5A and B: (A) Anterior segment photographs of a patient presenting as first onset disciform keratitis; (B) Patient with recurrent disciform keratitis

TABLE 2.3: Suggested treatment guidelines

Type of keratitis	Suggested regime	Choice of medications
Epithelial keratitis	Antiviral agents alone for 1–3 weeks Avoid topical steroids	Topical acyclovir or ganciclovir gel 0.15% or topical trifluridine 1% or Oral acyclovir 400 mg 5 x per day (Alternatives: Valacyclovir, famciclovir)
Stromal keratitis	Antiviral Plus topical steroids over at least 10 weeks	Topical acyclovir or oral acyclovir (Alternatives: Valacyclovir, famciclovir) and Topical prednisolone 1%
Endothelial keratitis	Antiviral for 1–2 weeks Plus topical steroids	Topical acyclovir or oral acyclovir (Alternatives: Valacyclovir, famciclovir) and Topical prednisolone 1%
Patients with high-risk of recurrence: • Multiple previous episodes of ocular HSV • Post-keratoplasty patients for HSV related scarring • Post cataract or laser in patient with known history of ocular HSV	Low dose oral antiviral treatment for at least 1 year	Oral Acyclovir 400 mg twice/day or Oral valacyclovir 500 mg once/day (Alternative: Famciclovir)

Prevention

Prevention of Recurrent HSV Keratitis

Recurrent herpetic keratitis is seen in about 32% of patients over 1 year.[7] It causes irregular astigmatism, corneal scarring and loss of vision. The HEDS 2 was conducted to look at the efficacy of low dose oral acyclovir in preventing recurrent herpetic keratitis.[7,54] The study found that a low dose of 400 mg oral acyclovir twice a day over 1 year reduced the risk of recurrent stromal keratitis by 50% in patients with a history of stromal keratitis. However, there was no significant difference in recurrence when compared to placebo at 6 months after stopping of treatment. The addition of high dosed (400 mg 5 times a day) oral acyclovir in the treatment of epithelial keratitis to patients already on treatment with topical antiviral agent did not prevent subsequent episodes of stromal keratitis.

Valacyclovir 500 mg once a day may be a more convenient alternative and has been shown to be as effective as oral acyclovir 400 mg twice a day in preventing recurrences of ocular HSV.[55]

Acyclovir resistance is seen in about 0.32% of immunocompetent individuals. This is higher among the immunocompromised, up to an estimate of 10.9%.[56,57] It is associated with thymidine kinase gene mutation. Cross resistance is seen in other medications such as valacyclovir, ganciclovir and famciclovir, which also rely on thymidine kinase phosphorylation.[58] Alternative medications would include foscarnet, cidofovir or trifluridine that work via a different mechanism.

HSV Vaccination

A randomized controlled trial conducted in 10 patients over 1 year investigated the use of a heat-shock inactivated HSV-1 vaccine. The vaccine was found to reduce the number and duration of HSV-1 related ocular recurrences.[59] Larger studies are necessary to establish the role of such vaccinations.

REFERENCES

1. Liesegang TJ. Epidemiology of ocular herpes simplex. Natural history in Rochester, Minn, 1950 through 1982. Arch Ophthalmol. 1989;107(8):1160-5.
2. Young RC, Hodge DO, Liesegang TJ, et al. Incidence, recurrence, and outcomes of herpes simplex virus eye disease in Olmsted County, Minnesota, 1976-2007: the effect of oral antiviral prophylaxis. Arch Ophthalmol 2010;128(9):1178-83. doi: 10.1001/archophthalmol.2010.187[published Online First: Epub Date]|.
3. Labetoulle M, Auquier P, Conrad H, et al. Incidence of herpes simplex virus keratitis in France. Ophthalmology 2005;112(5):888-95. doi: 10.1016/j.ophtha.2004.11.052[published Online First: Epub Date]|.
4. Serna-Ojeda JC, Ramirez-Miranda A, Navas A, et al. Herpes Simplex Virus Disease of the Anterior Segment in Children. Cornea. 2015;34 Suppl 10:S68-71. doi: 10.1097/ico.0000000000000559[published Online First: Epub Date]|.
5. Wilhelmus KR, Falcon MG, Jones BR. Bilateral herpetic keratitis. Br J Ophthalmol. 1981;65(6):385-7.
6. Souza PM, Holland EJ, Huang AJ. Bilateral herpetic keratoconjunctivitis. Ophthalmology 2003;110(3):493-6 doi: 10.1016/s0161-6420(02)01772-4[published Online First: Epub Date]|.
7. Oral acyclovir for herpes simplex virus eye disease: effect on prevention of epithelial keratitis and stromal keratitis. Herpetic Eye Disease Study Group. Arch Ophthalmol. 2000;118(8):1030-36. doi: 10.1001/archopht.118.8.1030[published Online First: Epub Date]|.

8. Fukuda M, Deai T, Higaki S, et al. Presence of a large amount of herpes simplex virus genome in tear fluid of herpetic stromal keratitis and persistent epithelial defect patients. Seminars in Ophthalmology. 2008;23(4):217-20. doi: 10.1080/08820530802111366[published Online First: Epub Date]|.
9. Kakimaru-Hasegawa A, Kuo CH, Komatsu N, et al. Clinical application of real-time polymerase chain reaction for diagnosis of herpetic diseases of the anterior segment of the eye. Japanese Journal of Ophthalmology. 2008;52(1):24-31. doi: 10.1007/s10384-007-0485-7[published Online First: Epub Date]|.
10. Burcea M, Gheorghe A, Pop M. Incidence of Herpes Simplex Virus Keratitis in HIV/AIDS patients compared with the general population. Journal of Medicine and Life. 2015;8(1):62-3.
11. Hodge WG, Margolis TP. Herpes simplex virus keratitis among patients who are positive or negative for human immunodeficiency virus: an epidemiologic study. Ophthalmology. 1997;104(1):120-4.
12. Young TL, Robin JB, Holland GN, et al. Herpes simplex keratitis in patients with acquired immune deficiency syndrome. Ophthalmology. 1989;96(10):1476-9.
13. Prabriputaloong T, Margolis TP, Lietman TM, et al. Atopic disease and herpes simplex eye disease: a population-based case-control study. American Journal of Ophthalmology. 2006;142(5):745-9. doi: 10.1016/j.ajo.2006.06.050[published Online First: Epub Date]|.
14. Carr DJ, Harle P, Gebhardt BM. The immune response to ocular herpes simplex virus type 1 infection. Exp Biol Med. (Maywood). 2001;226(5):353-66.
15. Liu S, Pavan-Langston D, Colby KA. Pediatric herpes simplex of the anterior segment: characteristics, treatment, and outcomes. Ophthalmology. 2012;119(10):2003-8. doi: 10.1016/j.ophtha.2012.05.008[published Online First: Epub Date]|.
16. Hou YC, Chen CC, Wang IJ, et al. Recurrent herpetic keratouveitis following YAG laser peripheral iridotomy. Cornea. 2004;23(6):641-2.
17. Huang SC, Wu WC, Tsai RJ. Recurrent herpetic keratitis induced by laser iridectomy: case report. Changgeng Yi Xue Za Zhi. 1999;22(3):515-9.
18. Yoon KC, Im SK, Park HY. Recurrent herpes simplex keratitis after verteporfin photodynamic therapy for corneal neovascularization. Cornea. 2010;29(4):465-7. doi: 10.1097/ICO.0b013e3181b53310[published Online First: Epub Date]|.
19. Reed SY, Shin DH, Birt CM, et al. Herpes simplex keratitis following argon laser trabeculoplasty. Ophthalmic Surgery. 1994;25(9):640.
20. Jain V, Pineda R. Reactivated herpetic keratitis following laser in situ keratomileusis. Journal of Cataract and Refractive Surgery. 2009;35(5):946-8. doi: 10.1016/j.jcrs.2008.11.065[published Online First: Epub Date]|.
21. Kymionis GD, Portaliou DM, Bouzoukis DI, et al. Herpetic keratitis with iritis after corneal crosslinking with riboflavin and ultraviolet A for keratoconus. Journal of Cataract and Refractive Surgery. 2007;33(11):1982-4. doi: 10.1016/j.jcrs.2007.06.036[published Online First: Epub Date]|.
22. Al-Qarni A, AlHarbi M. Herpetic Keratitis after Corneal Collagen Cross-Linking with Riboflavin and Ultraviolet-A for Keratoconus. Middle East African Journal of Ophthalmology. 2015;22(3):389-92. doi: 10.4103/0974-9233.159777[published Online First: Epub Date]|.
23. Yuksel N, Bilgihan K, Hondur AM. Herpetic keratitis after corneal collagen cross-linking with riboflavin and ultraviolet-A for progressive keratoconus. International Ophthalmology. 2011;31(6):513-5. doi: 10.1007/s10792-011-9489-x[published Online First: Epub Date]|.
24. Barequet IS, Wasserzug Y. Herpes simplex keratitis after cataract surgery. Cornea. 2007;26(5):615-7. doi: 10.1097/ICO.0b013e318033a708[published Online First: Epub Date]|.

25. Patel NN, Teng CC, Sperber LT, et al. New-onset herpes simplex virus keratitis after cataract surgery. Cornea. 2009;28(1):108-10. doi: 10.1097/ICO.0b013e318182262c[published Online First: Epub Date]|.
26. Remeijer L, Doornenbal P, Geerards AJ, et al. Newly acquired herpes simplex virus keratitis after penetrating keratoplasty. Ophthalmology. 1997;104(4):648-52.
27. Rezende RA, Uchoa UB, Raber IM, et al. New onset of herpes simplex virus epithelial keratitis after penetrating keratoplasty. American Journal of Ophthalmology. 2004;137(3):415-9. doi: 10.1016/j.ajo.2003.09.057[published Online First: Epub Date]|.
28. Mannis MJ, Plotnik RD, Schwab IR, et al. Herpes simplex dendritic keratitis after keratoplasty. American Journal of Ophthalmology. 1991;111(4):480-4.
29. Sterk CC, Jager MJ, Swart-vd Berg M. Recurrent herpetic keratitis in penetrating keratoplasty. Doc Ophthalmol. 1995;90(1):29-33.
30. Cockerham GC, Bijwaard K, Sheng Z-M, et al. Primary graft failure: A clinicopathologic and molecular analysis. Ophthalmology. 2000;107(11):2083-90. doi: http://dx.doi.org/10.1016/S0161-6420(00)00361-4[published Online First: Epub Date]|.
31. Foster CS, Barney NP. Systemic acyclovir and penetrating keratoplasty for herpes simplex keratitis. Doc Ophthalmol. 1992;80(4):363-9.
32. van Rooij J, Rijneveld WJ, Remeijer L, et al. Effect of oral acyclovir after penetrating keratoplasty for herpetic keratitis: a placebo-controlled multicenter trial. Ophthalmology. 2003;110(10):1916-9. discussion 19 doi: 10.1016/s0161-6420(03)00798-x[published Online First: Epub Date]|.
33. Goodfellow JF, Nabili S, Jones MN, et al. Antiviral treatment following penetrating keratoplasty for herpetic keratitis. Eye (London, England) 2011;25(4):470-4. doi: 10.1038/eye.2010.237[published Online First: Epub Date]|.
34. Barney NP, Foster CS. A prospective randomized trial of oral acyclovir after penetrating keratoplasty for herpes simplex keratitis. Cornea. 1994;13(3):232-6.
35. Ghosh S, Jhanji V, Lamoureux E, et al. Acyclovir therapy in prevention of recurrent herpetic keratitis following penetrating keratoplasty. American Journal of Ophthalmology. 2008;145(2):198-202. doi: 10.1016/j.ajo.2007.10.005[published Online First: Epub Date]|.
36. Wilhelmus KR. Antiviral treatment and other therapeutic interventions for herpes simplex virus epithelial keratitis. The Cochrane Database of Systematic Reviews 2015;1:Cd002898 doi: 10.1002/14651858.CD002898.pub5[published Online First: Epub Date]|.
37. Collum LM, McGettrick P, Akhtar J, et al. Oral acyclovir (Zovirax) in herpes simplex dendritic corneal ulceration. The British Journal of Ophthalmology. 1986;70(6): 435-8.
38. Collum LM, Akhtar J, McGettrick P. Oral acyclovir in herpetic keratitis. Transactions of the ophthalmological societies of the United Kingdom. 1985;104 (Pt 6):629-32.
39. Christophers J, Clayton J, Craske J, et al. Survey of Resistance of Herpes Simplex Virus to Acyclovir in Northwest England. Antimicrobial Agents and Chemotherapy. 1998;42(4):868-72.
40. Holland EJ, Schwartz GS. Classification of herpes simplex virus keratitis. Cornea. 1999;18(2):144-54.
41. Russell RG, Nasisse MP, Larsen HS, et al. Role of T-lymphocytes in the pathogenesis of herpetic stromal keratitis. Investigative ophthalmology and visual science 1984;25(8):938-44.
42. Metcalf JF, Kaufman HE. Herpetic stromal keratitis-evidence for cell-mediated immunopathogenesis. American Journal of Ophthalmology. 1976;82(6):827-34.
43. Wilhelmus KR, Gee L, Hauck WW, et al. Herpetic Eye Disease Study. A controlled trial of topical corticosteroids for herpes simplex stromal keratitis. Ophthalmology. 1994;101(12):1883-95; discussion 95-6.

44. Poirier RH, Kingham JD, de Miranda P, et al. Intraocular antiviral penetration. Archives of Ophthalmology. (Chicago, Ill : 1960). 1982;100(12):1964-7.
45. Rao SN. Treatment of herpes simplex virus stromal keratitis unresponsive to topical prednisolone 1% with topical cyclosporine 0.05%. American Journal of Ophthalmology. 2006;141(4):771-2. doi: 10.1016/j.ajo.2005.11.042[published Online First: Epub Date]|.
46. Heiligenhaus A, Steuhl KP. Treatment of HSV-1 stromal keratitis with topical cyclosporin A: a pilot study. Graefes Arch Clin Exp Ophthalmol. 1999;237(5):435-8.
47. Gunduz K, Ozdemir O. Topical cyclosporin as an adjunct to topical acyclovir treatment in herpetic stromal keratitis. Ophthalmic Research. 1997;29(6):405-8.
48. Knickelbein JE, Hendricks RL, Charukamnoetkanok P. Management of herpes simplex virus stromal keratitis: an evidence-based review. Survey of Ophthalmology. 2009;54(2):226-34. doi: 10.1016/j.survophthal.2008.12.004[published Online First: Epub Date]|.
49. Heiligenhaus A, Li H, Hernandez Galindo EE, et al. Management of acute ulcerative and necrotising herpes simplex and zoster keratitis with amniotic membrane transplantation. The British Journal of Ophthalmology. 2003;87(10):1215-9.
50. Shi W, Chen M, Xie L. Amniotic membrane transplantation combined with antiviral and steroid therapy for herpes necrotizing stromal keratitis. Ophthalmology. 2007;114(8):1476-81. doi: 10.1016/j.ophtha.2006.11.027[published Online First: Epub Date]|.
51. Collum LM, Logan P, Ravenscroft T. Acyclovir (Zovirax) in herpetic disciform keratitis. The British Journal of Ophthalmology. 1983;67(2):115-8.
52. Power WJ, Hillery MP, Benedict-Smith A, et al. Acyclovir ointment plus topical betamethasone or placebo in first episode disciform keratitis. The British Journal of Ophthalmology. 1992;76(12):711-3.
53. Porter SM, Patterson A, Kho P. A comparison of local and systemic acyclovir in the management of herpetic disciform keratitis. The British Journal of Ophthalmology. 1990;74(5):283-5.
54. Acyclovir for the prevention of recurrent herpes simplex virus eye disease. Herpetic Eye Disease Study Group. The New England journal of medicine. 1998;339(5):300-6. doi: 10.1056/nejm199807303390503[published Online First: Epub Date]|.
55. Miserocchi E, Modorati G, Galli L, et al. Efficacy of valacyclovir vs acyclovir for the prevention of recurrent herpes simplex virus eye disease: a pilot study. American Journal of Ophthalmology. 2007;144(4):547-51. doi: 10.1016/j.ajo.2007.06.001 [published Online First: Epub Date]|.
56. Danve-Szatanek C, Aymard M, Thouvenot D, et al. Surveillance network for herpes simplex virus resistance to antiviral drugs: 3-year follow-up. Journal of Clinical Microbiology. 2004;42(1):242-9.
57. Stranska R, Schuurman R, Nienhuis E, et al. Survey of acyclovir-resistant herpes simplex virus in the Netherlands: prevalence and characterization. Journal of clinical virology : the official publication of the Pan American Society for Clinical Virology. 2005;32(1):7-18. doi: 10.1016/j.jcv.2004.04.002[published Online First: Epub Date]|.
58. Morfin F, Thouvenot D. Herpes simplex virus resistance to antiviral drugs. Journal of clinical virology : the official publication of the Pan American Society for Clinical Virology. 2003;26(1):29-37.
59. Pivetti-Pezzi P, Accorinti M, Colabelli-Gisoldi RA, et al. Herpes simplex virus vaccine in recurrent herpetic ocular infection. Cornea. 1999;18(1):47-51.

Chapter 3

Recent Advances in Management of Ocular Surface Disorders

Jayesh Vazirani, Virender Sangwan, Govinda Jha

INTRODUCTION

The ocular surface plays a critical, though often under recognized role in maintaining visual function. More importantly, disturbances of the ocular surface have protean manifestations, leading not only to symptomatic distress and impairment of visual function but also having significant impact on the overall quality of life of the patient. The ocular surface unit includes adnexal structures such as the eyelids and meibomian glands, the lacrimal secretory and drainage systems, the tear film as well as the outer coat of the eyeball that is comprised by the conjunctiva, limbus and the cornea. The management of ocular surface disorders requires an understanding of the role that each of these components plays in health and disease, and has led to the emergence of a distinct sub-specialty within ophthalmology in recent years. Herein, we attempt to enumerate some of the advances made in recent times in the diagnosis and therapy of ocular surface disorders (Table 3.1). We have chosen to discuss these in the context of major clinical entities that comprise the bulk of ocular surface disorders. We hope, that this approach helps readers to make more informed decisions and provides them with updates regarding diagnostic and therapeutic options.

Advances in Diagnosis of Dry Eye

The diagnosis of dry eye disease has traditionally rested on symptoms as reported by the patient as well as examination findings such as tear film break up time, Schirmer testing and ocular surface staining characteristics. To this were later

TABLE 3.1: Recent advances in management of dry eye disease

Diagnostic
- Measurement of tear film matrix metalloproteinase-9 (MMP-9) levels

Therapeutic
- Lifitegrast
- Rebamipide
- Diquafosol
- LipiFlow
- Intense pulsed light therapy

added techniques such as non-invasive meibography, optical coherence tomography of the tear film and tear film osmolarity testing. However, there is no universally agreed upon "gold standard" objective test to diagnose dry eye.

A lot of recent work has focused on determination of tear film cytokine profile in dry eye and detection of pro-inflammatory markers in the tear film. One such molecule that has received particular attention is matrix metalloproteinase-9 (MMP-9). Mouse models of dry eye have shown elevated MMP-9 levels in the tear film. Normal levels of MMP-9 in human tears range from 3 to 41 ng/mL. A rapid diagnostic test that can measure MMP-9 levels in the tear film is now commercially available for use in clinics (InflammaDry, Rapid Pathogen Screening, Inc, Sarasota, Florida, USA). The test is read as a color change to red in the strip provided, with clearly positive results when MMP-9 levels are >40 ng/mL in the tear film sample, and fainter shades of red with levels of 30–40 ng/mL.[1] A couple of clinical studies have reported sensitivity >80% and specificity >90% with this test, when compared to clinical assessment for diagnosing dry eye disease.[2,3] In contrast to this, another recent study found no difference in dry eye profiles between subjects who tested positive or negative for MMP-9 in the tear film using this test.[4]

Raised levels of MMP-9 in the tear film may not be diagnostic of dry eye, as the marker is nonspecific, and can be elevated in conditions such as contact lens wear, vernal keratoconjunctivitis and conjunctivochalasis. The test, therefore, should at best be taken as complementary to other methods of diagnosis. A potential implication of assessing inflammatory activity in the tear film may be in determining the utility of anti-inflammatory medication such as cyclosporine, corticosteroids and doxycycline. However, more studies are needed to assess the prognostic value, if any, of MMP-9 testing in predicting response to anti-inflammatory therapy. Overall, the test is an addition to the tools available for evaluation of patients with dry eye in the clinic.

Novel Therapies for Dry Eye

Lifitegrast is an integrin antagonist that blocks interaction between two cell surface proteins (lymphocyte function-associated antigen 1 and intercellular adhesion molecule), and aims to tackle T-cell mediated inflammation on the ocular surface.[5] In a phase 3 clinical study, a twice daily dose of lifitegrast was found to significantly improve corneal fluorescein and conjunctival lissamine green staining when compared to placebo, along with improvement in subjective symptoms.[6] In another phase 3 study involving adult with use of artificial tears, lifitegrast-treated subjects experienced greater improvement in eye dryness compared to placebo-treated subjects. However, there was no difference in corneal staining between groups.[7] If proven to be effective in further clinical studies, lifitegrast would provide another option for addressing ocular surface inflammation in dry eye, in addition to topical steroids and cyclosporine.

Rebamipide is a drug used in treatment of gastric ulcers and gastritis. It is believed to increase mucin levels, as well as have cytoprotective and anti-inflammatory effects.[8] Interest in rebamipide as an agent for treating dry eye has grown in recent years. Preclinical studies with an ophthalmic solution of rebamipide have shown increased ocular surface mucin levels, as well as favorable effects on the corneal and conjunctival epithelium. Clinical studies have shown that use of 2% rebamipide ophthalmic solution leads to significant improvements in both objective signs of dry eye such as ocular surface staining as well as subjective symptoms such as dryness and foreign body sensation.[9,10] Rebamipide 2% ophthalmic solution is now commercially available in various markets around the world.

Diquafosol is a P2Y$_2$ receptor agonist that promotes tear film and mucin secretion from the conjunctival epithelium and goblet cells.[11] It has been compared in randomized clinical trials with placebo and sodium hyaluronate solution in treatment of dry eye.[12,13] Other than this, multiple studies have assessed the utility of diquafosol alone or in combination with sodium hyaluronate in treating dry eye. A systematic review of randomized control trials involving diquafosol found that improved ocular staining scores in all trials, as well as improvement in symptoms in a majority of trials.[14] In summary, it seems to be a well-tolerated drug which may lead to some improvement in objective signs and subjective symptoms of dry eye.

Other novel treatments for dry eye associated with meibomian gland dysfunction (MGD) have been proposed and tried in recent times. An automated device that provides thermal pulses to the meibomian glands (LipiFlow, TearScience Inc., Morrisville, NC, USA) is now available. It consists of a single 12-minute treatment, in which an "activator" is applied to the eyelids. The rear part of this device provides direct heat to the meibomian glands, while the front part simultaneously compresses the glands. Results of the treatment are comparable to a conventional three month regimen of manual warm compresses with lid massage, which make it difficult to justify the associated costs of the treatment.[15] Likewise, different versions of intense pulsed light therapy are being tried in the treatment of MGD, putatively addressing the telangiectasia associated with the condition. Data on this therapy are too scant at the moment to make a definitive judgment on its efficacy.[16]

Recent Advances in Management of Limbal Stem Cell Deficiency

The understanding of limbal stem cell deficiency (LSCD) has evolved over decades, and the condition still presents a formidable challenge to the ocular surface specialist. A plethora of causes can lead to LSCD, which in itself can have myriad manifestations. Therapeutic options for LSCD, which were initially quite limited, have come a long way in recent years. We provide updates on two modalities that are now widely used in management of LSCD—cell-based therapies and keratoprosthesis surgery (Table 3.2).

Cell-based therapies for LSCD include direct limbal transplantation techniques such as conjunctival limbal autografts (CLAU) and keratolimbal allograft (KLAL), as well as cultivated limbal epithelial transplantation (CLET), which involves ex-vivo cultivation of cells from a small piece of donor limbus.[17] Wherever facilities are available, CLET has largely supplanted CLAU and KLAL as the technique of choice for limbal stem cell transplantation due to the minimal risk of iatrogenic LSCD at the donor site. In 2015, the European Commission has granted marketing approval to Holoclar® (a commercial name for CLET as promoted by an Italian firm), making it the first authorized stem-cell treatment in

TABLE 3.2: Management of limbal stem cell deficiency

Cell based therapies
- European approval for CLET—Holoclar®
- Simple limbal epithelial transplantation (SLET)

Keratoprosthesis surgery
- Improvements in Type-1 KPro
- LVP-KPro

the European Union. It is authorized as a therapy for moderate to severe LSCD in adults due to physical or chemical injury.

Simple limbal epithelial transplantation (SLET) is a novel, inexpensive, single-stage technique for limbal stem cell transplantation that combines the advantages of both CLAU and CLET. As with CLET, a very small piece of donor limbal tissue is harvested. However, rather than being subjected to ex-vivo cultivation in an expensive stem cell laboratory, the limbal biopsy is cut up into multiple small transplants that are directly placed over the recipient corneal surface, using amniotic membrane as a scaffold for epithelial growth. Thus, SLET may be viewed as a form of "in-vivo" expansion of cells.[18] Long-term results indicate that SLET is as good as or better than CLET in terms of successful restoration of the ocular surface as well as improvement in visual acuity in eyes with unilateral LSCD.[19,20] As the technique is easy to learn, repeatable, requires no expensive infrastructure and can be performed in a single stage, it has the potential to transform the management of LSCD, as it greatly improves access to cell-based therapy for patients across the world. In our view, this is the single most important game-changing development in the management of ocular surface diseases in recent years (Figs 3.1A and B).

Keratoprosthesis surgery for cases of severe ocular surface disease including LSCD has been performed for several years now. The most commonly used device worldwide is the Boston type 1 keratoprosthesis, and incremental improvements in both design as well as postoperative regimens have led to steadily improving device retention rates and lower complication rates (Figs 3.2A and B).[21] The type 1 design has recently been modified to provide a longer anterior extension with

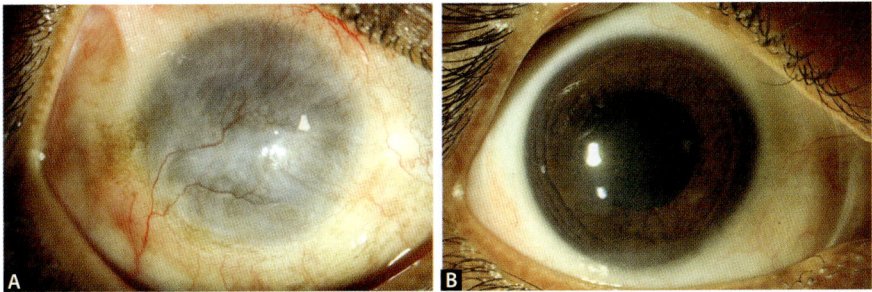

Figs 3.1A and B: (A) An eye with total limbal stem cell deficiency; (B) Completely epithelized surface post simple limbal epithelial transplantation (SLET)

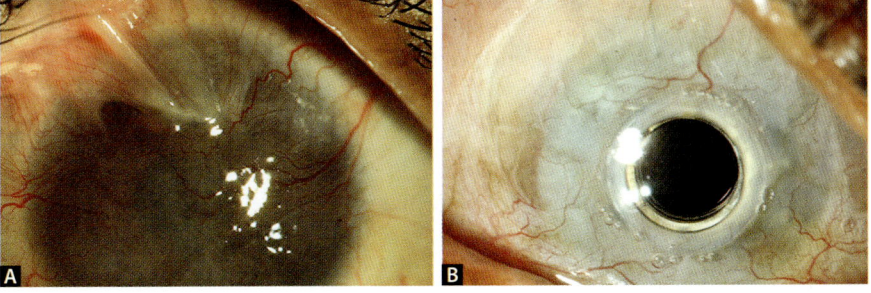

Figs 3.2A and B: (A) An eye with total limbal stem cell deficiency with a wet surface; (B) The same eye, post implantation of type 1 Boston KPro under existing ocular surface pannus

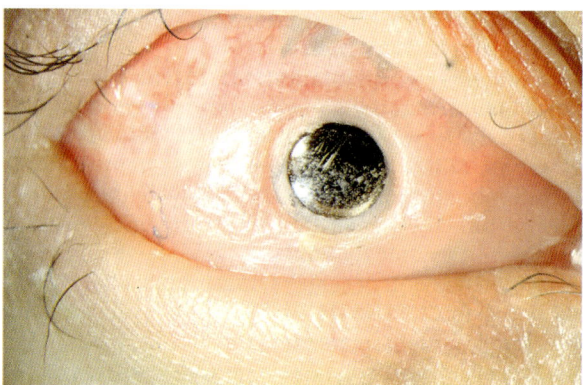

Fig. 3.3: LVP-Kpro implanted under mucous membrane in an eye with total limbal stem cell deficiency and dry surface

a flange, which enables implantation under a mucous membrane graft or ocular surface pannus. This modified device, known as the LVP-Kpro, can be used even in severely dry eyes with LSCD, overcoming a limitation of the type 1 Kpro (Fig. 3.3). Initial results in eyes with LSCD post Stevens-Johnson syndrome (SJS) appear promising, and long-term outcomes are awaited.[22]

Recent Advancements in Management of Other Ocular Surface Disorders (Table 3.3)

Topical chemotherapy for ocular surface squamous neoplasia (OSSN) has become increasingly popular in recent years. Mitomycin-C has been used for several years either as primary therapy or after surgical excision of OSSN for positive margins or recurrences. Interferon alpha-2b (IFNα-2b) administered as eye drops has found to be effective in treatment of OSSN, and is generally believed to have less ocular surface toxicity than Mitomycin-C. Therapy with IFNα2b is as efficacious as surgical excision for OSSN when used in the appropriate setting.[23] A recent study has also found topical 5-fluorouracil to be effective and well tolerated for treatment of OSSN.[24] On the diagnostic front, ultra high-resolution anterior segment optical coherence tomography (UHR-OCT) seems to be a promising tool for evaluating ocular surface lesions such as OSSN, which has distinctive features allowing differentiation from other pathologies.[25]

Topical tacrolimus drops or ointment in concentrations ranging from 0.01% to 0.1% have been found to be effective in controlling symptoms and signs of vernal keratoconjunctivitis (VKC).[26-28] Tacrolimus ointment for ophthalmic use is now commercially available in India, and provides another option for treatment of VKC.

The utility of amniotic membrane (AM) application on the ocular surface and eyelid margins in acute Stevens-Johnson syndrome (SJS) has been discussed and

TABLE 3.3: Showing measures in the treatment of ocular surface disorders

- Topical chemotherapy for ocular surface squamous neoplasia (OSSN)
- Topical tacrolimus for vernal keratoconjunctivitis (VKC)
- Amniotic membrane application in acute Stevens-Johnson syndrome (SJS)
- Umbilical cord serum for corneal epithelial healing

debated extensively in recent times. Reports suggest that AM application in acute SJS limits inflammation and may prevent long-term sequelae such as corneal scarring, vascularization and limbal stem cell deficiency. A grading system for ocular involvement in acute SJS has been proposed, and AM application is recommended in moderate to severe cases.[29,30] Umbilical cord serum (UCS) is rich in growth factors, and is believed to promote corneal epithelial healing. Application of UCS has been found to help corneal epithelial healing in acute ocular chemical burns as well as after keratoplasty.[31,32]

SUMMARY

A lot of exciting developments have been taking place in both diagnostic and therapeutic spheres in the realm of ocular surface disorders. Recent trends portend exciting times ahead for ocular surface specialists dealing with complex disorders affecting the eye.

REFERENCES

1. Lanza NL, Valenzuela F, Perez VL, Galor A. The Matrix Metalloproteinase 9 Point-of-Care Test in Dry Eye. Ocul Surf. 2016;14(2):189-95.
2. Sambursky R, Davitt WF 3rd, Friedberg M, Tauber S. Prospective, multicenter, clinical evaluation of point-of-care matrix metalloproteinase-9 test for confirming dry eye disease. Cornea. 2014;33:812-8.
3. Sambursky R, Davitt WF 3rd, Latkany R, et al. Sensitivity and specificity of a point-of care matrix metalloproteinase 9 immunoassay for diagnosing inflammation related to dry eye. JAMA Ophthalmol. 2013;131:24-8.
4. Lanza NL, McClellan AL, Batawi H, et al. Dry Eye Profiles in Patients with a Positive Elevated Surface Matrix Metalloproteinase 9 Point-of-Care Test Versus Negative Patients. Ocul Surf. 2016;14(2):216-23.
5. Perez VL, Pflugfelder SC, Zhang S, Shojaei A, Haque R. Lifitegrast, a Novel Integrin Antagonist for Treatment of Dry Eye Disease. Ocul Surf. 2016;14(2):207-15.
6. Sheppard JD, Torkildsen GL, Lonsdale JD, et al.; OPUS-1 Study Group. Lifitegrast ophthalmic solution 5.0% for treatment of dry eye disease: results of the OPUS-1 phase 3 study. Ophthalmology. 2014;121:475-83
7. Tauber J, Karpecki P, Latkany R, et al. OPUS-2 Investigators. Lifitegrast ophthalmicsolution 5.0% versus placebo for treatment of dry eye disease: results of the randomized phase III OPUS-2 study. Ophthalmology. 2015;122:2423-31.
8. Kashima T, Itakura H, Akiyama H, Kishi S. Rebamipide ophthalmic suspension for the treatment of dry eye syndrome: a critical appraisal. Clin Ophthalmol. 2014;8:1003-10.
9. Kinoshita S, Awamura S, Oshiden K, Nakamichi N, Suzuki H, Yokoi N. Rebamipide Ophthalmic Suspension Phase II Study Group. Rebamipide (OPC-12759) in the treatment of dry eye: a randomized, double-masked, multicenter, placebo-controlled phase II study. Ophthalmology. 2012;119(12):2471-8.
10. Kinoshita S, Oshiden K, Awamura S, Suzuki H, Nakamichi N, Yokoi N; Rebamipide Ophthalmic Suspension Phase 3 Study Group. A randomized, multicenter phase 3 study comparing 2% rebamipide (OPC-12759) with 0.1% sodium hyaluronate in the treatment of dry eye. Ophthalmology. 2013;120(6):1158-65.
11. Keating GM. Diquafosol ophthalmic solution 3 %: a review of its use in dry eye. Drugs. 2015;75(8):911-22.
12. Matsumoto Y, Ohashi Y, Watanabe H, et al. Efficacy and safety of diquafosol ophthalmic solution in patients with dry eye syndrome: a Japanese phase 2 clinical trial. Ophthalmology. 2012;119(10):1954-60.

13. Takamura E, Tsubota K, Watanabe H, et al. A randomized, double-masked comparison study of diquafosol versus sodium hyaluronate ophthalmic solutions in dry eye patients. Br J Ophthalmol. 2012;96(10):1310-5.
14. Wu D, Chen WQ, Li R, Wang Y. Efficacy and safety of topical diquafosol ophthalmic solution for treatment of dry eye: a systematic review of randomized clinical trials. Cornea. 2015;34(6):644-50.
15. Finis D, Hayajneh J, König C, Borrelli M, Schrader S, Geerling G. Evaluation of an automated thermodynamic treatment (LipiFlow®) system for meibomian gland dysfunction: a prospective, randomized, observer-masked trial. Ocul Surf. 2014;12(2):146-54.
16. Craig JP, Chen YH, Turnbull PR. Prospective trial of intense pulsed light for the treatment of meibomian gland dysfunction. Invest Ophthalmol Vis Sci. 2015;56(3):1965-70.
17. Vazirani J, Mariappan I, Ramamurthy S, Fatima S, Basu S, Sangwan VS. Surgical Management of Bilateral Limbal Stem Cell Deficiency. Ocul Surf. 2016;14(3):350-64.
18. Sangwan VS, Basu S, MacNeil S, Balasubramanian D. Simple limbal epithelial transplantation (SLET): a novel surgical technique for the treatment of unilateral limbal stem cell deficiency. Br J Ophthalmol. 2012;96(7):931-4.
19. Vazirani J, Ali MH, Sharma N, et al. Autologous simple limbal epithelial transplantation for unilateral limbal stem cell deficiency: multicentre results. Br J Ophthalmol. 2016;100(10):1416-20.
20. Basu S, Sureka SP, Shanbhag SS, Kethiri AR, Singh V, Sangwan VS. Simple Limbal Epithelial Transplantation: Long-Term Clinical Outcomes in 125 Cases of Unilateral Chronic Ocular Surface Burns. Ophthalmology. 2016;123(5):1000-10.
21. Aldave AJ, Sangwan VS, Basu S, et al. International results with the Boston type I keratoprosthesis. Ophthalmology. 2012;119(8):1530-8.
22. Basu S, Sureka S, Shukla R, Sangwan V. Boston type 1 based keratoprosthesis (Auro Kpro) and its modification (LVP Kpro) in chronic Stevens Johnson syndrome. BMJ Case Rep. 2014.
23. Nanji AA, Moon CS, Galor A, Sein J, Oellers P, Karp CL. Surgical versus medical treatment of ocular surface squamous neoplasia: a comparison of recurrences and complications. Ophthalmology. 2014;121(5):994-1000.
24. Joag MG, Sise A, Murillo JC, et al. Topical 5-Fluorouracil 1% as Primary Treatment for Ocular Surface Squamous Neoplasia. Ophthalmology. 2016 Mar 27. pii: S0161-6420(16)00316-X.
25. Thomas BJ, Galor A, Nanji AA, et al. Ultra high-resolution anterior segment optical coherence tomography in the diagnosis and management of ocular surface squamous neoplasia. Ocul Surf. 2014;12(1):46-58.
26. Labcharoenwongs P, Jirapongsananuruk O, Visitsunthorn N, Kosrirukvongs P, Saengin P, Vichyanond P. A double-masked comparison of 0.1% tacrolimus ointment and 2% cyclosporine eye drops in the treatment of vernal keratoconjunctivitis in children. Asian Pac J Allergy Immunol. 2012;30(3):177-84.
27. Pucci N, Caputo R, di Grande L, et al. Tacrolimus vs. cyclosporine eyedrops in severe cyclosporine-resistant vernal keratoconjunctivitis: A randomized, comparative, double-blind, crossover study. Pediatr Allergy Immunol. 2015;26(3):256-6.
28. Shoughy SS, Jaroudi MO, Tabbara KF. Efficacy and safety of low-dose topical tacrolimus in vernal keratoconjunctivitis. Clin Ophthalmol. 2016;10:643-7.
29. Sharma N, Thenarasun SA, Kaur M, et al. Adjuvant Role of Amniotic Membrane Transplantation in Acute Ocular Stevens-Johnson syndrome: A Randomized Control Trial. Ophthalmology. 2016;123(3):484-91.

30. Gregory DG. New Grading System and Treatment Guidelines for the Acute Ocular Manifestations of Stevens-Johnson Syndrome. Ophthalmology. 2016 Jun 11. pii: S0161-6420(16)30232-9.
31. Sharma N, Singh D, Maharana PK, et al. Comparison of Amniotic Membrane Transplantation and Umbilical Cord Serum in Acute Ocular Chemical Burns: A Randomized Controlled Trial. Am J Ophthalmol. 2016 May 19. pii: S0002-9394(16)30221-5.
32. Kamble N, Sharma N, Maharana PK, et al. Evaluation of the Role of Umbilical Cord Serum and Autologous Serum Therapy in Reepithelialization After Keratoplasty: A Randomized Controlled Clinical Trial. Eye Contact Lens. 2016 May 18.

Chapter 4

Intraocular Tuberculosis

Arshee Ahmed, B Sowkath Ali, Jyotirmay Biswas

INTRODUCTION

Intraocular tuberculosis (IOTB) is a form of extra-pulmonary tuberculosis, which is caused by the bacillus *Mycobacterium tuberculosis* (Mtb). It is noteworthy that a single organism produces such varied clinical features in a single organ and also that it is rarely isolated from samples which make a definitive diagnosis of this disease elusive in most of the cases.

EPIDEMIOLOGY

According to the WHO Global Tuberculosis Report 2015,[1] out of the 9.6 million new tuberculosis cases in 2014, 58% were in the South-East Asia region and Western Pacific regions. India, Indonesia and China had the largest number of cases (23,10% and 10% of the global total respectively). The WHO has now moved from STOP-TB Strategy (2006–2015) to END-TB Strategy (2016–2035) and aims to attain a world free of TB. India's TB control program is on track as far as reduction in disease burden is concerned. There was 50% reduction in mortality rate by 2013 as compared to 1990 levels. Similarly, there was also a 55% reduction in TB prevalence rate compared to 1990 levels.[2]

PATHOGENESIS

Mycobacterium tuberculosis is an obligate, aerobic, non-motile, non-spore-bearing, slow-growing bacterium. Human beings are the only natural host for this organism. It spreads via inhalation of aerosolized droplets when infected patients cough or sneeze. It usually affects organs with high regional oxygen content like the apices of the lungs, kidneys, bones, meninges and the choroid. The choroid is known to have one of the highest blood flow rates in the human body.

IOTB has been postulated to have pathogenetic mechanisms similar to other forms of extrapulmonary TB. These include the following stages:
1. Bacterial dissemination
   Mycobacterium tuberculosis is engulfed by alveolar macrophages and transported to hilar lymph nodes leading to priming of T cells. Macrophages/dendritic cells carrying *Mycobacterium tuberculosis* or even free bacteria may disseminate to different parts of the eye.
2. Localization in ocular tissues
   Amongst various ocular tissues wherein the bacilli gets lodged, RPE is most suited among different cell types to harbor *Mycobacterium tuberculosis*

3. Bacterial reactivation and initiation of inflammation
   Mycobacterium tuberculosis can remain latent for long periods of time. What factors can lead to reactivation is not known.

Tuberculosis and Uveitis

In patients with latent TB, antigenic mimicry between tubercular and retinal antigens could be a potential cause of uveitis. This hypothesis is supported by cytokine analysis of TB-associated uveitis that showed significantly increased interleukin-6 (IL-6) and other chemokines, but not IL-12, tumor necrosis factor-α (TNF-α) and interferon-γ (IFN-γ) that characterize active TB.[3]

Clinical Features

Ocular manifestations of tuberculosis are shown below (Fig. 4.1).
1. Anterior uveitis
   - Unilateral or bilateral
   - Usually granulomatous; can be non-granulomatous
   - Cornea- mutton fat keratic precipitates
   - AC–cells, flare, fibrinoid reaction
   - Iris nodules (Fig. 4.2) angle nodules
   - Posterior synechiae, peripheral anterior synechiae
   - Complicated cataract
   - Ciliary body granulomata.
2. Intermediate uveitis
   - Low grade, chronic uveitis
   - Vitritis
   - Snowball opacities
   - Snow banking
   - Peripheral vascular sheathing
   - Peripheral retinochoroidal granuloma.
3. Posterior uveitis
   - Choroidal tubercles
     – Unilateral or bilateral

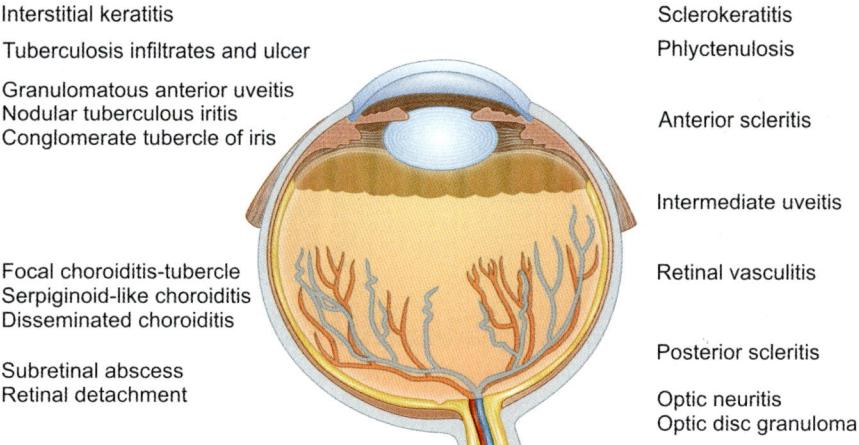

Fig. 4.1: Various anterior and posterior segment manifestations of tuberculosis

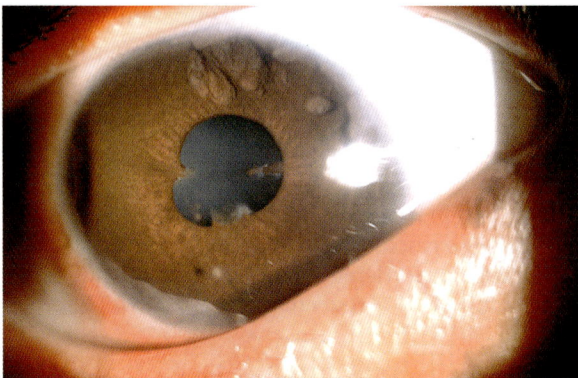

Fig. 4.2: A 21-year-old female patient with tubercular anterior uveitis showing mutton fat keratic precipitates, iris nodules, broad posterior synechiae and peripheral anterior synechiae

- Tubercles measure between 0.5–3 mm in diameter
- Overlying serous retinal detachment
- Respond well to ATT
- Heal leaving behind pale atrophic areas with variable pigmentation.
- Tuberculoma
    - Large, solitary mass
    - Upto 14 mm in diameter (Figs 4.3A and B)
    - Overlying hemorrhages, retinal folds, serous retinal detachment
    - Respond well to ATT and corticosteroids.
- Serpiginous-like choroiditis
    - Important to differentiate it from serpiginoid choroiditis
    - Chronic inflammation of the retinal pigment epithelium, choriocapillaries

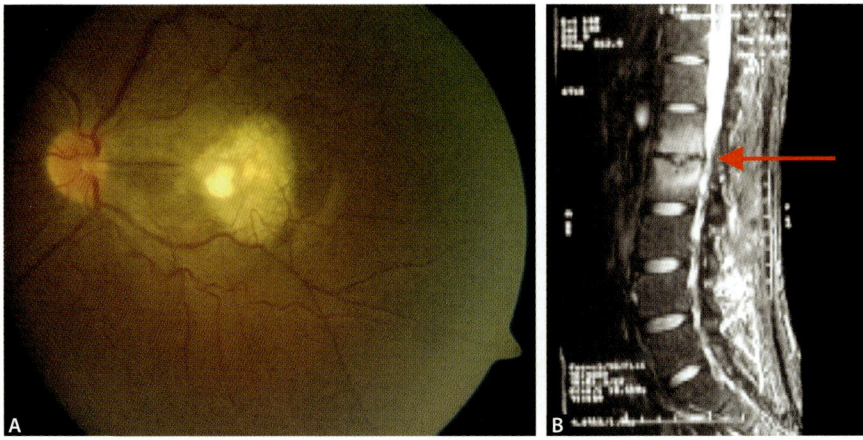

Figs 4.3A and B: A patient who was a known case of spinal tuberculosis presented with blurred vision in the left eye. (A) Fundus photograph of the left eye showing tubercular granuloma involving the macula; (B) MRI scan of the spine showing heterogenous, hyperintense signals from L1-L2 vertebrae with loss of intervening inter-vertebral disc morphology

- Immune-mediated hypersensitivity reaction in the presence of a few acid-fast bacteria in the choroid or retinal pigment epithelium
- Seen in TB-endemic countries
- Significant vitritis
- Presence of multifocal lesions in posterior pole, juxtapapillary region —gray-white lesions with ill-defined edges, spread centrifugally with multiple recurrences
- FFA shows early hypofluorescence and late hyperfluorescence
- Responds well to combination of ATT and corticosteroids
- Can show paradoxical worsening when treatment is initiated with ATT.[4]

- Subretinal abscess
  - Solitary, yellowish-white, circumscribed mass-like subretinal lesion
  - Often associated with overlying retinal hemorrhages
  - Vitritis
  - Can be diagnosed with the help of aqueous or vitreous samples subjected to PCR, microbial evaluation including smear, culture
  - Treatment must include ATT along with corticosteroids as this lesion responds very well to ATT.[5]

- Retinal vasculitis
  - Cause remains speculative; infective or hypersensitivity response to tubercular antigens
  - Predominantly venular involvement; occlusive vasculitis
  - Vitreous infiltrates (vitritis)
  - Retinal hemorrhages (Figs 4.4A and B)
  - Neovascularization leading to recurrent vitreous hemorrhage
  - Tractional retinal detachment
  - Neuroretinitis
  - Treatment with ATT, corticosteroids, and panretinal photocoagulation to the capillary non-perfusion areas as determined on FFA.

- Eales' disease: An idiopathic vasculitis; affects healthy adults, mostly men, in third to fourth decade of life, characterized by periphlebitis, capillary nonperfusion, neovascularization, recurrent vitreous hemorrhages, and fibrovascular proliferation. Absence of intraocular inflammation and

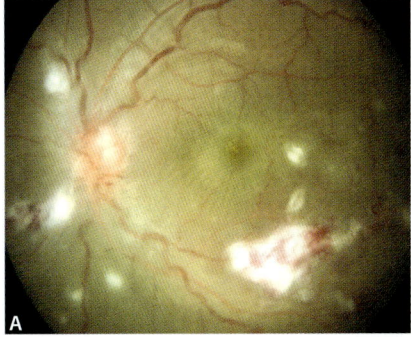 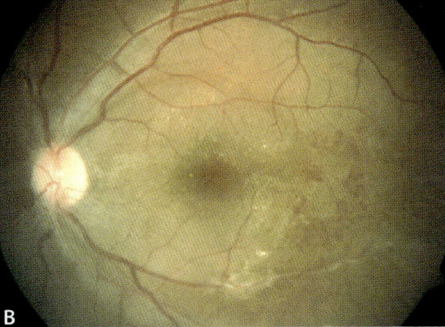

Figs 4.4A and B: Patient with tubercular retinal vasculitis, tested positive on Mantoux test and QuantiFERON TB Gold test with positive findings on HRCT-Chest. (A) Pretreatment fundus photograph of the left eye showing disc edema, cotton wool spots, hemorrhages, ILM folds; (B) Post-treatment with ATT and corticosteroids, vasculitis resolved leaving behind sheathing of the infer-temporal arcade vessel

absence of healed or active choroiditis lesions are important differentiating features from tuberculosis vasculitis. Biswas et al.[6] detected the *Mycobacterium tuberculosis* genome by PCR detection in a significant number of vitreous fluid specimens with Eales' disease, thus suggesting a possible association of *Mycobacterium tuberculosis* in the pathogenesis of Eales' disease.
- Optic nerve involvement
  - Contiguous spread from choroid or hematogenous spread from the primary focus
  - Optic neuritis, ONH granuloma/tubercle, retrobulbar neuritis, neuroretinitis, opticochiasmatic arachnoiditis.
- Endophthalmitis and panophthalmitis
  - Patients with subretinal abscesses can develop endophthalmitis due to treatment with corticosteroids without ATT because of rapid multiplication of bacilli along with liquefaction necrosis.
  - Scleral involvement can lead to panophthalmitis ending in globe perforation.

Pathology

Various ocular structures have been noted to be involved in specimens obtained from enucleated eyes like sclera, cornea, conjunctiva, iris, ciliary body, vitreous adjacent to pars plana ciliaris, retina and choroid.

The histopathology of ocular involvement characteristically reveals granulomatous inflammation with central caseous necrosis, and shows occasional acid-fast organisms. The granulomatous response consists of abundant epithelioid, histiocytes, occasional giant cells of langhans type, and peripheral mononuclear cells, primarily made up of lymphocytes.[3]

The disease should be differentiated from syphilis, leprosy, sarcoidosis, tumors, etc. (Table 4.1).

Diagnostic Techniques (Table 4.2)

- Immunologic
  - Tuberculin skin test (Mantoux test, PPD test)
  - Interferon-g release assays (QuantiFERON-TB GOLD or T-SPOT TB)
- Radiologic
  - Chest X-ray
  - Chest computer-assisted tomography
  - Positron emission tomography PET/CT.

TABLE 4.1: Showing differential diagnosis of tuberculosis

Infectious	Noninfectious	Neoplasia
Syphilis	Sarcoidosis	Retinoblastoma
Leprosy	Serpiginous choroiditis	Malignant melanoma
Toxoplasmosis	Sympathetic ophthalmia	Lymphoma
Histoplasmosis	Vogt–Koyanagi–Harada disease	Metastatic tumor
Borreliosis	Acute posterior multifocal placoid pigment epitheliopathy	
Brucellosis		
Herpetic retinochoroiditis	Punctate inner choroidopathy	
	Multifocal choroiditis and panuveitis	

TABLE 4.2: Diagnostic modalities for intraocular tuberculosis

Type		Principle	Advantages	Disadvantages
Immunologic	Tuberculin skin test (Mantoux test)	Skin hypersensitivity test for mycobacterial antigens	Low cost Wide availability Larger induration-more specific	Not specific Does not distinguish between latent and active TB May be positive with BCG vaccination/exposure to atypical mycobacteria Maybe negative in immunosuppressed states/children/extrapulmonary or miliary TB difficulties in test administration and interpretation may lead to false results
	Interferon-γ release assays (QFT-G, T-SPOT TB)	Interferon-γ release test after in vitro stimulation of patients' lymphocytes with *M. tuberculosis* specific antigens	More specific marker of *M. tuberculosis* infection/previous exposure Not influenced by BCG vaccination or exposure to atypical mycobacteria Not as subject to biases and errors of placement and reading as the TST	Higher cost Not widely available Possibly more sensitive to detect latent infection than TST but does not distinguish it from disease May be negative or indeterminate in immunosuppressed states Problems in collecting or transporting blood specimen may decrease the accuracy
Radiologic	Chest X-ray	Look for evidence of pulmonary involvement, either active or healed infection	Low cost and wide availability Useful when a suggestive pattern is found (e.g. upper lobe infiltrates and cavitation, Ghon's focus, miliary disease)	Not specific for tuberculosis Other infectious/granulomatous/lymphoproliferative/occupational disorders may lead to similar patterns Low sensitivity, especially for detection of lymphadenopathy A normal result does not exclude ocular tuberculosis
	CT scan of chest	Look for evidence of pulmonary involvement, either active or healed (postinflammatory)	More sensitive than chest radiograph Modality of choice for detection of lymphadenopathy and for tuberculomas	Higher cost and greater radiation exposure than chest X-ray Not specific for tuberculosis A normal result does not exclude ocular tuberculosis
	PET-CT scan			

Contd...

Contd...

Bacteriologic	Smear	Identify the presence of stained acid-fast bacilli in various clinical samples	Rapid and widely-available method Useful especially in specimens with large bacillary load	Low sensitivity (e.g. for sputum, detection threshold is >5,000 bacilli/mL) Other acid-fast organisms are also identified through this method
	Culture	Detects growth of *M. tuberculosis* after seeding of clinical samples in culture media	Gold standard. Unequivocal proof of microorganism viability Allows identification and drug sensitivity testing	Expensive and cumbersome needs long time for growth May not be widely available Results may take up to 6–8 weeks in solid media
Molecular	Nucleic acid amplification tests	Detects presence of *M. tuberculosis* genomic DNA in clinical samples after amplification (e.g. various PCR techniques)	High specificity Better sensitivity than microscopy Fast results Allows identification and investigation of genetic resistance patterns	Higher cost and limited availability. Variable sensitivity Inferior sensitivity for non-respiratory specimens (not established for ocular samples). Does not allow ruling out tuberculous etiology Detects only DNA (more prone to contamination and microorganisms may not be viable or may be dormant)
	LAMP	Based on the novel loop-mediated isothermal amplification (LAMP) platform; for detection of *Mycobacterium tuberculosis* complex, *Mycobacterium avium*, and *Mycobacterium intracellulare*	Fast, easy operation without sophisticated equipment, results visible to naked eye, robust to inhibitors and reaction conditions that usually adversely affect PCR results, simple enough to use in small-scale hospitals, primary care facilities, and clinical laboratories in developing countries	
Histologic	Histopathology	Stained tissue sections with evidence of granulomatous inflammation (especially with caseous necrosis) support the diagnosis. Finding of AFB in this setting is diagnostic	Allows the observation of the extent of tissue damage	Risks related to invasive procedure to obtain tissue specimen Other microrganisms/noninfectious entities may also lead to granulomatous inflammation Low sensitivity for AFB detection

Source: Daniel V. Vasconcelos-Santos, Manfred Zierhut, Narsing A Rao. Strengths and Weaknesses of Diagnostic Tools for Tuberculous Uveitis, Ocular Immunology and Inflammation. 2009;17(5):351-355.[7]

- Bacteriologic
    - Smear
    - Culture.
- Molecular
    - Nucleic acid amplification tests.
- Histologic
    - Histopathology.

Ancillary Investigations

- ***Fundus Fluorescein Angiography (FFA):*** It is a very useful technique to study the various presentations of IOTB including Tb-serpiginous-like choroiditis, tubercles, tuberculomas, retinal vasculitis and inflammatory choroidal neovascular membranes. Active choroiditis lesions demonstrate hypofluorescence in early phases with hyperfluorescence in the late phases. Serpiginous-like choroiditis, shows an initial hypofluorescent active edge with late hyperfluorescence and diffuse staining of the active advancing edge. In cases of vasculitis, the presence of areas of capillary non-perfusion and neovascularization can be picked up on FFA determining the need and extent of panretinal photocoagulation. Inflammatory CNVM can be diagnosed by the classical appearance of early lacy hyperfluorescence and intense leak with fuzziness of borders in late stages.
- ***Indocyanine Green Angiography (ICG):*** This angiography is useful in determining the extent of the choroidal lesion and the stage of disease and in evaluating treatment results. Herbort et al.[8] suggested that hypofluorescent lesions seen in all phases of ICGA represent full-thickness choroidal granulomas or atrophic lesions. ICGA changes are reversible and therefore, help in monitoring the disease.
- ***Wide-field Imaging (WFI):*** It is especially useful in cases with vasculitis involving the peripheral vessels, usually veins in patients with Eales' disease. Standard field FFA can miss the abnormalities in the peripheral retina. But with WFI, capillary non-perfusion areas in the periphery can be picked up earlier, preventing complications like neovascularization and bleeding.
- ***Fundus Autofluorescence (FAF):*** It is a novel, non-invasive technique which can help in differentiating active from inactive choroiditis. Gupta A and Biswas J[9] described the serial FAF pattern of serpiginous choroiditis and reported that in the initial phases the lesion appears hyperfluorescent. Sharpening of the hyper-autofluorescent borders indicated healing of the lesions. Completely healed lesions showed hypo or absence of fluorescence (Figs 4.5A and B).
- ***Optical Coherence Tomography:*** OCT It helps in the assessment of macular complications like cystoid macular edema and inflammatory CNVM in these cases. Also, entities that may mimic tubercles like CSCR and choroidal tumors can be excluded.
  Enhanced-depth imaging-OCT (EDI) of active Tb-SLC lesions demonstrated infiltration of the choroid, elevation of the RPE-Bruch's membrane complex and focal increase of choroidal thickness.[10] These findings are not seen in non-infectious SC and can help in differentiating between the two entities.
- ***Ultrasound (USG):*** It is a helpful tool in diagnosis and follow-up of choroidal mass lesions like subretinal abscess, which characteristically show an anechoic space within the mass on A-scan. Tuberculomas can be

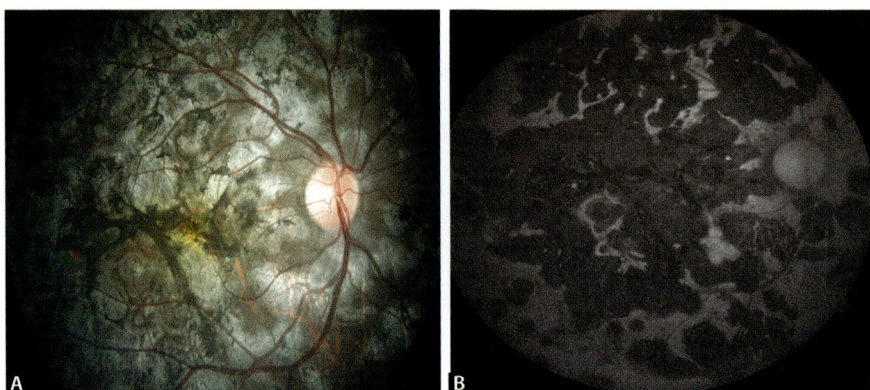

Figs 4.5A and B: A 22-year-old male patient with positve QuantiFERON TB- Gold test presented with features of (A) Healed multifocal choroiditis; (B) Fundus autofluorescence shows complete absence of autofluorescence indicating healed lesions

differentiated from malignancies like retinoblastomas, malignant melanomas and metastatic tumors.
- **Ultrasound Biomicroscopy (UBM):** It is a useful tool to study eyes with hypotony in patients with chronic uveitis and poor media clarity to assess the pars plana region. It can also pick up granulomas in this region.
- **Fine Needle Aspiration Cytology (FNAC):** Samples can be taken for histopathology or for techniques like PCR in cases, which present with diagnostic dilemmas.

Challenges in Diagnosis

The diagnosis of IOTB remains a challenging issue because each of the tests available has its strengths and weaknesses as discussed above and because TB infection can present with features of any type of extraocular or intraocular inflammation. Gupta A et al.[11] have proposed the classification of IOTB (Table 4.3) comprising of confirmed IOTB, probable IOTB and possible IOTB. These guidelines offer a greater degree of "certainty" of diagnosis as IOTB largely remains a presumptive diagnosis, as unequivocal evidence of infection is often not available. There are some signs which are consistent with intraocular tuberculosis; they are:

Presence of cells in anterior chamber or vitreous along with:
1. Broad posterior synechiae
2. Retinal perivasculitis with or without discrete choroiditis/scar
3. Multifocal serpiginoid choroiditis
4. Choroidal granuloma
5. Optic disc granuloma
6. Optic neuropathy.

Approach for the diagnosis of tuberculous uveitis in immunocompetent individuals[12] is shown in a flow chart below.

Showing diagnosis of tuberculous uveitis in immunocompetent individuals (Flowchart 4.1).[12]

Intraocular Tuberculosis

TABLE 4.3: The proposed classification of intraocular tuberculosis

Clinical diagnostic group	Case definition criteria
Confirmed IOTB (Both 1 and 2)	1. At least one clinical sign suggestive of IOTB 2. Microbiological confirmation of MTB from ocular fluids/tissues

Probable IOTB (1,2, and 3 together)	1. At least one clinical sign suggestive of IOTB (and other etiologies excluded)
	2. Evidence of chest X-ray consistent with TB infection or clinical evidence of extraocular TB or microbiological confirmation from sputum or EO sites
	3. At least one of the following:
	   a. Documented exposure to TB
	   b. Immunological evidence TB infection

Possible IOTB (1,2, and 3 together) OR (1 and 4)	1. At least one clinical sign suggestive of IOTB (and other etiologies excluded)
	2. Chest X-ray not consistent with TB infection and no clinical evidence of EOTB
	3. At least one of the following:
	   a. Documented exposure to TB
	   b. Immunological evidence TB infection
	4. Evidence of chest X-ray consistent with TB infection or clinical evidence of EO TB but none of the characteristics given in 3

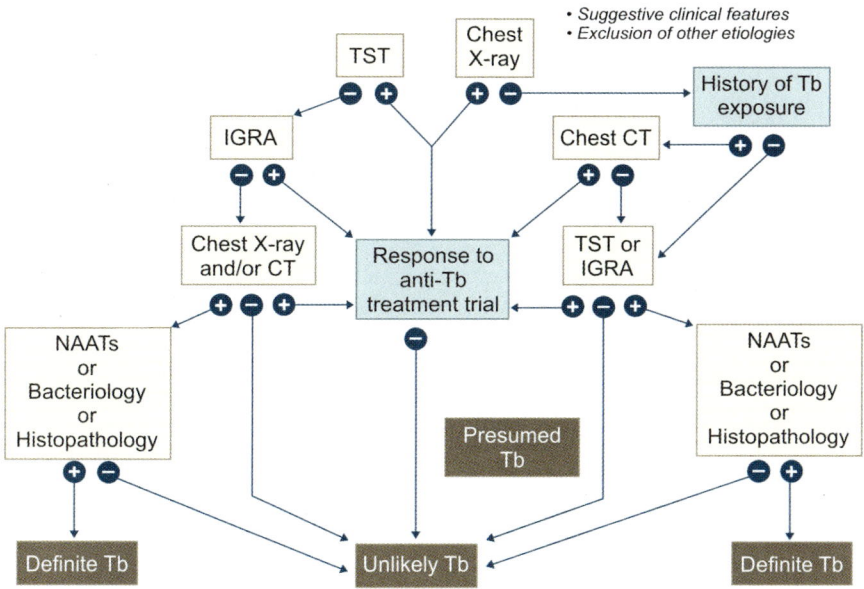

Flowchart 4.1: Uveitis in immunocompetent patient

Abbreviations: TST, tuberculin skin test; IGRA, interferon-gamma release assay; CT, computer-assisted tomography; TB, tuberculosis. Anti-TB treatment for 8 weeks; presumed and definite TB require treatment for 6 months
Source: Ang, et al. Diagnosis of Ocular Tuberculosis. Ocular Immunol Inflamm. 2016;5:1-9.

MANAGEMENT

Tuberculosis is a readily curable disease with highly effective treatment. The management of ocular TB includes medical management of the disease on the same lines as other forms of extrapulmonary TB and surgical management to treat complications developing due to chronic ocular disease.

Medical Management

Anti-tubercular therapy has been known to eliminate latent TB and decreases a person's lifetime risk of developing active TB by 90%.[13]

Majority of patients with uveitis secondary to presumed Tb have underlying latent TB so treatment with timely ATT helps in reducing recurrences. In a study by Bansal et al.[14] the addition of ATT significantly improved the 5-year probability of no recurrence of inflammation in their cohort.

Treatment is instituted in two distinct phases—the first intensive phase involves the use of 4 drugs—isoniazid, rifampicin, pyrazinamide and ethambutol. After use for 2–3 months, only isoniazid and rifampicin are continued for another 6–9 months. The CDC recommends prolonged therapy for tuberculosis of any site that is slow to respond and thus, patients with intraocular TB may require prolonged therapy.[15]

Along with the initiation of ATT, low dose oral steroids are also commenced for a period of 4–6 weeks as they help in reducing the damage to ocular tissues, which can happen due to, delayed hypersensitivity.

Essential first-line anti-TB drugs:

1. **Isoniazid:** It is a prodrug; activation of isoniazid produces oxygen-derived free radicals (superoxide, hydrogen peroxide, and peroxynitrite) and organic free radicals that inhibit the formation of mycolic acids of the bacterial cell wall, causing DNA damage and, subsequently, the death of the bacillus. It has a bactericidal effect on rapidly growing bacilli, but has a limited effect on slow-growing (generally intracellular) and intermittently growing (generally extracellular) bacilli.
2. **Rifampicin:** It inhibits the gene transcription of mycobacteria by blocking the DNA-dependent RNA polymerase, which prevents the bacillus from synthesizing messenger RNA and protein, causing cell death. It is a bactericidal drug that kills growing, metabolically active bacilli, as well as bacilli in the stationary phase, during which metabolism is reduced.
3. **Pyrazinamide:** It is a prodrug; enters the bacillus passively, is converted into pyrazinoic acid by pyrazinamidase, and reaches high concentrations in the bacterial cytoplasm due to an inefficient efflux system. Pyrazinoic acid decreases the intracellular pH to levels that cause the inactivation of enzymes-such as fatty acid synthase I, which plays a fundamental role in synthesizing fatty acids-and, consequently, the impairment of mycolic acid biosynthesis. It is also bactericidal and is particularly potent in elimination of persistent bacilli in the sporadic multiplication phase which are responsible for bacteriological relapse.
4. **Ethambutol:** It interferes with the biosynthesis of arabinogalactan, the principal polysaccharide on the mycobacterial cell wall. It acts on intracellular and extracellular bacilli, principally on rapidly growing bacilli.

Side effects of anti-tubercular drugs are well documented. Dose associated hepatotoxicity can be prevented by regular monitoring of liver-function tests. Other commonly seen side effects include cutaneous reactions, gastrointestinal intolerance, hematological reactions and renal failure.

TABLE 4.4: Ocular side-effects of antitubercular drugs

Drug	Side-effect
Isoniazid	Optic neuritis, optic atrophy
Ethambutol	Optic neuritis, acquired red-green dyschromatopsia, central scotomas, disk edema, peripapillary splinter hemorrhages, optic atrophy, retinal edema pigmentary changes at fovea (rare)
Rifabutin	Severe acute anterior uveitis (hypopyon uveitis), corneal endothelial deposits, inflammatory vitreous exudates and opacities

Side effects caused by these drugs are listed in Table 4.4.

A baseline ophthalmic examination including visual acuity, visual fields and color vision should be documented for all patients before starting ethambutol. In case of any ocular side effect the drug should be stopped immediately. Vision improves spontaneously in many cases. Parenteral hydroxocobalamin can be considered for a 10–28 week period for those who do not improve spontaneously.

The emergence of MDR-TB (multidrug resistance) and XDR-TB (extremely drug resistant) entails the use of next generation drugs for extended periods. About 8–10 drugs have to be used for 18–24 months. Additional agents include ethionamide, kanamycin, cycloserine, rifabutin, fluoroquinolones, interferon-γ and linezolid.

Surgical Management

Complications may arise due to longstanding ocular disease leading to non-clearing vitreous hemorrhage, tractional retinal detachment, etc. Both the conditions need surgical intervention—vitrectomy.

Research and Development[2]

- A diagnostic platform called the GeneXpert Omni is in development. It is meant for testing for TB and rifampicin-resistant TB using XpertMTB/RIF cartridges. It is supposed to be smaller, lighter and less expensive than current platforms.
- A next generation cartridge called Xpert-Ultra is in development and intends to replace the XpertMTB/RIF cartridge. It could potentially replace culture as the primary diagnostic tool for TB.
- Eight new or re-purposed anti-TB drugs are in advanced phases of clinical development. For the first time in six years, an anti-TB drug (TBA-354) is in Phase I trials.
- Several new TB treatment resistant regimens are being tested for use in drug-susceptible and/or drug-TB in Phase II or Phase III trials.
- Fifteen vaccine candidates are in clinical trials; emphasis has shifted from children to adolescents and adults.

REFERENCES

1. TB India 2015-RNTCP-Annual status report; page 22.
2. WHO Global tuberculosis report 2015; page 8.
3. Basu S, Wakefield D, Biswas J, Rao NA. Pathogenesis and Pathology of Intraocular Tuberculosis. Ocul Immunol Inflamm. 2015;23(4):353-7.

4. Gupta V, Gupta A, Arora S, et al. Presumed tubercular serpiginous like choroiditis: clinical presentation and management. Ophthalmology. 2003;110,1744-9.
5. Majumder PD, Biswas J, Bansal N, Ghose A, Sharma H. Clinical Profile of Patients with Tubercular Subretinal Abscess in a Tertiary Eye Care Center in Southern India. Ocul Immunol Inflamm. 2016:1-5. [Epub ahead of print]
6. Biswas J, Sharma T, Gopal L, et al. Eales' disease—an update. Surv Ophthalmol. 2002;47:197-214.
7. Daniel V. Vasconcelos-Santos, Manfred Zierhut, Narsing A Rao. Strengths and Weaknesses of Diagnostic Tools for Tuberculous Uveitis, Ocular Immunology and Inflammation. 2009;17(5):351-5.
8. Herbort CP, LeHoang P, Guex-Crosier Y. Schematic interpretation of indocyanine green angiography in posterior uveitis using a standard angiographic protocol. Ophthalmology. 1998;105:432-40.
9. Gupta A, Biswas J. Fundus autofluorescence imaging to document evolution, progression and healing pattern of serpiginous choroiditis. Oman J Ophthalmol. 2014;7(2):100-101.
10. Rifkin LM, Munk MR, Baddar D, Goldstein DA. A new OCT finding in Tuberculous serpignous-like choroidopathy. Ocul Immunol Inflamm. 2015;23(1):53-8.
11. Gupta A, Sharma A, Bansal R, Sharma K. Classification of Intraocular Tuberculosis. Ocul Immunol Inflamm. 2015;23(1):7-13.
12. Ang M, Vasconcelos DV, Sharma K, et al. Diagnosis of Ocular Tuberculosis. Ocular Immunol Inflamm. 2016:1-9. [Epub ahead of print]
13. Centers for Disease Control and Prevention. Targeted tuberculin testing and treatment of latent tuberculosis infection. American Thoracic Society. MMWR Recomm Rep. 2000;49:1-51.
14. Bansal R, Gupta A, Gupta V, et al. Role of anti-tubercular therapy in uveitis with latent/manifest tuberculosis. Am J Ophthalmol. 2008;146:772-9.
15. Centers for Disease Control and Prevention (CDC): American Thoracic Society, MMWR Morb Mortal Wkly Rep. 2003;52(31):735-9.

Chapter 5

Ocular Sarcoidosis

Eliza Anthony, Parthopratim Dutta Majumder, Jyotirmay Biswas

INTRODUCTION

Sarcoidosis is a multisystem chronic granulomatous inflammatory disorder. It was first described by Jonathan Hutchinson in 1878. However in 1909 ocular involvement was first described by Schumacher in a patient with nodular iritis.[1]

EPIDEMIOLOGY

Prevalence of sarcoidosis varies among different countries and ethnic groups. It is found in African Americans and Caucasians of north eastern origin.[2] Prevalence varies from as low as 3.7:100,000 in Japan to as high as 28.2; 100,000 in Finland. The overall incidence of sarcoidosis is 6–10 per 100,000 with highest incidence between 20–40 years age group.[3] Although ocular sarcoidosis has bimodal pattern of incidence, first at 20–30 years of age and second at 50–60 years of age, systemic sarcoidosis typically affects young adults.[2,4] Ocular involvement is associated with predilection for female gender and African American race as compared to Caucasians.[2]

ETIOLOGY

Sarcoidosis is caused by an exaggerated T-cell immune response to multiple self and no-self antigens capable of generating Th1-mediated response in a genetically susceptible individual and not an immunodeficiency. No gene has been implicated yet in causation of sarcoidosis. HLADR17 and TNF polymorphism have been found to be very crucial in predicting disease severity and prognosis. In Lofgren's syndrome high levels of TNF-α, associated with TNFA2 allele is described as a good prognostic marker. Butyrophilin-like 2 gene located near LA-DRB1 region has been described as a susceptivity gene.[3] Agents implicated in the etiology of sarcoidosis are shown in Table 5.1.

Histopathologically, sarcoidosis is characterized by a non caseating granuloma with modified macrophages or epithelioid cells in the center surrounded by a rim of lymphocytes and fibroblasts.[3] Inclusion bodies like asteroids (contain lipoprotein; accumulation of cytoskeletal filaments; seen in 2–9%), Schaumann's bodies (concentric, blue calcified laminated structures; accumulation of oxidized lipid within the lysosomes; seen in 48–88% of cases), Wesenberg-Hamazaki bodies (yellow, ovoid, periodic acid-schiff positive inclusion bodies which are giant lysosomes; seen in 11–68% of lymph nodes with sarcoidosis) and deposits of

TABLE 5.1: Shows agents implicated in the eiology of sarcoidosis [3]

Sl No.	Infectious agents	Scientific evidence in literature
1.	Mycobacterium tuberculosis	Mycobacterial DNA and RNA is detected in sarcoid tissue but not isolated from culture from the sarcoid tissue. Although Mycobacterium tuberculosis catalases peroxidase (mKatG)-reactive, IFN-γ-expressing T-cells are found in patients with active sarcoidosis
2.	Propionibacterium acnes	Propionibacterium acnes rRNA and DNA has been demon-strated in sarcoid tissue
3.	Epstein barr virus (EBV)	Higher antibodies against EBV in sarcoid patients
4.	Herpes simplex virus (HSV)	Higher antibodies against HSV in sarcoid patients
5.	Helicobacter pylori (H. pylori)	Higher antibodies against H. pylori in sarcoid patients
6.	Association with hepatitis C	Sarcoidosis is known to occur following INF-γ and antiviral therapy for hepatitits C treatment
7.	INF-γ	Sarcoidosis is known to occur following INF-γ therapy for hepatitits C treatment

immunoglobulins can also be seen.[5] Kveim-Siltzbach test is reported positive in almost all patients who have hilar lymphadenopathy, in absence of parenchymal involvement and erythema nodosum. Test is recorded as positive when a papule size ranging from a few millimeters to 1.5 cm is seen in biopsy proven patient, 4–6 weeks after subcutaneous injection of a suspension derived from spleen of a sarcoidosis patient.[5]

Immunohistochemical studies reveal presence of CD4⁺T cells admixed with epithelioid cells in the center of cellular infiltrate. A high CD4/CD8 T cell ratio is found in bronchoalveolar lavage (BAL) of patients with sarcoidosis.[3]

CLINICAL FEATURES

Systemic Sarcoidosis

Systemic sarcoidosis is frequently asymptomatic, incidentally detected on a routine chest radiography and can also manifest as a severe disease. Patient may present with respiratory symptoms or constitutional symptoms like fever, malaise, weight loss and fatigue. Disease can have a self-limiting or a chronic course. It affects multiple organs including lungs (90–95%), lymph nodes (15–40%), skin (15–20%), eyes (12–20%), heart, liver, muscle and bones.[2,3] Mortality rate is as high as 6% attributed mainly due to respiratory, neurological and cardiovascular involvement.[6]

Pulmonary Sarcoidosis involves Lung or Mediastinal Lymph Nodes

Stages of pulmonary sarcoidosis.[3]
Stage 1. Bilateral hilar lymphadenopathy without parenchymal involvement
Stage 2. Bilateral hilar involvement with parenchymal involvement
Stage 3. Pulmonary infiltrates including cystic change without hilar lympha-denopathy.

Heerfordt's syndrome (uvea parotid fever) comprises fever, uveitis, parotid swelling and facial palsy. *Acute Lofgren's syndrome* consists of erythema nodosum, arthritis and hilar lymphadenopathy. Skin involvement occurs in 25% of patients including manifestations like erythema nodosum, lupus pernio (indurated violaceous plaque usually seen on face), subcutaneous granulomas and nodules, maculopapular lesions, hyper or hypopigmented plaques and necrotizing cutaneous vasculitis. There could be generalized lymphadenopathy or localized enlargement of lymph nodes in the thoracic area. In case of liver involvement elevated liver enzymes can be demonstrated.[3] Although cardiac sarcoidosis is a very fatal form it is usually under diagnosed. It is seen in less than 5% of sarcoidosis patients. It can manifest as heart block with arrhythmias, congestive heart failure and pericardial abnormalities. Some studies have shown that peripheral chorioretinal atrophic lesions are associated with increased risk of cardiac disease which may require need for implantation of pacemaker.[3,6] About 20% of patients have joint involvement in sarcoidosis. Approximately, 5–26% of sarcoidosis patients have neurological involvement comprising of cranial nerve palsies, encephalopathy, hypothalamic and pituitary disorders. Neurological involvement could be secondary to direct sarcoid tissue infiltration or due to compressive effect of cerebral mass. In children less than 4 years of age, sarcoidosis manifests as a triad of rash, uveitis and arthritis. In older children it can have multisystem involvement. Often sarcoidosis in children is misdiagnosed as juvenile chronic arthritis.[3]

Ocular Sarcoidosis

Ocular involvement in sarcoidosis is observed in more than 25–60% of patients diagnosed with sarcoidosis. According to few reports ocular involvement can be as high as 90%.[7] Typical clinical presentation in case of ocular sarcoidosis is bilateral granulomatous uveitis. It is presenting sign in 10–20% of patient and is the most common intraocular manifestations seen in almost 2/3rd of patients. Most common extraocular involvement is the lacrimal gland.[2]

Sarcoidosis is usually bilateral and virtually involves almost all structures of eyeball. The anterior segment involvements are summarized in Table 5.2.

TABLE 5.2: Showing anterior segment involvements in sarcoidosis

1. Eyelid and conjunctival granulomas
2. Lacrimal gland involvement
3. Keratoconjunctivitis sicca
4. Nongranulomatous anterior uveitis
5. Mutton fat keratic precipitates (Fig. 5.1)
6. Iris and pupillary nodules/iris mass
7. Raised in intraocular pressure
8. Tent-shaped peripheral anterior synechiae
9. Nodules in trabecular meshwork
10. Intermediate uveitis (16–38%)[8,9]

Posterior Segment Involvement

Posterior segment involvement is seen in 25% of ocular sarcoidosis cases and in 5% of cases it is the only manifestation. It is shown in Table 5.3.

TABLE 5.3: Showing involvement of posterior segment in sarcoidosis

1. Snowballs or string of pearls vitreous opacities and vitritis (3–62%)[10-12]
2. Active or atrophic multifocal peripheral chorioretinal lesions[11](Fig. 5.2) and panuveitis I 9–13% cases[9-13]
3. Choroidal granuloma (Fig. 5.3).
4. Nodular and/or segmental periphlebitis with candle wax dripping (Fig. 5.4), and occlusive retinal vasculitis in 9–34%[10-12]
5. Retinal macroaneurysm
6. Hemorrhagic retinopathy with branch or central retinal venous occlusions
7. Acute posterior multifocal placoid pigment epitheliopathy and retinal pigment epithelial detachments
8. Optic nerve involvement is found in 7–34% patients.[9,10] Optic disk nodules (Fig. 5.5)/granuloma/optociliary shunts/dilated collateral veins on the optic nerve head and optic atrophy may occur either due to direct sarcoid tissue infiltration or compression by a cerebral mass
9. Neurological manifestations include cranial nerve palsies, encephalopathy, chiasmal syndromes, motility disorders, disorders of the hypothalamus and pituitary gland

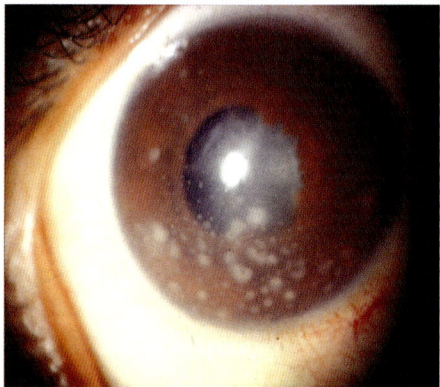

Fig. 5.1: Showing anterior granulomatous uveitis with mutton fat keratic precipitates on corneal endothelium

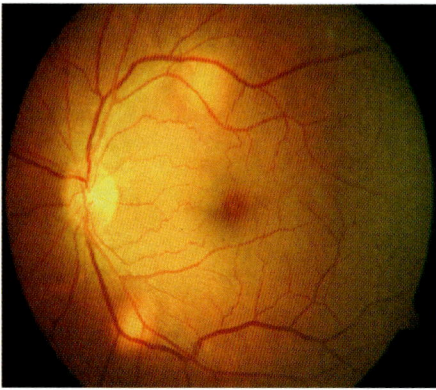

Fig. 5.2: Multifocal chorioretinal lesions

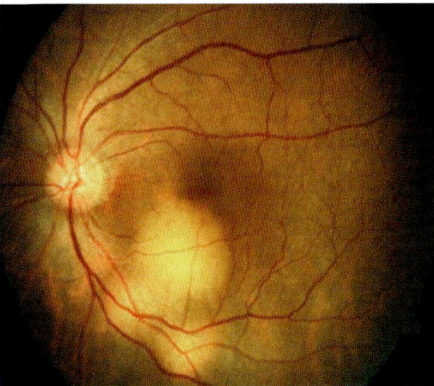

Fig. 5.3: Sarcoid nodule/granuloma

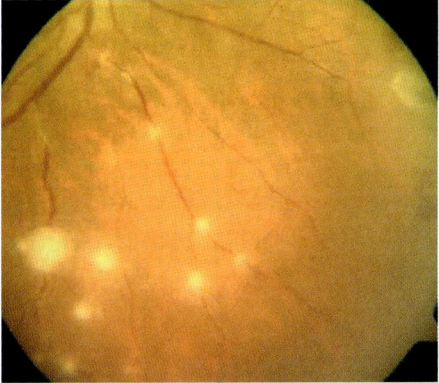

Fig. 5.4: Sarcoid vasculitis with candle wax drippings

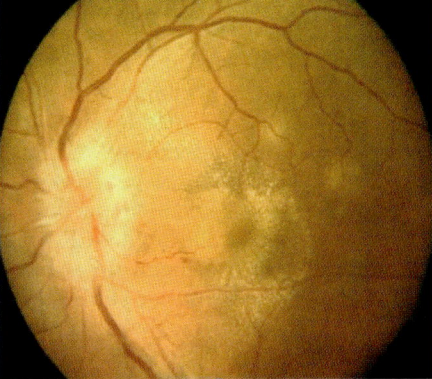

Fig. 5.5: Optic nerve head sarcoid granuloma

DIAGNOSIS

The clinical signs and laboratory investigations considered in diagnostic criteria proposed by International Workshop of Ocular Sarcoidosis, 2006(3) are described in Table 5.4.

TABLE 5.4: Showing criteria for the international diagnosis of sarcoidosis

1.	Biopsy supported diagnosis with compatible uveitis	Definitive ocular sarcoidosis
2.	Biopsy not done, bilateral hilar lymphadenopathy with compatible uveitis	Presumed ocular sarcoidosis
3.	Biopsy not done; chest radiograph normal; 3 suggestive signs out of 7 and 2 positive investigations	Probable ocular sarcoidosis
4.	Biopsy negative ; 4 suggestive ocular signs and 2 positive investigations	Possible ocular sarcoidosis

A. Clinical Signs of Sarcoidosis[3]

- Mutton fat keratic precipitates and/or iris nodules at pupillary margin or on stroma
- Trabecular meshwork nodules and/or tent-shaped peripheral anterior synechiae
- Snowballs/string of pearls in vitreous or vitreous opacities
- Multifocal peripheral chorioretinal lesions (active or atrophic)
- Nodular and/or segmental periphlebitis with or without candle wax exudates and/or macroaneurysms
- Optic disk nodule/granuloma and /or solitary choroidal nodule
- Bilateral inflammation (evident on clinical examination or on imaging)

B. Laboratory Investigations for Suspected Sarcoidosis

- Negative tuberculin test in a patient who has received BCG vaccination or who had a positive Mantoux test
- Elevated serum angiotensin-converting enzyme (ACE) and/or elevated serum lysozyme
- Chest X-ray-bilateral hilar lymphadenopathy
- Abnormal liver enzyme tests (any two of alkaline phosphatase, aspartate transaminase, alanine transaminase)
- HRCT chest in patients with normal chest radiograph
    - ACE is produced by the macrophages of the sarcoid granuloma. ACE levels are elevated in 60–90% of patients with active sarcoidosis.[5] Although ACE levels can be normal in early stages of disease or when the epithelioid cell number is not large enough to cause an elevation as in ocular sarcoidosis. Normal ACE level in serum is approximately 55 units/liter, but serum ACE levels are age dependent. Serum ACE levels are higher in age group less than 21 years as compared to age group above 21 years. Its 84% sensitive and 95% specific, when ACE levels above 50 units/liter are considered.[14] Elevated ACE levels in tears of patient with ocular sarcoidosis has also been described although it is not a specific test for sarcoidosis.[15] Another study has reported one patient with normal serum ACE but elevated levels in aqueous humor.[16]
    - Lysozyme is important in patients who are on ACE inhibitors. ACE and lysozyme can be elevated in uveitis caused by other disease also.[5] It is secreted by epitheloid cells of the sarcoid granuloma. Other laboratory investigations include hypercalcemia, hypercalciuria, elevated erythrocyte sedimentation rate, C-reactive protein and elevated alkaline phosphatase. Hypercalcemia can be presented alone but hypercalcemia is always associated with hypercalciuria.[17] Serum surfactant protein-D(SPD) is a new marker which was reported to be significantly elevated in sarcoidosis than in other uveitis etiologies.[18]

Ocular Complications

- Ocular complications include CME, cataract, glaucoma, retinal ischemia, optic disk edema, vascular occlusions, retinal and optic disk neovascularization, vitreous hemorrhage and retinal detachment. Inflammatory neovascular membrane has also been reported in few studies. Band-shaped keratopathy is observed in chronic cases.[2,3]

Differential Diagnosis of Ocular Sarcoidosis[2]

- The differential diagnosis of sarcoidosis is listed in Table 5.5.
- Among the list tuberculosis, syphilis, VKH, birdshot retinochoroidopathy and primary intraocular lymphoma can present with choroidal granulomas
- Granulomatous uveitis may be seen in VKH, tuberculosis, syphilis, toxoplasmosis, herpetic uveitis and multiple sclerosis.

TABLE 5.5: Showing the differential diagnosis of sarcoidosis

Vogt-Koyanagi-Harada syndrome (VKH)	Sympathetic ophthalmia
Multifocal choroiditis	Primary intraocular lymphoma
Tuberculosis	Syphilis
Lyme disease	Birdshot retinochoroidopathy
Herpetic uveitis	Toxoplasmosis
Multiple sclerosis	Blau syndrome
Juvenile rheumatoid arthritis in children	

Role of Ancillary Investigations in Diagnosis of Ocular Sarcoidosis

Radiological Examination

Approximately 50–89% of patients with systemic sarcoidosis presents with bilateral hilar lymphadenopathy (Fig. 5.6) HRCT chest (Fig. 5.7) is more sensitive in detecting hilar lymphadenopathy than chest radiography[19] and is also superior to transbronchial lung biopsy (TBLB) in diagnosis. Elderly age, posterior synechiae

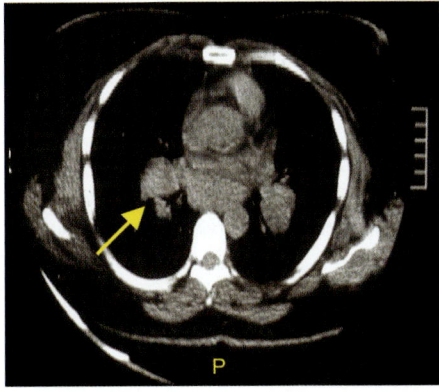

Fig. 5.6: HRCT chest showing bilateral hilar lymphadenopathy (arrow)

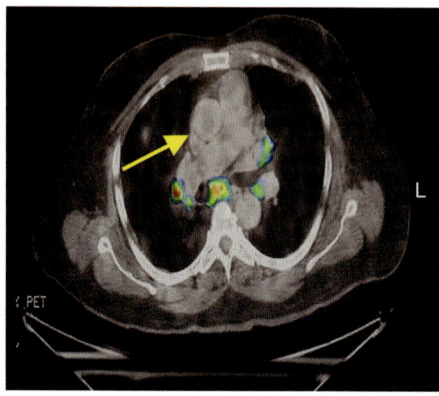

Fig. 5.7: PETCT showing metabolically active multiple lymph nodes (arrow) in the right

and peripheral multifocal chorioretinitis are significantly associated with HRCT findings indicative of sarcoidosis.[20] However, the hilar lymphadenopathy can be present in ocular tuberculosis also. HRCT chest can show enlargement of right paratracheal lymph nodes, aortic plutonic window lymph nodes and mediastinal lymph nodes. However lymph nodes are more discrete in sarcoidosis in contrast to conglomerate nature in ocular tuberculosis. Fissural, subfissural nodule, micronodules with lymphangitic spread, which implies peribronchovascular, subpleural and interlobular septal distribution, are characteristically described in ocular sarcoidosis. Apical fibrosis is seen in tuberculosis. Few studies have described lymph node necrosis in case of which tuberculosis has to be ruled out especially in endemic areas. Alveolar densities and patchy ground glass opacities are reversible changes, while honeycombing, architectural distortion, bullae, and tractional bronchiectasis are irreversible changes seen in sarcoidosis. In cases where HRCT shows necrosis of lymph nodes it is important to rule out tuberculosis especially in endemic areas like India.[21]

Newer modalities like whole body positron emission tomography (PET) scan, cardiac MRI can also provide additional useful information.[21] PET scans are superior to Ga scan. It helps in identifying the inflammation foci for diagnostic biopsy and to follow up disease activity in cases with extraocular sarcoidosis[6] (Fig. 5.7).

Gallium (Ga) citrate scanning is a nonspecific test in which uptake of radioactive isotope gallium 67 is assessed and graded in the lacrimal gland, salivary gland, thorax, spleen, liver and eyes, 48–72 hours after injection.[3] Ga uptake of lacrimal and parotid gland is referred as panda pattern[22] and the parahilar, infrahilar and right paratracheal lymph nodes uptake has been referred as lambda pattern.[23]

Pulmonary Function Test

Pulmonary function test (PFT) is more sensitive (70%) in cases with positive radiographic evidence and helps in initial diagnosis and follow up of patients with pulmonary involvement.[5]

Bronchoalveolar Lavage and Vitreous Cytology

CD4/CD8 ratio greater than 3.5 in BAL and in vitreous infiltrating lymphocytes (vitreous cytology) has 94% and 100% specificity and 53 % and 96.3% sensitivity respectively in predicting diagnosis of sarcoidosis[3] but it is not pathognomic.[5]

Transbronchial Lung Biopsy

Transbronchial lung biopsy (TBLB) also yield higher positive rates in presence of positive radiographic findings. When four biopsies are obtained at each bronchoscopy, the diagnostic yield increases to 90%.[24]

Tissue Biopsy

Biopsy supported diagnosis is definitive diagnosis for ocular sarcoidosis. It can be obtained from conjunctiva, lacrimal gland or from skin tissue. Conjunctival biopsy gives positive yield in 14–40.4% cases. Lower lid is retracted and 1 cm long and 3 mm wide conjunctival specimen is obtained from the stretched conjunctiva.[5] Lacrimal gland biopsy is done in patient with clinically enlarged lacrimal gland and in cases with positive Ga uptake by the gland. Skin biopsy from the skin lesions like lupus perniomaculopapular rashes and subcutaneous nodules can also be taken to confirm the ocular diagnosis of sarcoidosis.[5]

Indocyanine Angiography and Fluorescein Angiography

Indocyanine angiography helps to detect occult choroidal lesions.[3] Fluorescein angiography shows retinal vascular leakage, early blocked fluorescence and late staining of choroidal granulomas, retinal pigment epithelium window defects and cystoid macular edema (CME).[2]

Negative Mantoux Test

It is due to cutaneous anergy[25] that is the compartmentalization of immune response due to competitive depletion of the T-helper cells from the site of delayed type hypersensitivity reaction to the site of granuloma. Cutaneous anergy is seen with other skin antigens also.[5]

TREATMENT

Corticosteroids

Mainstay of therapy for systemic and ocular sarcoidosis is corticosteroids. Mild anterior uveitis is managed with topical steroids and cycloplegics. For resistant and severe cases, orbital disease, posterior uveitis and in neovascularization periocular and/or systemic steroids are used.[5] Intravenous steroids are useful in very severe disease which has optic nerve or macular involvement. In cases of CME intravitreal steroids or sustained release steroid drug delivery devices like that of dexamethasone and fluocinolone acetonide implants have been found useful.[2]

Immunosuppressives

Immunomodulatory therapy may be used in cases, which are unresponsive to corticosteroids. Methotrexate, mycophenolate mofetil, cyclosporine and azathioprine have been used successfully in treatment of sarcoidosis.[2] Methotrexate is most frequently used. Low dose methotrexate (10–20 mg/week) is an effective as well as safe treatment.[26]

Biologicals—rituximab and infliximab have been reported to be successful in treating sarcoidosis.[2]

Intravitreal anti-VEGFs are administered for the treatment of inflammatory neovascular membranes in sarcoidosis.[2]

Pan retinal photocoagulation to ischemic areas detected on fluorescein angiography, in cases of retinal neovascularization, shows good response.[5]

Secondary glaucoma unresponsive to medical management may need trabeculectomy and cryoablative therapy.[11,27] Laser trabeculoplasty and conventional filtering procedures have not shown good results and therefore trabeculectomy with the use of antimetabolites or seton drainage devices might be necessary.

Large sarcoid iris nodules may require sometimes surgical excision if they fail to respond to corticosteroids.[5]

Prognosis of Ocular Sarcoidosis

Early treatment offers a good prognosis. Poor visual prognosis is seen in chronic posterior or panuveitis, presentation at older age, delay in presentation and in cases with complications like glaucoma, cataract and CME.[2]

CONCLUSION

Ocular sarcoidosis is a potentially blinding disease that demands early diagnosis and an aggressive management. It is seen in more than 25–60% of patients diagnosed with sarcoidosis. Ocular signs are variable and can involve any part of eye and orbital structures, and thus it is very important to have a careful examination, strong suspicion, complete review of system and appropriate investigations may help to make the correct diagnosis.

REFERENCES

1. Schumacher G. Fall von beiderseitiger iridocyclitis chronica bei boeckschem multiplem benignem sarkoid. Munch Med Wochenschr. 1909;56:2664.
2. Sen HN, Nussenblatt RB. Sarcoidosis associated uveitis. Color atlas and synopsis of clinical ophthalmology wills eye institute-uveitis. Lipincott Williams and Wilkins. 2012;65-71.
3. Babu K. Uveitis: Ocular Sarcoidosis. An Update. Springer India; 2016;133-41.
4. Rothova A. Ocular involvement in sarcoidosis. Br J Ophthalmol. 2000;84:110-6.
5. Capella MJ, Foster CS. Sarcoidosis. Diagnosis and treatment of uveitis. Jaypee Highlights. 2013;967.
6. Dianne Liu, Andrea D. Birnbaum. Update on Sarcoidosis. Curr Opin Ophthalalmol. 2015;26:512-6.
7. Babu K, Kini R, Mehta R, Abraham MP, Subbakrishna DK, Murthy KR. Clinical profile of ocular sarcoidosis in a south Indian patient population. Ocul Immunol Inflamm. 2010;18(5):362.
8. Obenauf CD, Shaw HE, Sydnor CF, Klintworth GK. Sarcoidosis and its ophthalmic manifestations. Am J Ophthalmol. 1978;86(5):648-55.
9. Hunter DG, Foster CS. Ocular manifestation of sarcoidosis. In: Albert DM, Jackobiec FA (Eds). Principles and practice ofophthalomolgy. Philadelphia: WB Sauders. 1994;443-50.
10. Jabs DA, John CJ. Ocular involvement in chronic sarcoidosis. Am J Ophthalmol. 1986;102(3):297-301.
11. Dana MR1, Merayo-Lloves J, Schaumberg DA, Foster CS. Prognosticators for visual outcome in sarcoid uveitis. Ophthalmology. 1996;103(11):1846-53.
12. Rothova A, Alberts C, Glasius E, Kijlstra A, Buitenhuis HJ, Breebaart AC. Risk factors for ocular sarcoidosis. Doc Ophthalmol. 1989;72(3-4):287-96.

13. Crick RP, Hoyle C, Smellie H. The eyes in sarcoidosis. Br J Ophthalmol. 1961;45(7): 461-81.
14. Baarsma GS, La Hey E, Glasius E, de Vries J, Kijlstra A. The predictive value of serum angiotensin converting enzyme and lysozyme levels in the diagnosis of ocular sarcoidosis. Am J Ophthalmol. 1987;104(3):211-7.
15. Immonen I, Friberg K, Sorsila R, Fyhrquist F. Concentration of angiotensin-converting enzyme in tears of patients with sarcoidosis. Acta Ophthalmol (Copenh). 1987;65(1):27-9.
16. Weinreb RN, Sandman R, Ryder MI, Friberg TR. Angiotensin-converting enzyme activity in human aqueous humor. Arch Ophthalmol. 1985;103(1):34-6.
17. Costabel U, Teschler H. Biochemical changes in sarcoidosis. Clin Chest Med. 1997;18(4):827-42.
18. Kitaichi N, Kitamura M, Namba K, Ishida S, Ohno S. Elevation of surfactant protein D, a pulmonary disease biomarker, in the sera of uveitis patients with sarcoidosis. Jpn J Ophthalmol. 2010;54(1):81-4.
19. Chung YM, Lin YC, Liu YT, Chang SC, Liu HN, Hsu WH. Uveitis with biopsy-proven sarcoidosis in Chinese—a study of 60 patients in auveitis clinic over a period of 20 years. J Chin Med Assoc. 2007;70(11):492-6.
20. Clement DS, Postma G, Rothova A, Grutters JC, Prokop M, de Jong PA. Intraocular sarcoidosis: association of clinical characteristics of uveitis with positive chest high-resolution computed tomography findings. Br J Ophthalmol. 2010;94(2): 219-22.
21. Babu K, Sai BS, Mariamma P. High Resolution Chest Tomography in the Diagnosis of Ocular Sarcoidosis in High TB Endemic Population. Ocul Immunol Inflmm. 2016;00(00):1-6.
22. Sulavik SB, Spencer RP, Weed DA, Shapiro HR, Shiue ST, Castriotta RJ. Recognition of distinctive patterns of gallium-67 distribution in sarcoidosis. J Nucl Med. 1990;31(12):1909-14.
23. Sulavik SB, Spencer RP, Palestro CJ, Swyer AJ, Teirstein AS, Goldsmith SJ. Specificity and sensitivity of distinctive chest radiographic and/or 67Ga images in the noninvasive diagnosis of sarcoidosis. Chest. 1993;103(2):403-9.
24. Gilman MJ, Wang KP. Transbronchial lung biopsy in sarcoidosis. An approach to determine the optimal number of biopsies.Am Rev Respir Dis. 1980;122(5):721-4.
25. Boeck C. Nochmals zur clinic und zur stellung des" Benignen Miliarlupoids".Arch dermatol Syph(Wien). 1916;121:707-41.
26. Dev S, McCallum RM, Jaffe GJ. Methotrexate treatment for sarcoid-associated panuveitis. Ophthalmology. 1999;106:111-8.
27. Akova YA, Foster CS. Cataract surgery in patients with sarcoidosis-associated uveitis. Ophthalmology. 1994;101(3):473-9.

Chapter 6

Advances in Intravitreal Therapeutics in Uveitis

Parthopratim Dutta Majumder, Jyotirmay Biswas

Uveitis is often chronic and potentially sight threatening disorder and because of the chronic nature of the inflammation and associated risks of complications, the treatment of uveitis remains a challenge to the ophthalmologists. Corticosteroid remains mainstay of the treatment of non-infectious uveitis. Cases refractory to corticosteroids or patients intolerant to the corticosteroids are usually treated with second-line immunosuppressive drugs as steroid-sparing agents. Both corticosteroid and immunosuppressives are known to have many systemic side-effects.

Because of the considerable systemic side-effects associated with oral steroid and immunosuppressives the treatment of chronic cases of non-infectious uveitis is difficult. Proper and effective control of these chronic inflammation requires high doses of these immunomodulatory agents to achieve and sustain therapeutic intraocular levels which increases the risks of such potential side-effects, which can be life threatening in some cases. The risk of systemic toxicity with these medications can be considerably reduced with the local delivery of the drugs especially in conditions which are not associated with any systemic diseases and unilateral involvement. In this article we have tried to summarize the commonly intravitreal medications used in the management of non-infectious uveitis.

Intravitreal injections allow the drug to reach the desired target of action. The vitreous cavity acts like a reservoir where the desired levels of drugs can be maintained for relatively longer periods. The concentration of the drug in vitreous cavity achieved through this route is much higher than the concentrations obtained by the administration of drugs through other ways (i.e. topical, oral, intravenous). This route also minimizes possible systemic side effects associated with a drug. Over the last decade there has been an enormous progress in intravitreal medications for the treatment of uveitis.

Intravitreal Therapeutics in Noninfectious Uveitis

Intravitreal Triamcinolone Acetonide

Corticosteroids act by the suppression of prostaglandin and interleukin synthesis by inhibition of phospholipase A2, reduction of VEGF expression and stabilization of the blood–retinal barrier. Triamcinolone acetonide remains the most widely used intravitreal steroid in the management of non-infectious uveitis.

Triamcinolone acetonide is a minimally water-soluble corticosteroid injected intravitreally in suspension form and prolonged duration of action of this drug is because of its decreased water solubility. Mean half-life of triamcinolone is 18.6 days in nonvitrectomised patients and 3.2 days in post vitrectomy patient.[1] It has been estimated that a single intravitreal injection of triamcinolone acetonide, can yield a concentration of 0.22 ± 0.24 µg/mL in vitreous.[2] Desirable concentration of the drug are reported to last for 3 months in vitreous of nonvitrectomised eyes.

Intravitreal Triamcinolone Acetonide: At a Glance

- Synthetic steroid of the glucocorticoid family
- Molecular weight: 434.50[3]
- Empirical formula: $C_{24}H_{31}FO_6$[3]
- Physical property: commercially available as an ester, a white powder
- Solubility: minimally soluble in water but soluble in alcohol and chloroform
- Commonly used doses: 4 mg/0.1 mL and 2 mg/0.5 mL[4].

Intravitreal injections of triamcinolone acetonide (IVTA) have increasingly been reported as a treatment of intraocular inflammatory disease. It is most commonly used for chronic cystoid macular edema (CME) due to uveitis. Various studies have shown that a single intravitreal injection of 4 mg triamcinolone acetonide can effectively reduce CME and improve visual acuity in 50% to 70% of patients. In some patients, Intravitreal triamcinolone acetonide helped in reducing the need and dosage of the immunosuppressive therapy. However, the period of effectiveness of the medications remained variable; 3 to 6 months. Factors favoring better response to intravitreal triamcinolone acetonide include CME of less than 1 year duration, younger age, and nonvitrectomised eyes.[5]

One needs to monitor intraocular pressure following injection of triamcinolone. In a randomized controlled trial in patients with neovascular age related macular degenerations (ARMD), 42.7% of the eyes developed raised IOP following intravitreal triamcinolone; however, all were adequately controlled with topical antiglaucoma medication.[6] The risk of cataract formation also increases with repeat injections of IVTA. Endophthalmitis is also a major risk involved associated with intravitreal triamcinolone injections.

I-vation® (MK0140) is a helical sustained-release implant containing 0.925 µg triamcinolone acetonide and elutes drug for up to 2 years. The helical shape is designed to increase surface area available for drug diffusion. Phase 1 clinical trials of I-vation showed its effectiveness in treating diabetic macular edema (DME) though complications like increased IOP and cataract development were significant. Phase 2b trials of the implant were terminated.[7]

Fluocinolone Acetonide Sustained Drug Delivery Device

Fluocinolone acetonide is a low-solubility corticosteroid. The fluorine substitution at position 9 in the steroid nucleus greatly enhances activity of this molecule. However, it is relatively weaker corticosteroid when compared to triamcinolone acetonide and has a shorter half-life in vitreous.

Retisert® is a non-biodegradable sustained drug delivery device, which received the US Food and Drug Administration (FDA) approval in 2005 and became the first intravitreal device for the treatment of chronic noninfectious uveitis. It is composed of a central core containing either 0.59 mg of fluocinolone acetonide, compressed into a 1.5-mm drug core coated with an elastomer and designed to release therapeutic levels of the drug slowly. Release of the drug occurs through a diffusion port in the coating. These devices release the drug at approximately 0.59 microgram per day over a period of 30 months. The device is 5 mm long, 2 mm wide and 1.5 mm thick and inserted into the vitreous cavity and sutured to the sclera through a pars plana surgical technique.

Intravitreal Fluocinolone Acetonide: At a Glance

- Synthetic steroid of the fluorinated glucocorticoid family
- Molecular weight: 452.49[8]
- Empirical formula: $C_{24}H_{30}F_2O_6$[8]
- Physical property: odorless, white, crystalline powder
- Solubility: low aqueous solubility (1/24th of dexamethasone)[8]
- Commonly used doses: Retisert® Total dose 590 µg; Daily release 0.59 µg/day[8]
- Iluvien® Total dose 190 µg; daily release 0.19 µg/day.[8]

Fluocinolone acetonide sustained drug delivery device was found to significantly minimise inflammation and reduce intravitreal vascular endothelial growth factor (VEGF) levels. The recurrence of inflammation in patients with noninfectious posterior uveitis was significantly reduced following treatment with this non-biodegradable implant.[9,10] However, multicenter uveitis steroid treatment (MUST) trial, which compared the relative effectiveness of systemic therapy and fluocinolone acetonide implant for the treatment of noninfectious uveitis in 479 eyes over 2 years, found that both treatment groups were equally effective and in terms of improving visual acuity neither group was superior to the other. The implant group had an 80% risk of cataract surgery.

Rise of IOP is a major concern with Retisert®, 51% of patients had raised IOP that required anti glaucoma medication and at 3 years, 78% of the eyes required anti-glaucoma medications and approximately 40% required glaucoma filtering surgery. Also almost all the phakic patients developed cataract within 3 years of implantation of this device.[9,10]

Iluvien® (Alimera Sciences Inc., Alpharetta, GA; pSivida Inc., Watertown, MA) is another nonbiodegradable intravitreal implant containing fluocinolone acetonide. It is 3.5 mm long and 0.37 mm wide. Iluvien uses the same drug matrix as Retisert, but is thought to release a lower dose of drug (0.2 µg/day or 0.5 µg/day) than Retisert (nominally 0.59 µg/day) over a period of 18–36 months.[11] It is inserted with a 25-gauge needle. The implant received FDA approval for the treatment of diabetic macular edema (DME) in patients who have been previously treated with a course of corticosteroids and did not have a clinically significant rise in intraocular pressure.

Intravitreal Dexamethasone Implants

Dexamethasone is a highly potent corticosteroid, widely used for the treatment of systemic inflammatory conditions. Anti-inflammatory activity of dexamethasone is 6-fold greater than that of triamcinolone acetonide. Its hydrophilicity allows for higher vitreous concentration compared to other corticosteroid preparation, but it is shorter acting in the vitreous with a half-life of ~5 hour. This limitation in ocular pharmacokinetic of the drug has been overcome with the special design of drug delivery system.

Intravitreal Dexamethasone: At a Glance

- Synthetic steroid of the fluorinated glucocorticoid family

- Molecular weight: 516.404624 g/mol
- Empirical formula: $C_{22}H_{28}FNa_2O_8P$
- Physical property: odorless, white, crystalline powder
- Solubility: ethanol: soluble 1 mg/mL, Solubility in water (25°C): 10 mg/100 mL
- Commonly used doses: 0.7 mg (700 µg).

Ozurdex is intravitreal, biodegradable, sustained-release implant gradually delivers dexamethasone and it can be inserted in to the eye through a small pars plana incision or puncture. It is made of a solid biodegradable polymer composed of polylactic acid-co-glycolic acid (PLGA) matrix and as the implant erodes, it gradually releases 700 microgram of dexamethasone in to the vitreous. This PLGA matrix dissolves completely into lactic acid and glycolic acid. These products are in turn converted into CO_2 and H_2O which can be easily eliminated by ocular tissue. Dexamethasone was detected in the vitreous up to 6 months after insertion of this device.[12]

In a double-masked, randomized, controlled trial (HURON study), comparing the effect of two implant doses (0.7 mg and 0.35 mg) with sham injection, this implant found to effective in controlling vitreous inflammation and improving visual acuity.[12] Approximately half of the patients treated with the higher dose implant had a vitreous haze score of 0 at 8 weeks. This effect was maintained at 26 weeks. Compared to other intravitreal preparations of corticosteroid, the side effects associated with this implant were less. The incidence of cataract reported in the study was 15% but did not require any surgical intervention. With the exclusion of steroid responders from the study, incidence of raised IOP (which was defined as IOP≥ 25 mm Hg) was less than 10%.[12]

In a meta-analysis, Kidder et al.[13] compared the IOP rise following injection of IVTA 4 mg, fluocinolone acetonide implant 0.59 and 2.1 mg and dexamethasone 0.35 and 0.7 mg implant. Ocular hypertension developed in 32% of IVTA injected eyes, 66% and 79% in low and high dose fluocinolone acetonide implant and 11 and 15% in low and high dose dexamethasone implant.

Intravitreal Nonsteroidal Anti-inflammatory Drug (NSAID)

Ketorolac is a potent NSAID with known analgesic, anti-pyretic, and anti-inflammatory properties. Topical ketorolac has been found to be effective in reducing postoperative inflammation and macular edema. Ketorolac does not reach significant levels in the vitreous or retina after topical or systemic application.

Intravitreal ketorolac attains peak drug concentrations in the vitreous (234 µg/mL) and retina (280 µg/g) which is 100-fold greater than what can be achieved with topical or systemic administration.[14] Ketorolac's intraocular half-life is limited by its high water solubility and retinal concentration of the drug is below the inhibitory concentration of 50% for both isoforms of COX (COX-1 and COX-2) after 48 hours of intravitreal injection. Phase I trial of intravitreal ketorolac in ten patients showed some effect in treating intraocular inflammation and macular oedema.[15] However, a similar pilot study of another intravitreal NSAID Diclofenac showed no benefit in macular edema of various etiologies.[16]

Anti-vascular Endothelial Growth Factor (VEGF) Agents

The role of vascular endothelial growth factor (VEGF) in induction of inflammation, increasing vascular permeability and its role in uveitic cystoid macular edema has been well established. Anti-VEGF agents like bevacizumab, ranibizumab may be a supplementary off-label therapeutic option for persistent uveitis CME. However most of the studies failed to prove any statistical significant increase in visual acuity in patients with intravitreal application of these agents. These agents have been also used to treat choroidal neovascularization secondary to inflammatory conditions like toxoplasmosis, punctate inner choroidopathy, serpiginous choroiditis and multifocal choroiditis. The rate of cataract progression or IOP rise is much less with these agents. These are of particular use in those patients who are known to be steroid responders.[17] However it must be remembered that anti-VEGF agents have less anti-inflammatory effect and cannot be used as primary agents for the management of inflammatory CME.

Ranibizumab Port Delivery System is a novel port delivery system (filled with 150 µg of ranibizumab) which is designed to release 10 mg/mL over an extended period of time with a unique feature to refill the device. The device showed promising results and waiting for randomized control trial.[7]

Intravitreal Immunosuppressives

To overcome the side-effects such as progression of cataract, rise in IOP and relative shorter duration of actions of corticosteroids, various other medications have been tried for Intravitreal application in the management of intraocular inflammations.

Intravitreal Methotrexate

Methotrexate is a folate analog. It inhibits the enzyme dihydrofolate reductase, thereby inhibiting the production of tetrahydrofolate which in turn inhibits formation of thymidylate, leading to inhibition of DNA replication and RNA transcription. It acts both on T and B cells. Methotrexate has little action on resting cells. It is mainly active against rapidly dividing immune cells. Methotrexate has been used increasingly in ophthalmic disease, mainly systemically. Intravitreal methotrexate was used in the management of intraocular lymphomas associated with primary central nervous system lymphoma. Intravitreal methotrexate has been used in the treatment of uveitis also. The widely used dosage of intravitreal methotrexate is 400 µg of the drug in 0.1 mL. The duration of effect of intravitreal methotrexate has been estimated to be approximately 4 months.

Intravitreal methotrexate was found to be effective in reducing vitritis and uveitis macular oedema. According to a study reported by Taylor et al. there was significant improvement in visual acuity, which was statistically significant at the 3-month and 6-month follow-up examinations. In the same study the onset of effect was observed within 1 week and lasted approximately 4 months. No rise in IOP was encountered in patients with a history of steroid response.[18]

A larger collaborative multicenter study has showed promising result and intravitreal methotrexate may induce longer term remission in some patients.[19] In an animal model study, Deng et al.[20] that intravitreal MTX reduces the risk of development of endophthalmitis and concluded that intravitreal methotrexate can be a safer option for the treatment of refractory uveitis than intravitreal steroids. However corneal epithelial edema and risks of corneal endothelial decompensation is a serious and major side effect of intravitreal methotrexate.[21] However, in a prospective noncomparative interventional series of 21 eyes, authors did not observed any significant effect of intravitreal injection of 400 µg methotrexate on corneal endothelial cell measurements performed by specular microscopy.[22]

Recently a biodegradable intraocular micro-implant for sustained release of methotrexate was experimented on rabbit eyes and therapeutic concentration of the drug in the vitreous was detected for 33 days.[23] This implant can emerge as prospective alternative to current treatment protocols of repeated intravitreal

MTX injections in intraocular disorders such as primary intraocular lymphoma, and selected cases of non-microbial intraocular inflammation.

Intravitreal Use of Other Immunosuppressives

Sirolimus inhibits activation of T and B cells by blocking the response to interleukin-2. Sirolimus has potent immunosuppressive, antiangiogenic and antiproliferative properties. Due to its gastrointestinal and dermatological side effects, its systemic use has been limited and efficacy of the drug has been tried via the intravitreal route.[24] After intravitreal administration, the drug preparation forms a non-dispersive depot in the vitreous subsequently and dissolves slowly, and diffuses through the vitreous humor. A detectable ocular tissue level of Sirolimus has been reported after 60 days of single intravitreal administration. A multinational, multicenter, randomized, double-masked phase III trial (Study Assessing Double-masKed Uveitis tReAtment; SAKURA) assessed the safety and efficacy of intravitreal injections of three doses of sirolimus for the treatment of active, noninfectious uveitis of the posterior segment of the eye in 347 patients. The patients were randomized to three different treatment groups (for the doses of 44, 440 and 880 µg in a total volume of 20 µL). Each patient received three injections at days 1, 60 and 120. A vitreous haze score of 0 was reached by 23% in the 440 µg group. Changes in visual acuity were moderate and effects on macular thickness were small with the best results in macular edema patients without epiretinal membranes. Patients in the 440 µg group did better than in the 880 µg group with the least effectivity demonstrated with the low dose 44 µg.[25]

Cyclosporine works on T-cell by binding to an intracellular peptide known as cyclophilin which results in blockage of transcription and production of interleukins, activation of CD4 and CD8 T cells and production of other lymphokines such as interferon. Being a cytostatic drug (inflammation may recur when the drug is stopped); cyclosporin is generally used for a long time when administered systemically. Renal toxicity is a notorious side effect of this medication and often limits its use in the management of uveitis. In animal models, intravitreal cyclosporin has been reported to show satisfactory results in controlling intraocular inflammation. No toxic effects were reported in any animals treated with ≤100 mg of intravitreal cyclosporin.[26]

Intravitreal Use of Biologicals

Biologicals are a group of drugs which are directed mainly against specific cytokines or their receptors. These groups of drugs were introduced as an alternative therapy for refractory cases of uveitis about 15 years ago. Recently these agents have been used extensively systemically as well as for intravitreal application for the management of non-infectious uveitic conditions.

Infliximab is a genetically engineered monoclonal antibody to TNF-α. It reduces levels of interleukin-6 and chemokines, including macrophage chemoattractant protein-1, as well as adhesion molecules, such as intercellular adhesion molecule-1. Infliximab is found to effective as a short term immunosuppressive agent in noninfectious uveitis. However repeated infusions are often needed to prevent recurrences.

Intravitreal injection of 1.5 mg infliximab has been reported to show significant improvement in visual acuity, with a significant decrease in the central macular thickness and vitreous inflammation. The intravitreal application of the drug has shown promising results in patients with recurrent intraocular inflammation especially Behçet's disease and recalcitrant uveitis CME.[27] However intravitreal infliximab has been reported to cause intraocular inflammation in nonuveitic eyes when the drug was injected for either diabetic macular edema or neovascular age-related macular degeneration.

Adalimumab is an IgG monoclonal antibody to human necrosis factor. Adalimumab has an added advantage over infliximab as it is a fully humanized antibody. However intravitreal injection of this drug in uveitis CME failed to produce any significant improvement in vision or reduction of macular thickness.[28]

Intravitreal corticosteroids, though associated with potential side-effects such as cataract formation, rise of IOP and warranting surgical intervention in many cases, remain mainstay of intraocular therapy. Though there is increasing number of steroid sparing intravitreal medications, the need of moratorium on the clinical use of such agents has to be achieved and randomized; controlled trials would be required to confirm results and efficacy of these agents.

Intravitreal Therapeutics in Infectious Uveitis

Intravitreal Ganciclovir

The first intravitreal drug implant was developed for the local treatment of cytomegalovirus retinitis in HIV patients. The ganciclovir implant consists of 4.5 mg of ganciclovir as the active ingredient and 0.25% magnesium stearate as the inactive ingredient in a tablet coated with polyvinyl alcohol and hydrophobic ethylene vinyl acetate.

The implant releases 1 µg of ganciclovir per hour and has therapeutic effects over a period of eight months. Being a non-degradable and relatively large implant, the implant must be sutured to the wall of the globe in the area of the pars plana of the ciliary body through a 5.5-mm incision. It has to be removed usually after 6 months or if there are any complications such as endophthalmitis or retinal detachment. Vitrasert has been reported to offer superior control of CMV retinitis over systemic ganciclovir therapy.[29]

Intravitreal Clindamycin

Oral clindamycin has been widely used in the treatment of ocular toxoplasmosis. Though in animal studies clindamycin has been reported to reduce the number of tissue cysts, the drug has not been proven to prevent recurrent disease in humans.[30] Various authors reported the efficacy of intravitreal clindamycin and dexamethasone in patients with contraindication, intolerance, or a lack of response to traditional systemic anti-toxoplasma therapy.[31] Also systemic medications not be efficacious enough to control the infection in all cases of ocular toxoplasmosis.[32] In a prospective randomized single-blind clinical trial, intravitreal injection of clindamycin and dexamethasone was found to be as effective as conventional oral therapy in the treatment of ocular toxoplasmosis with fewer systemic side-effects.[33]

REFERENCES

1. Beer PM, Bakri SJ, Singh RJ, Liu W, Peters GB, Miller M. Intraocular concentration and pharmacokinetics of triamcinolone acetonide after a single intravitreal injection. Ophthalmology. 2003;110(4):681-6.
2. Inoue M, Takeda K, Morita K, Yamada M, Tanigawara Y, Oguchi Y. Vitreous concentrations of triamcinolone acetonide in human eyes after intravitreal or subtenon injection. Am J Ophthalmol. 2004;138(6):1046-8.

3. Tao Y, Jonas JB. Intravitreal triamcinolone. Ophthalmol J Int Z Für Augenheilkd. 2011;225(1):1-20.
4. Degenring RF, Jonas JB. Intravitreal injection of triamcinolone acetonide as treatment for chronic uveitis. Br J Ophthalmol. 2003;87(3):361.
5. Kok H, Lau C, Maycock N, McCluskey P, Lightman S. Outcome of intravitreal triamcinolone in uveitis. Ophthalmology. 2005;112(11):1916.e1-7.
6. Gillies MC, Simpson JM, Luo W, Penfold P, Hunyor ABL, Chua W, et al. A randomized clinical trial of a single dose of intravitreal triamcinolone acetonide for neovascular age-related macular degeneration: one-year results. Arch Ophthalmol Chic Ill 1960. 2003;121(5):667-73.
7. Wang J, Jiang A, Joshi M, Christoforidis J. Drug delivery implants in the treatment of vitreous inflammation. Mediators Inflamm. 2013;2013:780634.
8. Sadiq MA, Agarwal A, Soliman MK, Hanout M, Sarwar S, Do DV, et al. Sustained-release fluocinolone acetonide intravitreal insert for macular edema: clinical pharmacology and safety evaluation. Expert Opin Drug Saf. 2015;14(7):1147-56.
9. Jaffe GJ, Martin D, Callanan D, Pearson PA, Levy B, Comstock T, et al. Fluocinolone acetonide implant (Retisert) for noninfectious posterior uveitis: thirty-four-week results of a multicenter randomized clinical study. Ophthalmology. 2006;113(6):1020-7.
10. Callanan DG, Jaffe GJ, Martin DF, Pearson PA, Comstock TL. Treatment of posterior uveitis with a fluocinolone acetonide implant: three-year clinical trial results. Arch Ophthalmol Chic Ill 1960. 2008;126(9):1191-201.
11. Kane FE, Burdan J, Cutino A, Green KE. Iluvien: a new sustained delivery technology for posterior eye disease. Expert Opin Drug Deliv. 2008;5(9):1039-46.
12. Kuppermann BD, Blumenkranz MS, Haller JA, Williams GA, Weinberg DV, Chou C, et al. Randomized controlled study of an intravitreous dexamethasone drug delivery system in patients with persistent macular edema. Arch Ophthalmol Chic Ill 1960. 2007;125(3):309-17.
13. Kiddee W, Trope GE, Sheng L, Beltran-Agullo L, Smith M, Strungaru MH, et al. Intraocular pressure monitoring post intravitreal steroids: a systematic review. Surv Ophthalmol. 2013;58(4):291-310.
14. Barañano DE, Kim SJ, Edelhauser HF, Durairaj C, Kompella UB, Handa JT. Efficacy and pharmacokinetics of intravitreal non-steroidal anti-inflammatory drugs for intraocular inflammation. Br J Ophthalmol. 2009;93(10):1387-90.
15. Tsilimbaris MK, Tsika C, Kymionis GD. Intravitreal ketorolac for the treatment of chronic cystoid macular edema after cataract surgery. Ther Clin Risk Manag. 2016;12:177-82.
16. Soheilian M, Karimi S, Ramezani A, Peyman GA. Pilot study of intravitreal injection of diclofenac for treatment of macular edema of various etiologies. Retina Phila Pa. 2010;30(3):509-15.
17. Hazirolan D, Pleyer U. Think global—act local: intravitreal drug delivery systems in chronic noninfectious uveitis. Ophthalmic Res. 2013;49(2):59-65.
18. Taylor SRJ, Habot-Wilner Z, Pacheco P, Lightman SL. Intraocular methotrexate in the treatment of uveitis and uveitic cystoid macular edema. Ophthalmology. 2009;116(4):797-801.
19. Taylor SRJ, Banker A, Schlaen A, Couto C, Matthe E, Joshi L, et al. Intraocular methotrexate can induce extended remission in some patients in noninfectious uveitis. Retina Phila Pa. 2013;33(10):2149-54.
20. Deng SX, Penland S, Gupta S, Fiscella R, Edward DP, Tessler HH, et al. Methotrexate reduces the complications of endophthalmitis resulting from intravitreal injection compared with dexamethasone in a rabbit model. Invest Ophthalmol Vis Sci. 2006;47(4):1516-21.

21. Gorovoy I, Prechanond T, Abia M, Afshar AR, Stewart JM. Toxic corneal epitheliopathy after intravitreal methotrexate and its treatment with oral folic acid. Cornea. 2013;32(8):1171-3.
22. Ghasemi Falavarjani K, Golabi S, Hadavandkhani A. Effect of Intravitreal Injection of Methotrexate on Human Corneal Endothelial Cells. Cornea. 2016;35(2):217-9.
23. Manna S, Banerjee RK, Augsburger JJ, Al-Rjoub MF, Donnell A, Correa ZM. Biodegradable chitosan and polylactic acid-based intraocular micro-implant for sustained release of methotrexate into vitreous: analysis of pharmacokinetics and toxicity in rabbit eyes. Graefes Arch Clin Exp Ophthalmol Albrecht Von Graefes Arch Für Klin Exp Ophthalmol. 2015;253(8):1297-305.
24. Mudumba S, Bezwada P, Takanaga H, Hosoi K, Tsuboi T, Ueda K, et al. Tolerability and pharmacokinetics of intravitreal sirolimus. J Ocul Pharmacol Ther Off J Assoc Ocul Pharmacol Ther. 2012;28(5):507-14.
25. Pleyer U, Thurau SR. Sirolimus for the treatment of noninfectious uveitis. Expert Opin Pharmacother. 2016;17(1):127-35.
26. Grisolano J, Peyman GA. Retinal toxicity study of intravitreal cyclosporin. Ophthalmic Surg. 1986;17(3):155-6.
27. Sfikakis PP, Kaklamanis PH, Elezoglou A, Katsilambros N, Theodossiadis PG, Papaefthimiou S, et al. Infliximab for recurrent, sight-threatening ocular inflammation in Adamantiades-Behçet disease. Ann Intern Med. 2004;140(5):404-6.
28. Tsilimbaris M, Diakonis VF, Naoumidi I, Charisis S, Kritikos I, Chatzithanasis G, et al. Evaluation of potential retinal toxicity of adalimumab (Humira). Graefes Arch Clin Exp Ophthalmol Albrecht Von Graefes Arch Für Klin Exp Ophthalmol. 2009;247(8):1119-25.
29. Martin DF, Parks DJ, Mellow SD, Ferris FL, Walton RC, Remaley NA, et al. Treatment of cytomegalovirus retinitis with an intraocular sustained-release ganciclovir implant. A randomized controlled clinical trial. Arch Ophthalmol. 1994;112(12):1531-9.
30. Holland GN, Lewis KG. An update on current practices in the management of ocular toxoplasmosis 1, 2. Am J Ophthalmol. 2002;134(1):102-14.
31. Martinez CE, Zhang D, Conway MD, Peyman GA. Successful management of ocular toxoplasmosis during pregnancy using combined intraocular clindamycin and dexamethasone with systemic sulfadiazine. Int Ophthalmol. 1998-1999;22(2):85-8.
32. Lasave AF, Díaz-Llopis M, Muccioli C, Belfort R, Arevalo JF. Intravitreal clindamycin and dexamethasone for zone 1 toxoplasmic retinochoroiditis at twenty-four months. Ophthalmology. 2010;117(9):1831-8.
33. Baharivand N, Mahdavifard A, Fouladi RF. Intravitreal clindamycin plus dexamethasone versus classic oral therapy in toxoplasmic retinochoroiditis: a prospective randomized clinical trial. Int Ophthalmol. 2013;33(1):39-46.

Chapter 7

Current Role of Imaging in Glaucoma Management

*Malarchelvi Palani, Sangeetha Rajagopal,
Nivean Madhivanan, Murali Ariga*

Glaucoma is a progressive optic neuropathy with characteristic optic disc changes and corresponding visual field loss, for which elevated intraocular pressure is one of the main risk factor.[1] In glaucoma the structural damage usually precedes the functional deterioration and by the time white on white perimetry shows defect, about 40 to 45% of retinal ganglion cells (RGC) are lost. This is attributed to the fact that even if some RGC are lost, the surrounding ganglion cells subserving the same area would signal the presence of the target and there would be no functional visual field loss. Hence structural evaluations of the optic nerve head and retina are the key for the early diagnosis and follow-up of glaucoma patients. There are three predominant imaging technologies currently in use for the detection and progression of glaucoma, namely:
1. Scanning laser polarimetry—GDx.
2. Confocal scanning laser ophthalmoscopy—Heidelberg Retina Tomograph (HRT).
3. Optical coherence tomography.

These imaging technologies provide objective quantitative measurements of the posterior segment structures that are involved in glaucoma.

SCANNING LASER POLARIMETRY

Scanning laser polarimetry is an objective imaging technique of the retinal nerve fiber layer (RNFL), based on retardation of the polarized light.

Evolution

The earlier versions of the instrument were equipped with a fixed corneal compensator. This was not able to adjust for the variability of the corneal thickness among different individuals. Hence with the goal of providing more reliable and reproducible measurements of the RNFL thickness, the initial versions of the device have been upgraded several times. The new generation instrument has the GDx VCC (variable corneal compensation) and the latest has the GDx ECC (enhanced corneal compensation) both from Carl Zeiss Meditec, Dublin, CA, USA.[2]

Principle

The principle used in GDx is birefringence. The birefringent intraocular tissues are cornea, lens and retina. The variable corneal compensator in GDx VCC individually corrects for the polarization induced by the cornea and lens, improving the ability of GDx to discriminate between glaucomatous and healthy eyes. GDx ECC performs significantly better than GDx VCC in glaucoma detection in patients with more severe atypical retardation patterns as seen in eyes with high myopia.[3,4]

Interpretation of the GDx VCC Report (Figs 7.1 to 7.3)

Patient data: This contains the name, date of birth, gender, ethnicity of the patient with the ID number and date of examination.

Quality score: The image quality is shown in a box above the fundus image that ranges from scale 1 to 10. An ideal image quality score is from 7 to 10.

Fundus image: The fundus image is used to check the quality of the image, focus, illumination and proper centration of the black ring around the optic nerve head (ONH). The calculation circle is a fixed circle centered on the ONH. The band is 0.4 mm wide and has an outer diameter of 3.2 mm and an inner diameter of 2.4 mm which measures the temporal-superior-nasal-inferior-temporal (TSNIT) and nerve fiber indicator (NFI) parameters.

RNFL Thickness map: This is a color coded representation of the peripapillary RNFL thickness. Thick RNFLs are colored yellow, orange and red, while thinner

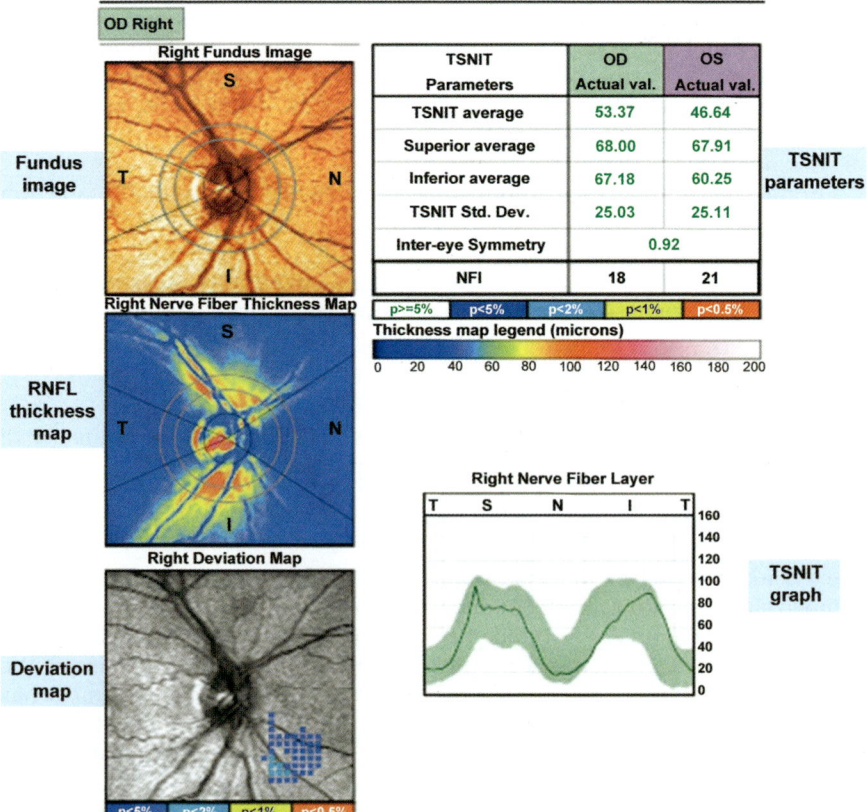

Fig. 7.1: Normal GDx VCC report—single eye

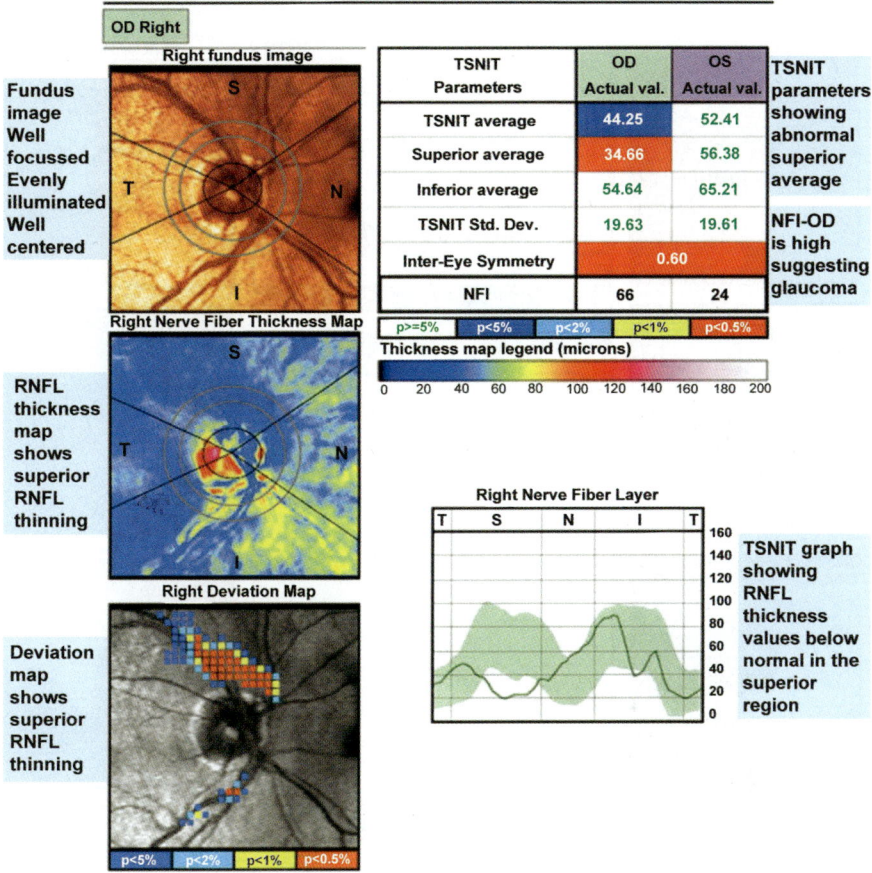

Fig. 7.2: Abnormal GDx VCC report—single eye

areas are colored blue and green. A typical normal scan of vertical bow-tie pattern is the one with brighter colors in the superior and inferior quadrants corresponding to the thicker RNFL superiorly and inferiorly.

Deviation map: This map compares patient's RNFL thickness with the values derived from normative database. The map is averaged into a grid 32 × 32 squares, where each square is compared with age-matched normative database.

TSNIT graph: This graph demonstrates the patient's RNFL thickness as a black line drawn over a green and purple shaded area of normality for the right and left eye respectively.

TSNIT symmetry graph: The graph overlays the individual TSNIT graphs of the right and left eye.

TSNIT comparison graph and serial analysis graph: These graphs compare two or more scans of the same eye obtained on different visits. They do not appear on regular printouts.

TSNIT Parameters

TSNIT average: The average RNFL thickness around the entire circle.
Superior average: The average RNFL thickness in the superior 120° region of the calculation circle.

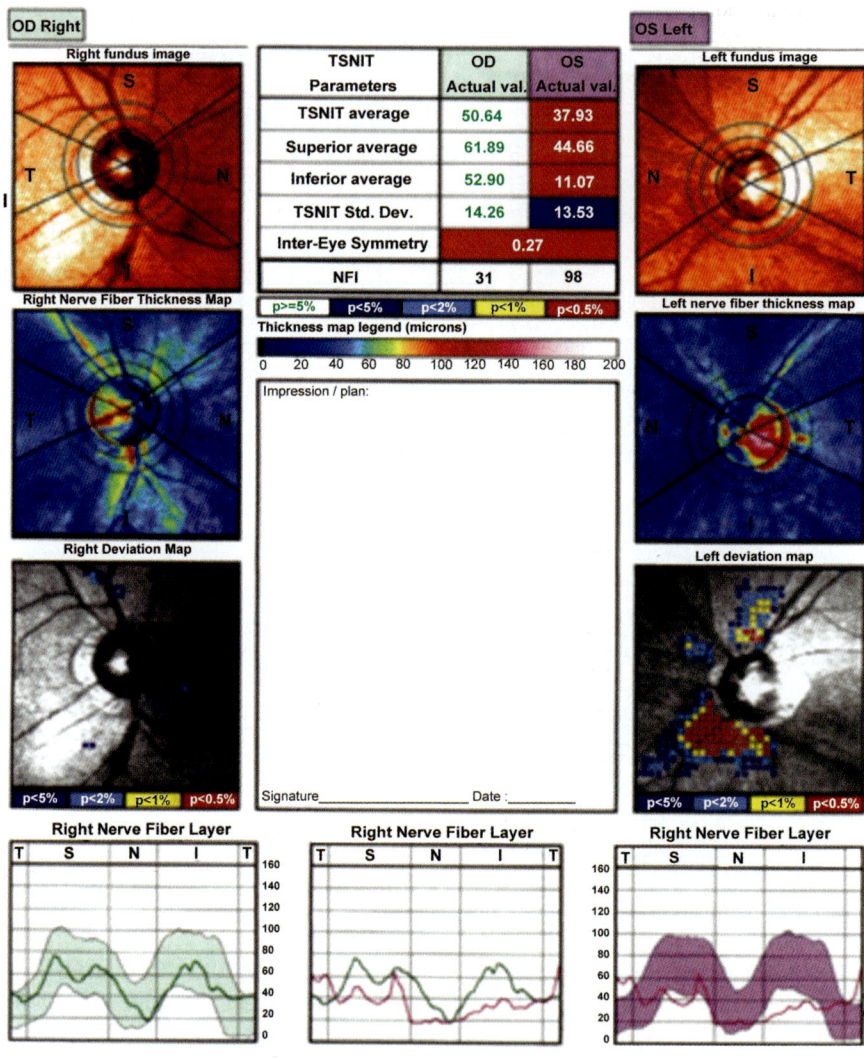

Fig. 7.3: Both eyes GDx VCC report: OD shows normal report. OS showing thinning of RNFL in the superior and inferior region, abnormal TSNIT (total, superior and inferior) average RNFL values, NFI <50, TSNIT graph below the normal suggesting glaucoma

Inferior average: The average RNFL thickness in the inferior 120° region of the calculation circle.

TSNIT standard deviation: It represents the standard deviation of the overall measurements—bigger the number healthier the eye.

Inter-eye symmetry: It is a correlation coefficient of the total measurement from both eyes. A value close to 1 indicates high symmetry between the eyes.

Nerve fiber indicator (NFI): It is a global measure based on the entire RNFL thickness map. It is calculated using an advanced form of neural network called a support vector machine. It ranges from 0 to 100. The higher NFI reflects towards patient being glaucomatous. GDx offers the following guidelines on the NFI interpretation:

- 1 to 30—Normal
- 31–50—Borderline
- 51+ —Abnormal

Diagnostic Accuracy

Sensitivity, specificity of GDx VCC in the early diagnosis of glaucoma ranges from 72 to 78% and 56 to 92% respectively.[5-8] The sensitivity of GDx VCC in the detection of glaucoma increased with the severity of glaucoma.

Strengths and Limitations

1. GDx is easy, rapid and simple to operate.
2. Does not require pupillary dilatation.
3. Good reproducibility.
4. This device can only provide RNFL data.
5. The technique does not measure the actual RNFL value, but an inferred value.
6. Measures RNFL at different locations for each patient.
7. GDx VCC does not differentiate true biological change from variability.
8. It has limited use in moderate or advanced glaucoma.
9. It is affected by anterior and posterior segment pathology, ocular surface disorder, macular pathology, large peripapillary atrophy,[9] cataract and refractive surgery.

CONFOCAL SCANNING LASER OPHTHALMOSCOPE

The confocal scanning laser ophthalmoscope (CSLO) is an imaging technology that is based on the principle of spot illumination and spot detection. HRT (Heidelberg Retinal Tomograph, Heidelberg Engineering, Germany) is the major commercially available instrument based on the principle of confocality. It gives a rapid and reproducible quantitative analysis of the optic disc parameters and RNFL.

Evolution

Confocal imaging procedures were initially developed over 30 years ago as a technique to provide optical sectioning of biologic and industrial specimens. Modified techniques have been used in ophthamology for in vivo corneal, retinal, and optic disc imaging. Since 1992, CSLO has been used for glaucoma diagnosis. The first commercially available instrument was the Heidelberg Retinal Tomograph which was studied extensively in the Ocular Hypertension Treatment Study (OHTS). However, it was highly operator dependant and required fine tuning of several manual settings. The current glaucoma practice uses the HRT II and HRT III which are designed to be more user friendly with high precision.

Principle

HRT and HRT II use a rapid scanning 670 nm diode laser based on the principle of confocality. The emitted beam is redirected in the X-axis and Y-axis along a plane of focus perpendicular to the optic axis (Z-axis) using two oscillating mirrors to obtain a 15° × 15°, two-dimensional image reflected from the surface of the retina and optic disc.

In the confocal optical system, a small diaphragm placed in front of the detector at a location which is optically conjugate to focal plane of illuminating system. A luminance detector measures the light reflected from each point in the image after passing through a confocal imaging aperture. This reflected light from the focal plane, is detected only if it focuses at the level of diaphragm.

The HRT II utilizes a higher resolution of 384 × 384 pixels and measures a 15 degree scan area with higher resolution than original HRT. A typical imaging session with HRT II is done in less than 7 seconds, including the prescan and 3 confocal scans. It has automatic quality control measures to detect scans that are interrupted by blinks and saccades and obtains three high quality scans. The software automatically aligns and averages the images to obtain a matrix of maximum height measurement.

Interpretation

The stepwise analysis of HRT is done in the following way (Figs 7.4 and 7. 5):
1. **Patient data:** This contains the name, date of birth, gender, ethnicity of the patient with the ID number and date of examination.
2. **Image quality:** If the standard deviation is equal to or less than 30 microns, it is acceptable, else the scan has to be repeated.

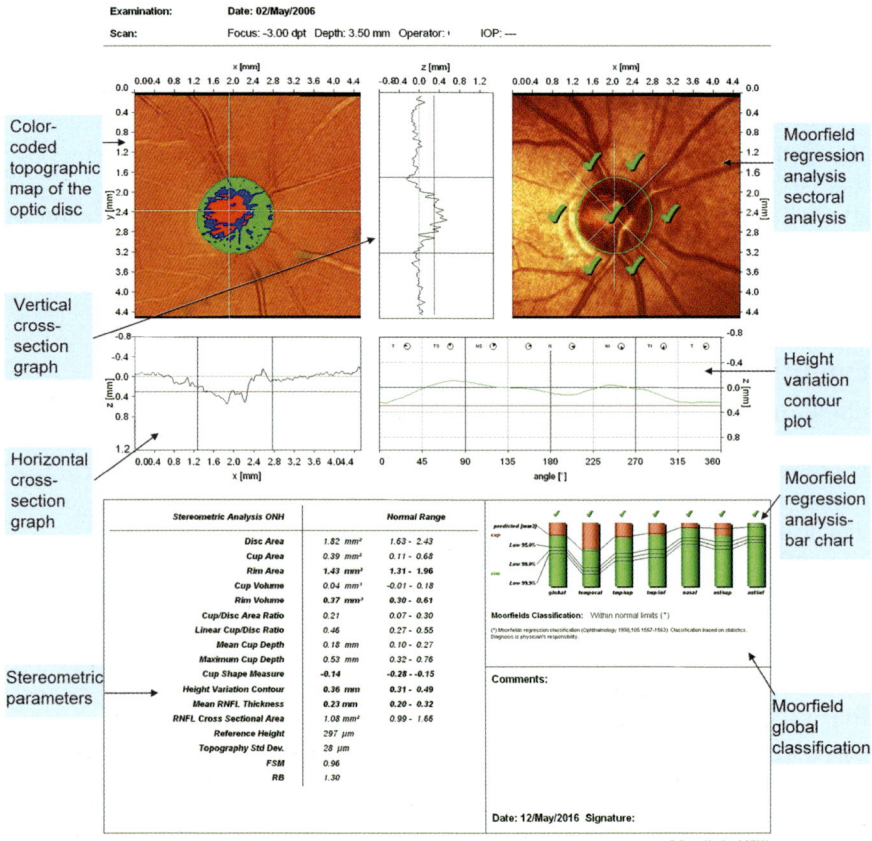

Fig. 7.4: HRT II single eye report

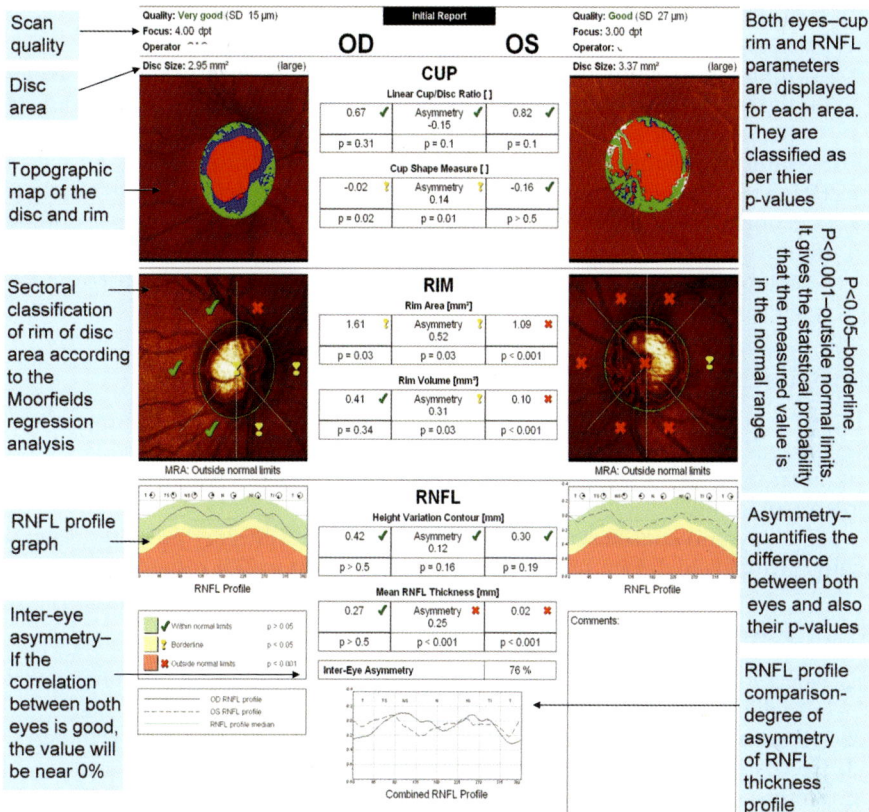

Fig. 7.5: HRT II both eyes report

3. **Optic disc size:** The position of the contour line in both the topographic image and in the reflectance image should be carefully evaluated. It should be placed at the inner margin of the disc margin, as the HRT parameters are calculated based on the location of the contour line. The optic disc is evaluated as small, average and large discs. The Moorfield's regression analysis (MRA) is valid only for disc size within a range of 1.2–2.8 mm.[2] Disc size outside this range may not be represented in database, and in such cases the interpretation must be done with caution.
4. **Structure of optic disc:** HRT gives a color coded topography map of the optic disc. The cup (red) and the rim (blue and green) are represented as overlay on the topographic image. This facilitates a quick qualitative assessment of the relation of rim tissue and cup, and detection of localized area of rim thinning.
5. **Stereometric parameters:** The disc area, rim area and C/D ratio are more useful at follow up visits to monitor progression.
6. **Moorfield's regression analysis:** It is able to identify the structural damage by comparing the patient's data to a normative database of Caucasian eyes (refractive error less than 6 diopters and disc size between 1.2–2.8 mm^2).
   – The analysis results for each sector are indicated as overlay on the reflectivity image.

- A bar diagram representing global as well as six sector analysis of neuroretinal rim to disc area ratio is also given.

  Individual values are classified as within normal limits if they are inside the 95% confidence interval for normality (green check), borderline if between 95% and 99.9% (yellow exclamation mark), and outside normal limits if outside the 99.9% confidence interval (red cross).
7. **Height variation contour plot:** It provides useful information about status of retinal nerve fibre layer. In normal subjects the plot usually has a double hump appearance, but has wide variability. When the RNFL is lost, the nerve fiber layer contour line represented in green line flattens and reaches the red reference plane.

Sensitivity and Specificity

HRT is found to be sensitive and specific for glaucoma detection[10] and progression. This imaging technology has been evaluated extensively in various studies. HRT has been used in CSLO study as an ancillary project of Ocular Hypertension Treatment Study.[11,12]

Sensitivity and specificity of HRT in the diagnosis of healthy eyes and glaucomatous visual field defects ranges from 77 to 92% and 81 to 97% respectively.[13-16]

Strengths and Limitations

1. Does not need pupillary dilatation though image quality is often improved with dilatation in dense cataracts.
2. Needs only low level of illumination improving patient comfort during the scan.
3. Normative database include a large, race specific normal subjects.
4. Sophisticated analysis software for glaucoma detection and progression.
5. Ability to monitor quality control during image acquisition.
6. Most of the measurement relies on the user-defined contour line for the reference plane. However in the recent HRT III, the contour line and the reference plane are not user defined.
7. The data are not reliable in disc sizes that are outside the normal range.
8. The stereometric measurements may be influenced by moderate changes in IOP.[17]

HEIDELBERG RETINAL TOMOGRAPHY III (FIG. 7.6)

This is the latest software version of Heidelberg Retinal Tomography. This is operator independent for contour line placement as it automatically fits the optic nerve head and the RNFL to that of a model optic disc. The technique provides stereometric data by applying an automatic model of the ONH shape.[18] These data are analyzed by a machine learning classifier and yields the Glaucoma Probability Score (GPS). This version uses GPS for analysis instead of MRA (Table 7.1).

Glaucoma probability score is more advantageous in detecting early stage glaucoma, but does not differentiate normal and ocular hypertensive eyes. It is more sensitive but less specific than MRA. The agreement between MRA and GPS agreement was low.[20]

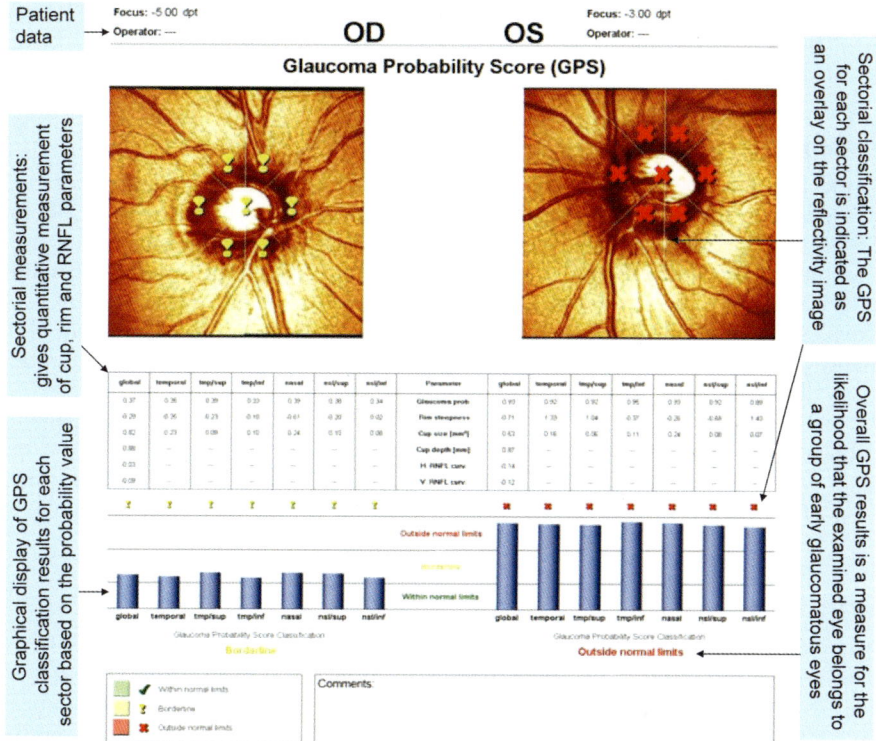

Fig. 7.6: HRT III: Glacuoma probabillity score
Sources: www.heidelbergengineering.com

TABLE 7.1: Showing glaucoma probability score and moorfield regression analysis

Glaucoma probability score	Moorfield regression analysis
Operator independent	Operator dependent
Normative database—733 patients of Caucasian descent, 215 patients of African descent, and 100 Indian participants	Normative database—112 normal Caucasian eyes
Analyzes the topographic image of the optic disc, including the cup size, cup depth, rim steepness and horizontal/vertical RNFL curvature	Analyzes the logarithmic relationship between the neuroretinal rim and optic disc areas
Reproducibility is not affected by refraction, disc size, disc characteristics like peripapillary atrophy or tilting, or the severity of the glaucoma[19]	Affected by refraction and disc size

OPTICAL COHERENCE TOMOGRAPHY

Optical coherence tomography is a non-invasive optical imaging technology that provides high-resolution, cross-sectional in vivo images of the retina. OCT has the ability to scan the following three distinctive ocular structures for the detection and progression of glaucoma.

- The peripapillary retinal nerve fiber layer
- The optic nerve head and
- The macular region.

Evolution

Optical coherence tomography (OCT) was first described by Huang and his associates in the year 1991.[21] OCT became popular in 2002 with the release of Stratus OCT, a time-domain technology (TD-OCT). Four years later, several companies started to release the next generation technology, spectral-domain OCT (SD-OCT). Currently, the most common commercially available SD-OCT devices are: Cirrus HD-OCT (Carl Zeiss Meditec, Dublin, CA, USA), RTVue-100 (Optovue Inc., Fremont, CA, USA), Spectralis OCT (Heidelberg Engineering, Heidelberg, Germany), and Topcon 3D-OCT 2000 (Topcon Corporation, Tokyo, Japan), Nidek RS-3000. The older time domain OCT machines are now being replaced by the spectral domain OCT for increased axial resolution, faster scanning speeds and improved reproducibility.[22,23] Ultrahigh speed swept source OCT, ultrahigh resolution OCT, adaptive optics OCT and polarization sensitive OCT are all on the horizon.

Principle of OCT

The OCT is based on the principle of low-coherence interferometry.[24] It uses non-contact transpupillary approach to capture the images. The TD-OCT is based on the ability to discriminate the retinal layers depending on the difference in the time delay of their reflections. In SD-OCT, a dispersive detector is used to break the optical beam into light beam of different wavelengths and the scan is obtained by analyzing the interference signal based on the wavelength of light.

This section will review the practical approach towards the role of OCT in glaucoma.

Normative Database

Each machine has different glaucoma scan patterns, proprietary software segmentation algorithms, and display outputs. The normative database which is utilized for comparison of the subject's measurement to that of the normal values varies from machine to machine. Thus the size, age limit, refractive error, ethnicity of a particular OCT machine's normative database can influence the interpretation of OCT results and the subsequent management by the clinician. Sometimes the results obtained may be statistically flagged abnormal who are not represented in the normative database. Review of literature revealed various studies conducted in different centers in India using the various spectral domain OCT machines. It revealed maximum RNFL thickness is in the inferior quadrant followed by superior, nasal and temporal quadrants supporting the ISNT rule. The mean nerve fiber layer thickness along the circumference was also comparable.[25-28]

Patient Data

Identification of the patient data including name, sex and in particular age is vital. The results are interpreted in comparison to the age-matched controls.

Scan Quality

Particular attention to the signal strength (SS) or the scan quality index (SQI) should be given. A poor signal strength or scan quality index may make the interpretation less reliable. Simple comparison of signal strength between different OCT machines may not be possible as each OCT machine and their versions might vary in their image processing strategy and data analysis.

Scan quality may be influenced by age, visual acuity and extent of media opacity. The signal strength can range from 1 to 10, with 10 being the maximum. Signal strength of more than 5 is considered desirable.

Scan Quality Index—Optovue iVue: The good scan quality index is indicated in green and the poor quality in red. The scan is said to be of poor quality when they are below 40 in retina scan; below 27 in ONH scan and below 32 in GCC scan.

Retinal Nerve Fiber Layer Analysis

SD-OCTs are capable of segmenting the RNFL layer around the ONH and measure the area between the internal limiting membrane and the RNFL border.

The RNFL thickness map is represented in a false color scale with thickness value in reference to the normative database progressing from blue to red.

The normal pattern is a symmetrical hourglass shape of bright colors in superior and inferior quadrants corresponding to thicker RNFL in superior and inferior quadrant and thinner RNFL in nasal and temporal quadrant (Figs 7.7A and B). The analysis of RNFL should include the following steps:
1. Focal defects of RNFL corresponding to fundus image
2. Diffuse loss
3. Superior-inferior asymmetry
4. Inter-eye asymmetry.

Deviation Map

The deviation map is an estimate of deviation of the subject's RNFL thickness profile compared to the age matched normative database. The thickness that falls below the normal range is color coded based on the probability of normality (Fig. 7.8).

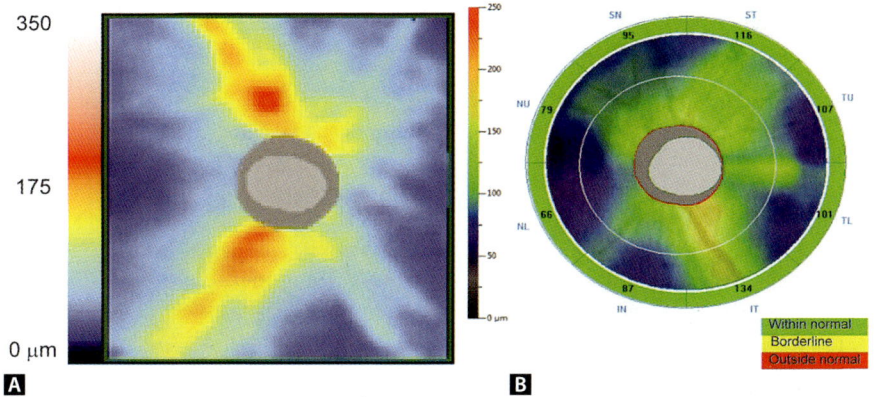

Figs 7.7A and B: (A) Zeiss Cirrus OCT—RNFL thickness map showing normal vertical hourglass pattern of RNFL thickness with bright colors in the superior and inferior quadrant; (B) Optovue-iVue OCT showing normal RNFL thickness map depicting the average thickness of RNFL in clock hour distribution

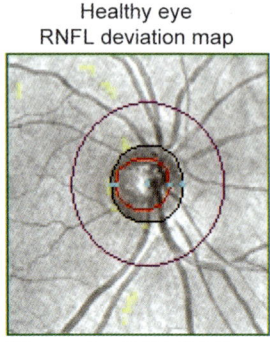 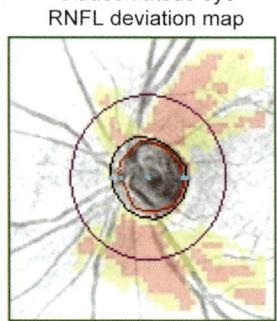

Fig. 7.8: Ziess Cirrus OCT—RNFL deviation map showing deviation of the subject's RNFL thickness profile compared to the age matched normative database. It is color coded based on the probability of normality when the values are less than normal range

TSNIT RNFL Thickness Profile

The temporal-superior-nasal-inferior-temporal (TSNIT) RNFL thickness profile is the linear representation of the RNFL thickness along the scan circle that starts temporally and then superiorly, nasally, inferiorly and ends temporally. As the RNFL is thicker in superior and inferior quadrants than nasally and temporally, the TSNIT thickness profile in a normal eye has a "double hump" pattern. When the subject's RNFL thickness follows the pattern of normal eye it falls in the green area (representing >95% of normal eyes), borderline loss if falling in yellow area (1–5% of normal eyes), and severe loss if falling in red (<1% of normal eyes) (Fig. 7.9).

The numerical data values of the RNFL parameters are given in the analysis. All the values are color coded according to the probability levels that are given in the print out (Fig. 7.10).

1. **Average RNFL thickness:** The average RNFL thickness around the entire RNFL calculation circle.
2. **Average superior RNFL:** The average RNFL thickness in the superior 120 degrees of the scan circle.
3. **Average inferior RNFL:** The average RNFL thickness in the inferior 120 degrees of the scan circle.

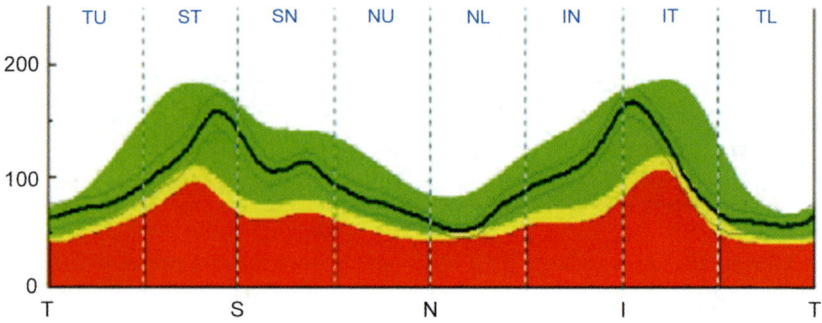

Fig. 7.9: Optovue-iVue OCT showing the TSNIT-RNFL thickness profile of a normal eye with the classic double-hump pattern

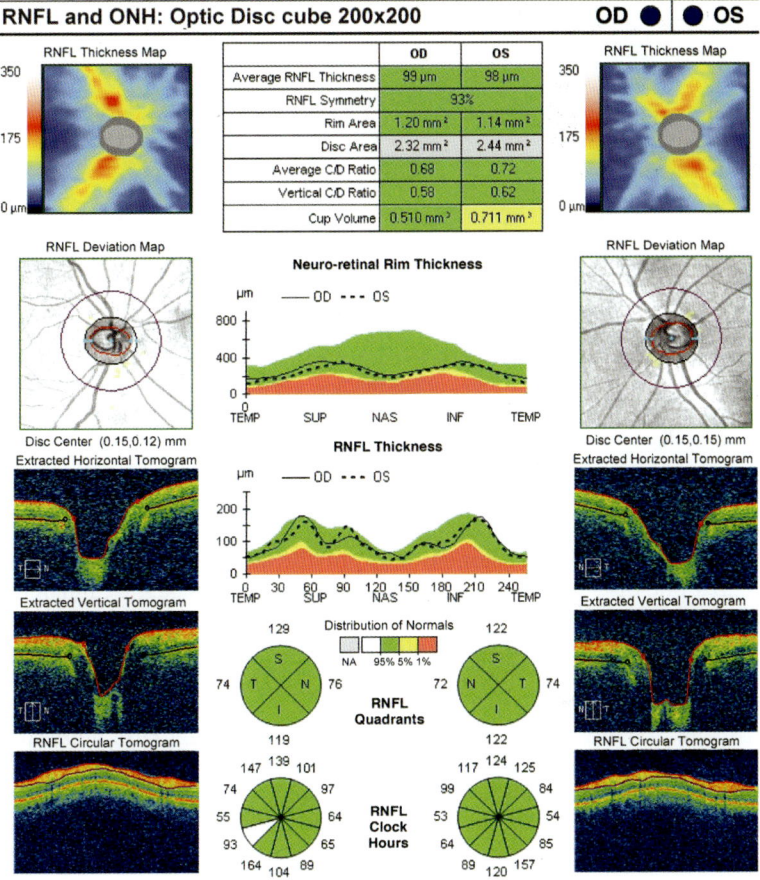

Fig. 7.10: Zeiss Cirrus OCT both eyes shows analysis of optic nerve head and peripapillary nerve fiber layers in a healthy patient

4. Superior-inferior difference calculates the difference between the average superior-inferior RNFL thickness
5. RNFL symmetry: Shows the percentage of RNFL symmetry between right and left eyes.
6. RNFL quadrants and RNFL clock hours: Shows the average thickness along the four quadrants and 12 clock hours.

The sensitivity and specificity of various RNFL parameters in Cirrus OCT is comparable to Stratus OCT.

Optic Nerve Head Analysis

The Stratus-OCT defines the ONH margin automatically as the termination of the retinal pigment epithelium. A straight line is drawn connecting the edges of the RPE and a parallel line is constructed 150 µm anterior to this line. The neuroretinal rim is identified as the area above this line, whereas the cup is the area located below this plane (Fig. 7.11A). A topographic image of the ONH is constructed with the optic disc borders, corresponding to the edges of the RPE, that shown in red and the cup shown in green (Fig. 7.11B).

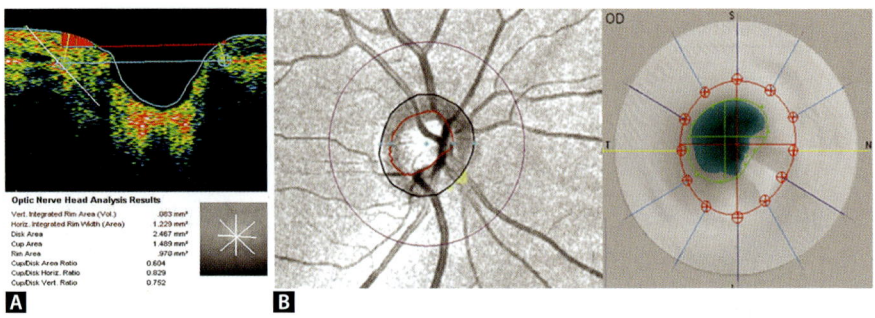

Figs 7.11A and B: (A) Optic nerve head analysis by Stratus OCT showing a straight line drawn connecting the edge of the RPE and a parallel line is constructed 150 μm anterior to this line. The neuro-retinal rim is identified as the area above this line and the cup is the area located below this plane; (B) A topographic image of the optic nerve head is constructed with the optic disc borders, corresponding to the edges of the RPE, shown in red and the cup is shown in green

The SD-OCT produces high-resolution three-dimensional volume of the ONH which can be automatically segmented to provide objective measurements of the optic cup, optic disc and the neuroretinal rim. The optic disc is delineated as the termination of Bruch's membrane[29] and then finds the shortest perpendicular distance to the internal limiting membrane (minimum band distance) to define the inner cup margin. Each SD-OCT provides several built-in scan pattern options for imaging the ONH.

The ONH parameters that are analyzed by SD-OCT are: Disc area, rim area, average CD ratio, cup volume, vertical and horizontal CD ratio.

Neuroretinal (NRR) rim thickness profile: This is a graphical representation of the NRR thickness along the temporal-superior-nasal-inferior-temporal (TSNIT) circle. It is interpreted in the same way as RNFL thickness profile.

Ganglion Cell Complex Analysis

The ganglion cell complex (GCC) (Fig. 7.12) includes:
1. Axons of retinal ganglion cells—nerve fiber layer
2. The cell bodies of the ganglion cells (RGC)—inner nuclear layer
3. The dendrite of retinal ganglion cells—inner plexiform layer.

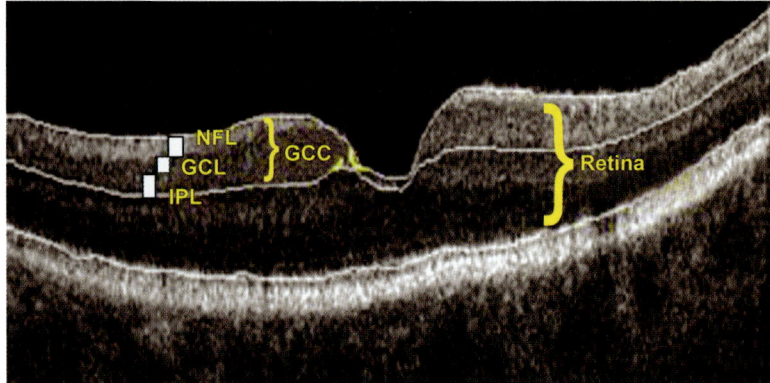

Fig. 7.12: SD-OCT of the macula illustrating the ganglion cell complex
Abbreviations: NFL, nerve fiber layer; GCL, ganglion cell layer; IPL, inner plexiform layer

Macula has the highest concentration of ganglion cells in the retina, approximately 50% of RGC of the entire retina.[30] Glaucoma affects the macular ganglion cells early in its course. The GCC becomes thinner as the ganglion cells die from glaucoma. Hence study of ganglion cell complex is very useful for the early detection and progression of glaucoma. GCC analysis directly measures the thickness of these 3 layers and provides an analysis of the percent loss of these layers compared to an extensive normative database. The results are presented as significant loss from normal which makes clinical interpretation straight forward. The macular GCC parameters are able to identify early glaucoma eyes and this ability is comparable to that of the disc and RNFL parameters.[31]

In a normal eye, thickness map contains a bright 'doughnut-shaped' circular band surrounding the macula representing thick GCC from the healthy ganglion cells. It is false color coded with the color scale present in the print out. The centre of the macula is thin due to absence of ganglion cells in fovea. The GCC deviation map or the GCC NDB reference map shows the amount of deviation of the subject's GCC thickness profile in macula from the normal values.

The Cirrus OCT (Fig. 7.13) gives the macular GCC thickness along six sectors (each 60 degree of the entire macular circle).

The optovue iVue macular GCC analysis (Fig. 7.14) has the parameter table showing the total, superior and inferior average GCC thickness. Focal loss volume (FLV) percentage indicates the focal loss volume indicating the amount of focal loss over the entire GCC map representing focal depressions. The FLV is the most accurate parameter to differentiate normal from glaucomatous eyes. GLV (global loss volume) percentage indicates the average GCC loss over the entire GCC map representing overall depression of the GCC thickness. FLV and GLV are analog to the total and pattern deviation maps in visual field tests.

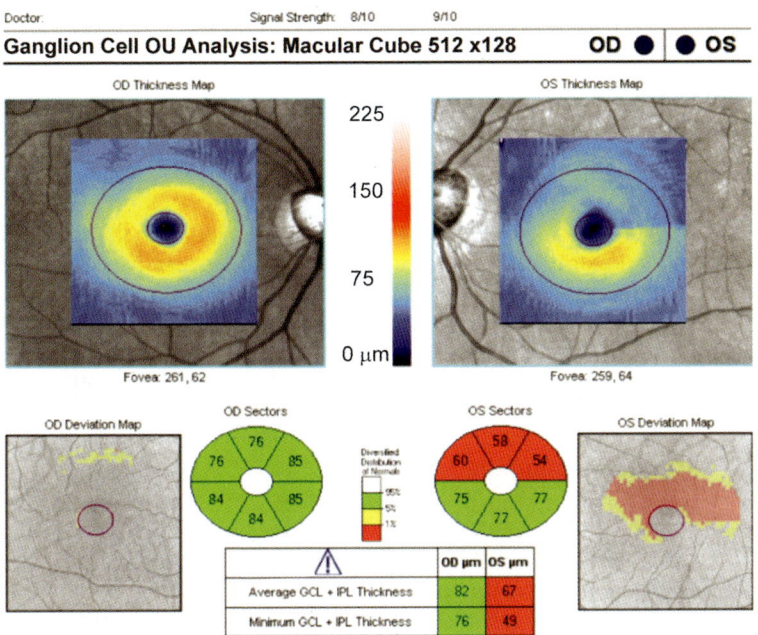

Fig. 7.13: Zeiss Cirrus OCT GCC analysis—OD shows the 'doughnut-shaped' thick GCC around macula in a normal eye. OS shows loss of GCC in the superior quadrant in a glaucomatous eye with corresponding changes in the GCC deviation map

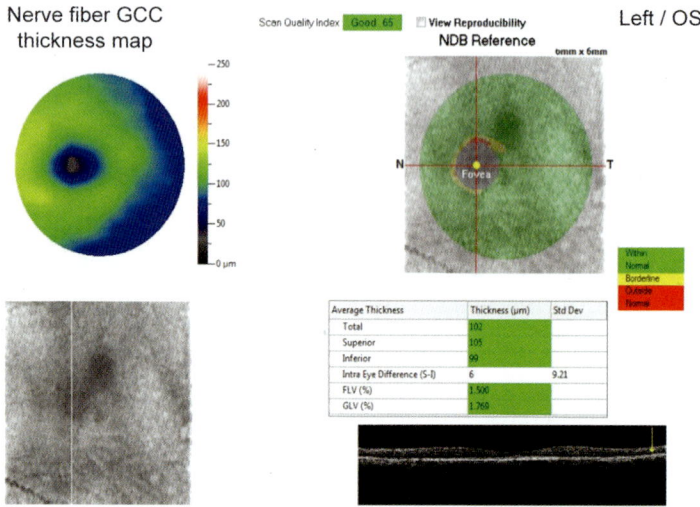

Fig. 7.14: Optovue-iVue GCC analysis showing the normal doughnut shaped thick GCC around the macula in a normal eye

Limitations of OCT in the Diagnosis of Glaucoma

1. Results are less reliable when the signal strength is poor.[32,33]
2. RNFL thickness values are affected by age,[34] axial length, disc size and tilt.
3. When the scan circle is not centered on the optic disc, it can lead to erroneous measurements.
4. During eye blinking or saccade when acquiring scan, the alignment of the scans is improper, leading to unreliable RNFL measurements.
5. Conditions that lead on to segmentation error should be ruled out[35] (e.g. ERM, disc edema).
6. Age-related loss can confound with the identification of glaucoma progression.

Floor-effect

The OCT is a very useful tool for assessing early to moderate glaucoma but in advanced glaucomatous disease, SD-OCT is clinically less useful due to the "floor-effect". The retinal nerve fiber layer is not only made up of retinal ganglion cells but also contains blood vessels and supporting cells like glial and Muller cells. So in advanced glaucomatous eye disease, the RNFL thickness levels off and rarely falls below 40 to 50 µm due to the assumed presence of the residual glial and non-neural tissue including the blood vessels.[36]

Role of Imaging in Follow-up

The detection of progression of glaucoma is critical as glaucoma is a slowly progressing optic neuropathy and thus identification of glaucomatous changes is essential for glaucoma management. These imaging instruments take multiple scans at baseline and at each follow-up, providing reproducible data of the optic nerve head and RNFL changes, both globally and regionally. The GDx- GPA, HRT – TCA and OCT–GPA are studied to be highly sensitive in detecting the glaucoma progression by the ONH and RNFL parameters especially in eyes showing progression based on stereophotographic images and visual field analysis than in non-progressing eyes.[37,38]

SCANNING LASER POLARIMETRY
Serial Analysis
The serial analysis printout has 5 elements (Fig. 7.15) that should be considered when assessing RNFL change over time.
1. Thickness map
2. Deviation map
3. Deviation from reference maps
4. Parameters
5. TSNIT graphs.

Serial analysis can compare up to four examinations. The first examination is the baseline or reference examination and follow-up examinations are compared to the baseline. The deviation from reference map displays the RNFL difference pixel by pixel of the follow-up examinations compared to the baseline examination. A colored rectangular box to the left side of the thickness map contains the date and quality score of each examination. The same color is used in the TSNIT graph to indicate the TSNIT curve of that examination.

The deviation from reference map shows the RNFL difference of the follow-up examination compared to the baseline examination. If the difference exceeds 20 microns, the pixel is color coded. The areas of RNFL change shown on the deviation from reference map will frequently correspond to the areas of loss detected by the deviation map. This is because the 'deviation map' shows loss compared to the normative database while the 'deviation from reference maps'

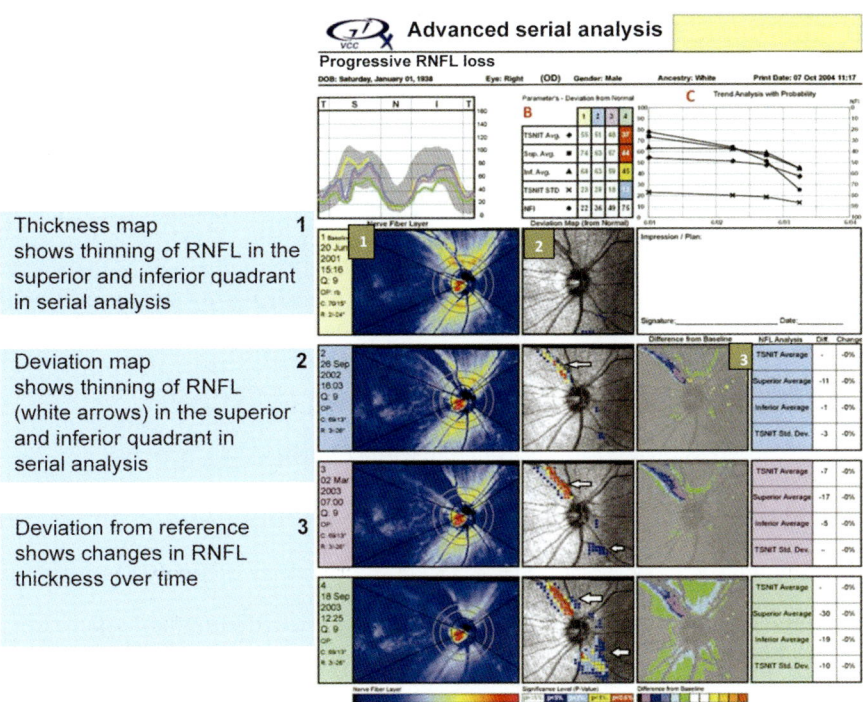

Fig. 7.15: GDx VCC serial analysis shows progressive RNFL loss as depicted in the trend analysis and nerve fiber layer analysis
Source: Carl Zeiss Meditec

shows RNFL change over time in the same eye. The TSNIT curves are overlaid on the shaded area representing the normal range for the patient's age. RNFL loss will result in a lower TSNIT curve on the follow-up examination compared to the baseline examination.

GDx-Guided Progression Analysis

The GDx VCC guided progression analysis (GPA) is a software that evaluates and compares progression over time and determines whether the difference is statistically significant. GDx GPA reports progression of glaucoma as:
1. "Possible progression" when significant change is detected once
2. "Likely progression" when significant reduction is detected in at least two consecutive examinations
3. "Possible increase" if an increase in RNFL thickness is detected.

Progression analysis has two modes–fast and extended mode. Fast mode is for analyzing data sets that include single measurements. It compares change to a predetermined average measurement variability derived from a sample population. In contrast, extended mode requires the mean of three measurements and GPA calculates the individual measurement variability of each eye for a selected patient. It measures and detects the progression based on three different parts of the analysis (Fig. 7.16).

1. **Image progression map:** Recognizes the change in the reflectance image. The minimal cluster size considered is 150 pixels which is 2% of the image size. Possible progression areas are shown in yellow, likely progression areas in red and possible increase areas in purple. It can detect narrower and deeper defects.
2. **TSNIT progression graph:** The ring around the optic nerve is divided into 64 equal segments and compared on follow-up. If three adjacent segments show significant change on follow-up, the progression is indicated. Areas between current baseline set and current examination that report significant change are displayed with possible progression in yellow, likely progression in red and possible increase in purple. This detects shallower and broader defects.
3. **Summary parameter charts:** The TSNIT average, superior average and inferior average are compared. On the chart, regression line is drawn to show likely progression and $P < 5\%$. This can detect diffuse changes in the RNFL. This parameter can also compare the rate of progression before and after treatment, thus helpful for guiding the treatment protocol.

CONFOCAL SCANNING LASER OPHTHALMOSCOPE

The two progression algorithms available with HRT are:
1. Trend analysis
2. Topographical change analysis.

HRT Trend Analysis (Fig. 7.17A)

The trend analysis compares the global and stereometric summary indices from the baseline examination to that of the follow-up visits. The analysis is represented graphically as the normalized change from the baseline over time. The changes in volume (red line) and area (blue line) of the neuroretinal rim are displayed as two independent lines. The changes in volume are represented in red triangles

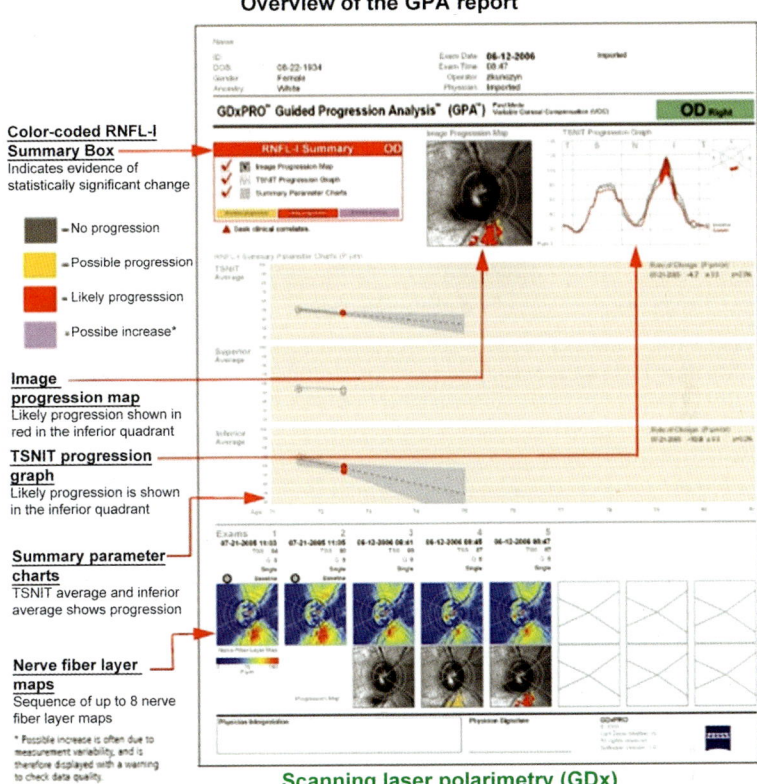

Fig. 7.16: Guided progression analysis for GDx shows likely progression depicted in red in the inferior quadrant suggestive of glaucoma progression

and the changes in area are represented in blue squares along the y-axis. The examination date is represented along the x-axis.

HRT Topographic Change Analysis (TCA) (Fig. 7.17B)

The TCA gives a quantitative change analysis within the disc margin contour and analyzes the changes in the topographical height of the HRT image at the super pixel level. The HRT images of at least three examinations (baseline and two or three follow-up exams) are compared. Before the analysis, these images are automatically aligned.

Change probability map: The statistical method estimates the probability of the difference in heights between the baseline and followup and generates a 'change probability map.' It shows significant and repeatable changes in picture elements over the topographic map, with red pixels representing height depression and green pixels representing significant elevation.

The TCA change summary parameters can be used to describe size and location of regions of change. The color intensity reflects the extent of change measured.

Studies suggest that HRT TCA analysis may be helpful in detecting more subtle change in glaucoma patients for assessing progression earlier than stereophotographic assessment and visual field analysis.[39]

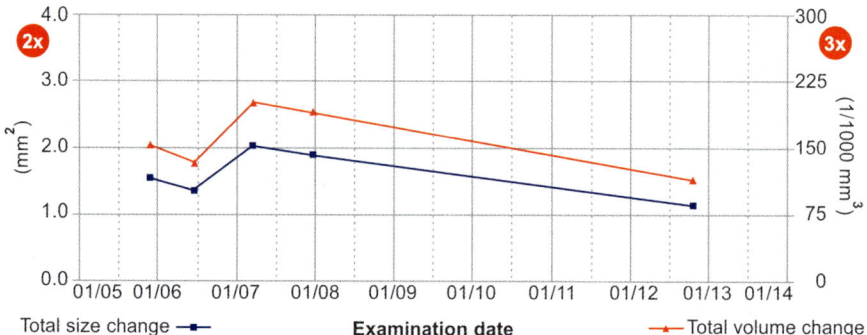

Fig. 7.17A: HRT II — Trend analysis — shows the development of the entity of all red marked clusters over time. Changes in volume and area are displayed separately as two independent lines

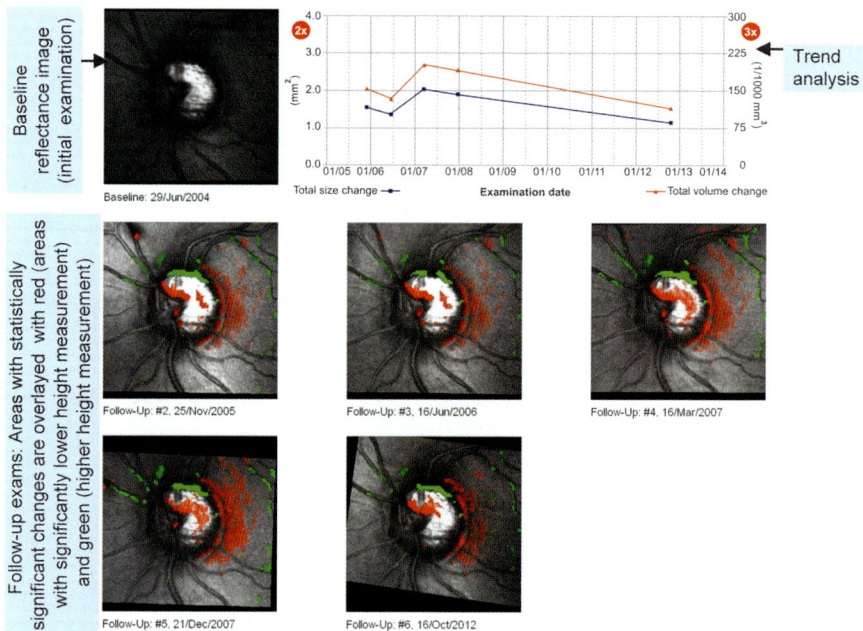

Fig. 7.17B: Topographic change analysis (TCA)

Limitation of HRT–TCA

The standard stereographic follow-up assessment of the optic disc examines nerve fiber layer defects, peripapillary hemorrhages and rim loss whereas the TCA analyzes the surface changes which is not easily identified by disc stereophotograph. This suggests that visual fields, stereophotographs and the TCA should be used in complementary fashion.

OPTICAL COHERENCE TOMOGRAPHY

Guided Progression Analysis

SD-OCT [40-46] is more sensitive in identifying progression than TD-OCT. [47-49]

Among the SD-OCT devices that are manufactured by several companies, only Cirrus OCT and Optovue-iVue currently offer progression analysis as part of their commercially available software. With guided progression analysis, Cirrus OCT can perform event analysis and trend analysis of RNFL thickness and ONH parameters. Event analysis assesses change from baseline compared to expected variability. If change is outside the range of expected variability, it is identified as progression. Trend analysis looks at the rate of change over time, using linear regression to determine rate of change. Figure 7.18 illustrates the interpretation of the Cirrus OCT guided progression analysis map.

The progression analysis offered by the Optovue-iVue (Fig. 7.19) includes side-by-side RNFL thickness measurements and overlay of the RNFL profiles for the consecutive scans. Similar reports are also provided for ganglion cell complex thickness (Fig. 7.20) along with thickness change plots. Changes are presented in a similar fashion for the ganglion cell complex of the macula. However, a formal statistical analysis of change over time is not currently included in the latest version of the software for this device (version 6.1).

Figures 7.21 to 7.31 illustrate clinical examples that depicting the structure—function correlation of the optic nerve head and the retina in the diagnosis and follow-up of glaucoma.

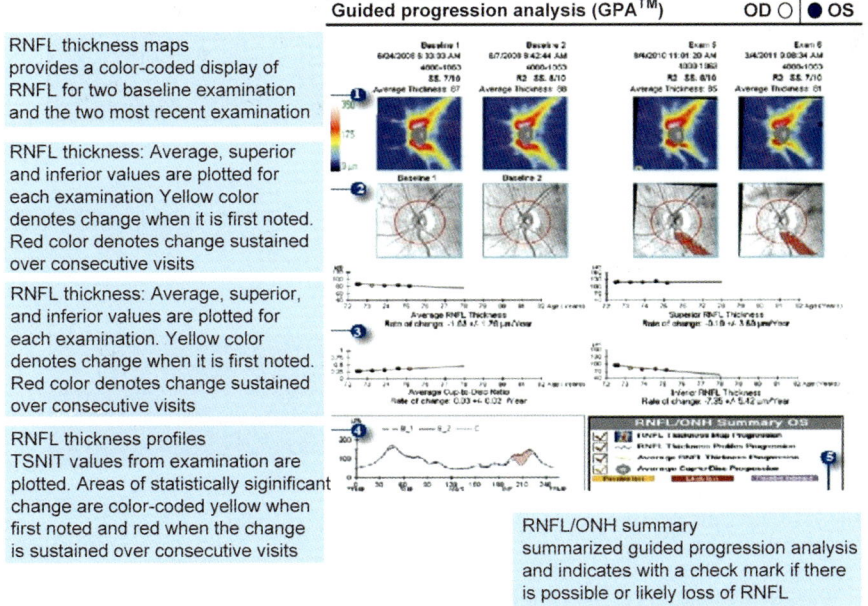

Fig. 7.18: Cirrus SD OCT-Guided progression analysis: RNFL thickness maps show gradual progression in the inferotemporal region (yellow and red sectors). The inferotemporal progression is also notable in the RNFL thickness profiles (red). Average RNFL thickness plots show statistically significant thinning in the overall, superior and inferior RNFL thickness.
Courtesy: www.zeiss.com

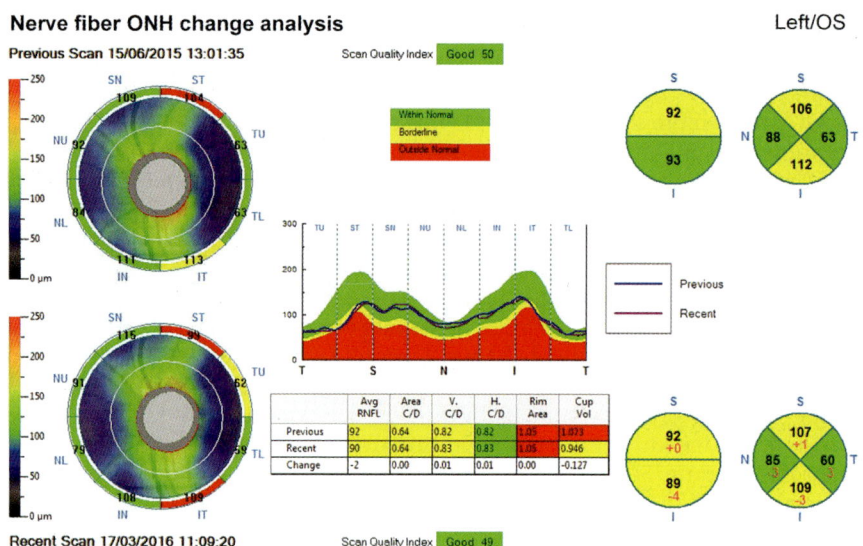

Fig. 7.19: Optovue-iVue progression analysis of RNFL parameters shows side by side RNFL thickness measurements and overlay of the RNFL profiles of the consecutive scans

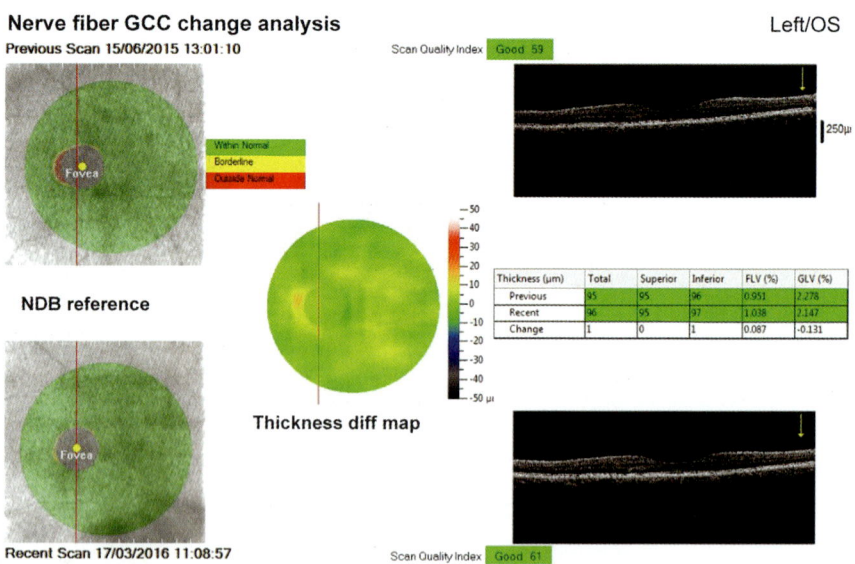

Fig. 7.20: Optovue-iVue progression analysis of ganglion cell complex

Figure 7.21 depicts the structure—function correlation of a diabetic patient with pre-perimetric glaucoma. He presented with intraocular pressure (IOP) of 26 mm Hg, central corneal thickness (CCT) of 501 μm, fundus examination showing vertical cup disc ratio (VCDR) of 0.7 with normal reliable visual fields by Humphrey visual field analyzer and thinning of RNFL at superotemporal quadrant by Optovue-iVue SD-OCT.

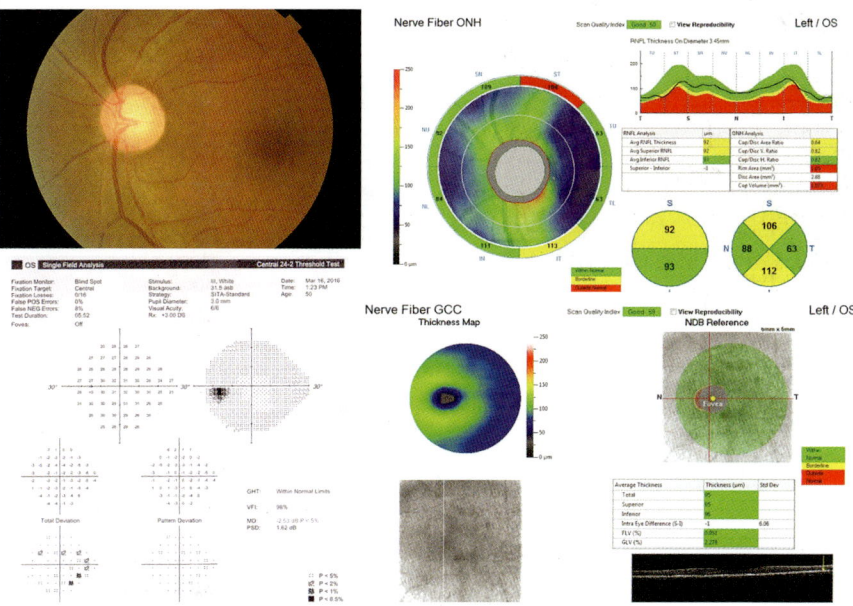

Fig. 7.21: Fundus photo, visual fields and OCT of a patient with pre-perimetric glaucoma

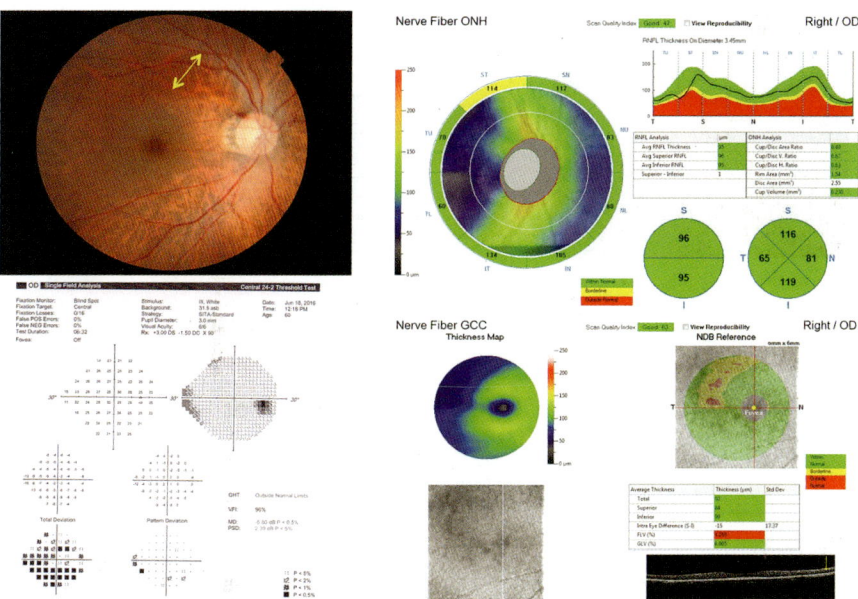

Fig. 7.22: Fundus photo shows disc hemorrhage with superior wedge-shaped RNFL defect and focal thinning of superotemporal neuroretinal rim. Visual field shows early field defect. OCT-ONH analysis shows borderline changes in the superotemporal quadrant with corresponding depression in the TSNIT graph and GCC thickness

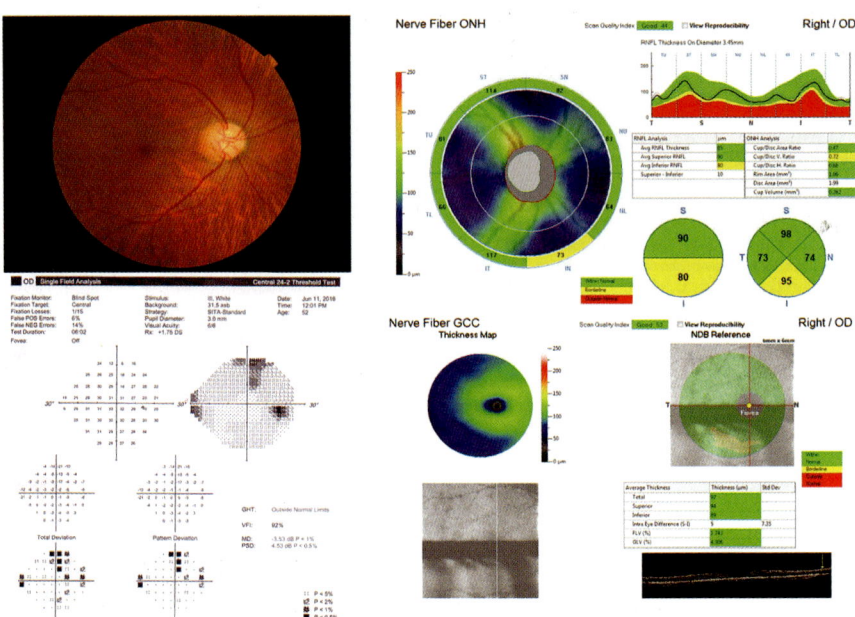

Fig. 7.23: Fundus photo shows myopic disc with thinning of inferior neuroretinal rim and early superior scotoma with borderline changes in OCT suggesting early glaucomatous damage

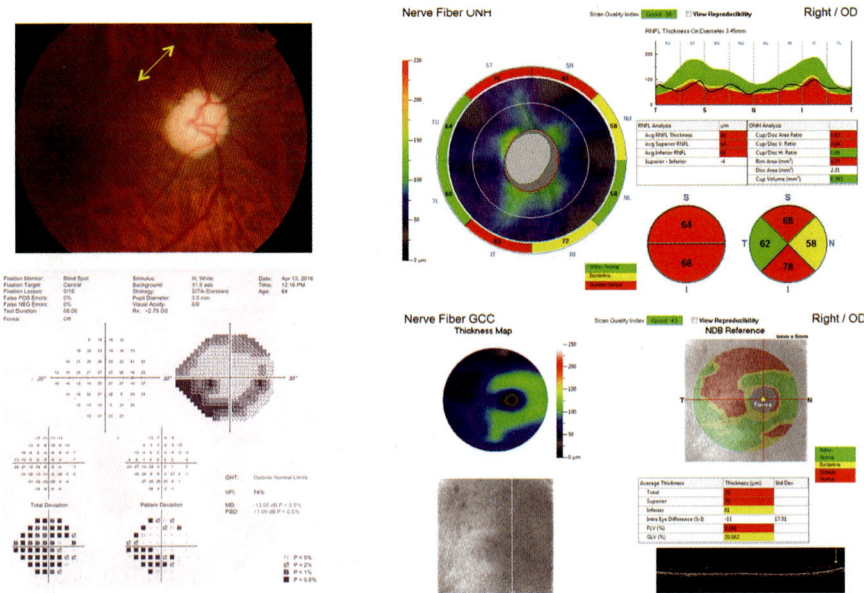

Fig. 7.24: Fundus photo shows superior wedge-shaped RNFL defect with thinning of superior and inferior neuroretinal rim. Visual field shows inferior arcuate scotoma with areas of depressed sensitivity along the superior area. OCT ONH analysis shows reduction in superior and inferior RNFL thickness with depressed TSNIT graph and corresponding reduction of GCC thickness

Figure 7.22 portrays the details of a patient with primary open angle glaucoma with IOP of 24 mm Hg, fundus showing VCDR 0.6 with disc hemorrhage, superior wedge-shaped RNFL defect and focal thinning of supero-temporal neuroretinal rim. Visual field shows early field defect. OCT-ONH analysis shows borderline changes in the supero-temporal quadrant with corresponding depression in the TSNIT graph and GCC thickness.

Figure 7.23 reveals fundus photograph showing myopic disc with thinning of inferior neuroretinal rim and early superior scotoma with borderline changes in OCT suggesting early glaucomatous damage.

Figure 7.24 shows the fundus photograph with increased VCDR, superior wedge-shaped RNFL defect with thinning of superior and inferior neuroretinal rim. Visual field shows inferior arcuate scotoma with areas of depressed sensitivity along the superior area. OCT-ONH analysis shows reduction in superior and inferior RNFL thickness with depressed TSNIT graph and corresponding reduction of GCC thickness.

Figure 7.25 depicts the structure-function correlation details of a patient with normotensive glaucoma. Patient was a diabetic and hypertensive on treatment. Fundus photograph shows inferior notching with peripapillary atrophy more in the inferior quadrant. Visual field shows superior arcuate scotoma. Nidek RS-3000 OCT ONH analysis shows reduction in RNFL thickness in the inferotemporal clock hour with corresponding depressed TSNIT graph.

Figure 7.26 depicts the structure-function details of an 18-year-old patient with myopia and pigmentary glaucoma. Fundus photograph shows VCDR 0.7

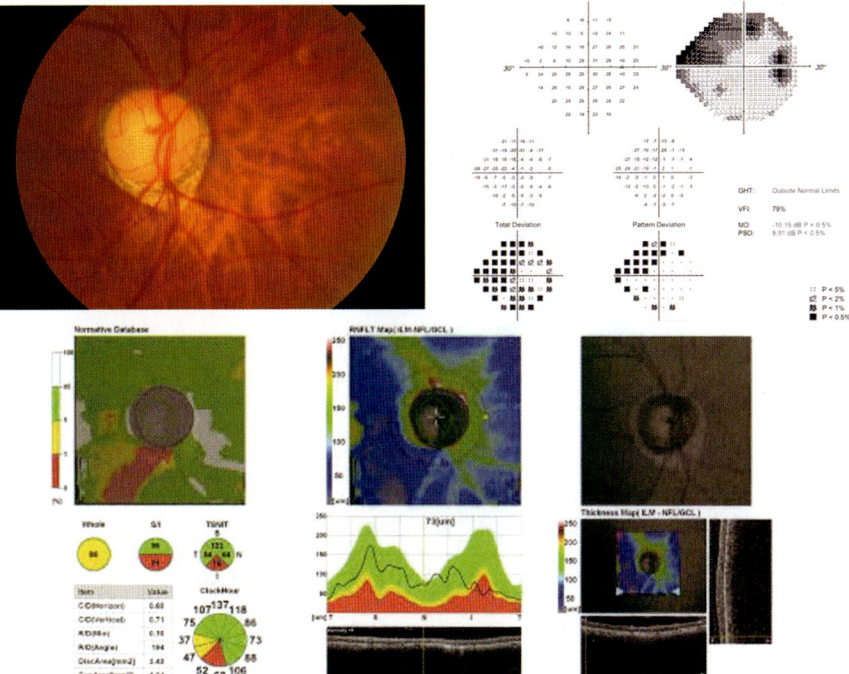

Fig. 7.25: Fundus photo shows inferior notching with peripapillary atrophy more in the inferior quadrant. Visual field shows superior arcuate scotoma. OCT ONH analysis shows reduction in RNFL thickness in the inferotemporal clock hour with corresponding depressed TSNIT graph.

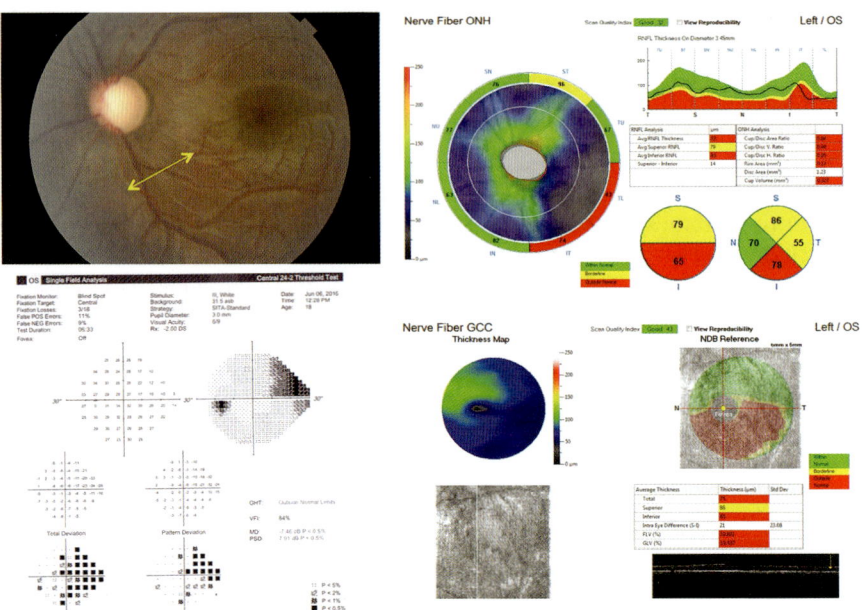

Fig. 7.26: Fundus photo shows VCD ratio 0.7 with wedge-shaped inferior RNFL defect. Visual field shows superior scotoma. OCT ONH analysis shows reduction in RNFL thickness in the inferior quadrant with corresponding depression in the TSNIT graph and reduction of GCC thickness

with wedge-shaped inferior RNFL defect. Visual field shows superior scotoma. Optovue-iVue OCT-ONH analysis shows reduction in RNFL thickness in the inferior quadrant with corresponding depression in the TSNIT graph and reduction of GCC thickness.

Figure 7.27 shows the details of a diabetic patient who came to the glaucoma clinic with IOP of 28 mm Hg in both eyes, right eye fundus photograph shows thinning of inferior neuroretinal rim. Visual field shows corresponding scotoma in the superior quadrant. OCT-ONH analysis depicts reduction of inferior RNFL thickness with corresponding depression in the TSNIT graph and NDB map.

Figure 7.28 reveals structure-function correlation of the same patient, left eye fundus photograph shows increased VCDR with thinning of inferior neuroretinal rim. Visual field shows superior arcuate scotoma. OCT-ONH analysis depicts reduction of inferior RNFL thickness with corresponding depression in the TSNIT graph and reduction of GCC thickness.

Figure 7.29 shows a fundus photograph of a patient depicting enlarged VCDR of 0.7 with thinning of superior and inferior neuroretinal rim. Visual field shows a corresponding superior and inferior arcuate scotoma. OCT-ONH analysis shows reduction in superior and inferior RNFL thickness with depressed TSNIT graph and corresponding reduction of GCC thickness is noted in the NDB map.

Figure 7.30 depicts the fundus photograph showing increased VCDR with thinning of superior and inferior neuroretinal rim. Visual field shows a corresponding superior arcuate scotoma with areas of depressed sensitivity along the inferior arcuate area. OCT-ONH analysis shows reduction in superior and inferior RNFL thickness with depressed TSNIT graph and corresponding reduction of GCC thickness.

Current Role of Imaging in Glaucoma Management

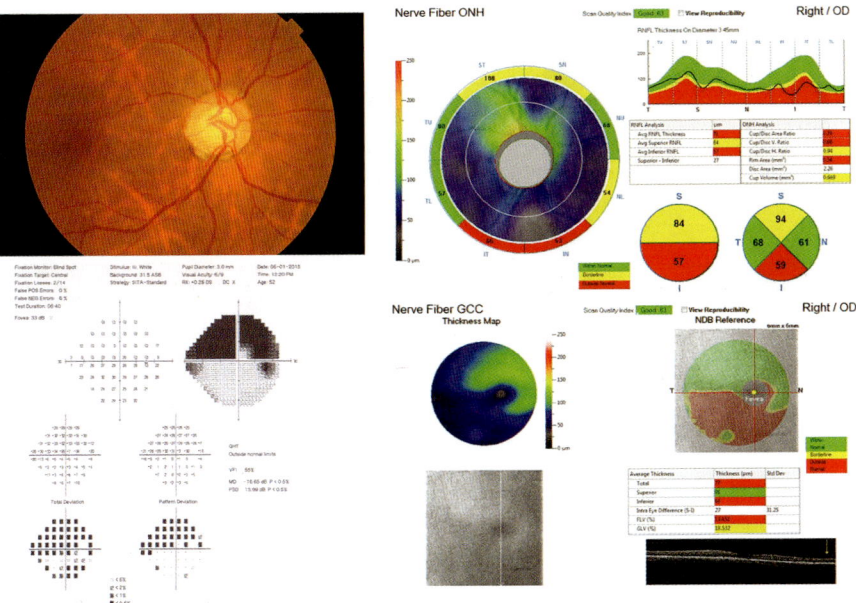

Fig. 7.27: Fundus photo shows thinning of inferior neuroretinal rim. Visual field shows scotoma in the superior quadrant. OCT ONH analysis depicts reduction of inferior RNFL thickness with corresponding depression in the TSNIT graph and NDB map

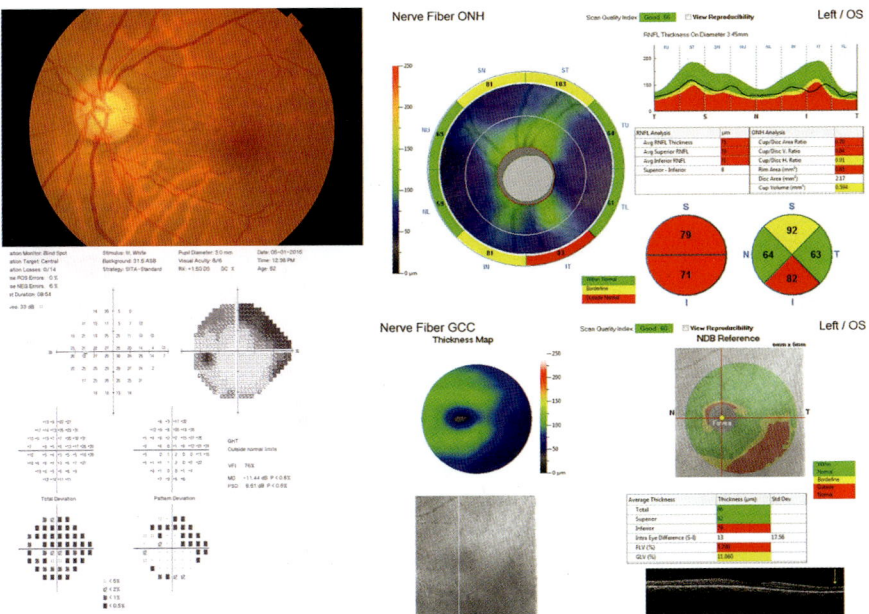

Fig. 7.28: Fundus photo shows increased VCD ratio with thinning of inferior neuroretinal rim. Visual field shows superior arcuate scotoma. OCT ONH analysis depicts reduction of inferior RNFL thickness with corresponding depression in the TSNIT graph and reduction of GCC thickness is noted in NDB map

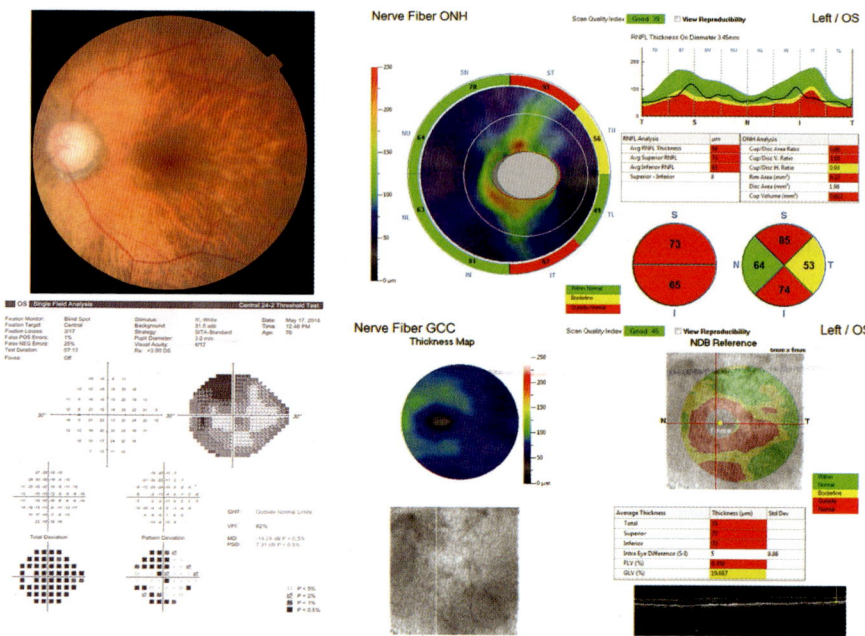

Fig. 7.29: Fundus photo shows enlarged VCD ratio of 0.7 with thinning of superior and inferior neuroretinal rim. Visual field shows a corresponding superior and inferior arcuate scotoma. OCT ONH analysis shows reduction in superior and inferior RNFL thickness with depressed TSNIT graph and corresponding reduction of GCC thickness is noted in NDB map

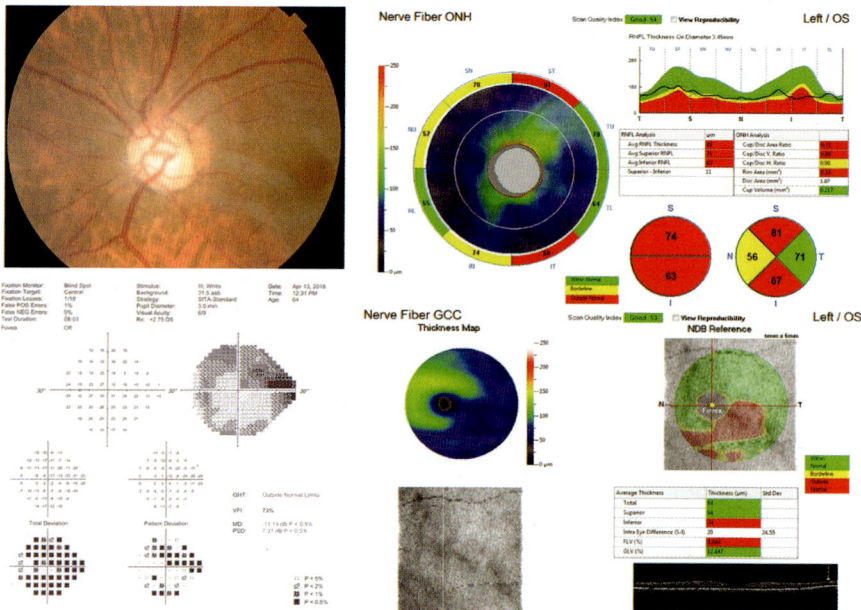

Fig. 7.30: Fundus photo shows increased VCD ratio with thinning of superior and inferior neuroretinal rim. Visual field shows a corresponding superior arcuate scotoma with areas of depressed sensitivity along the inferior arcuate area. OCT-ONH analysis shows reduction in superior and inferior RNFL thickness with depressed TSNIT graph and corresponding reduction of GCC thickness

Current Role of Imaging in Glaucoma Management

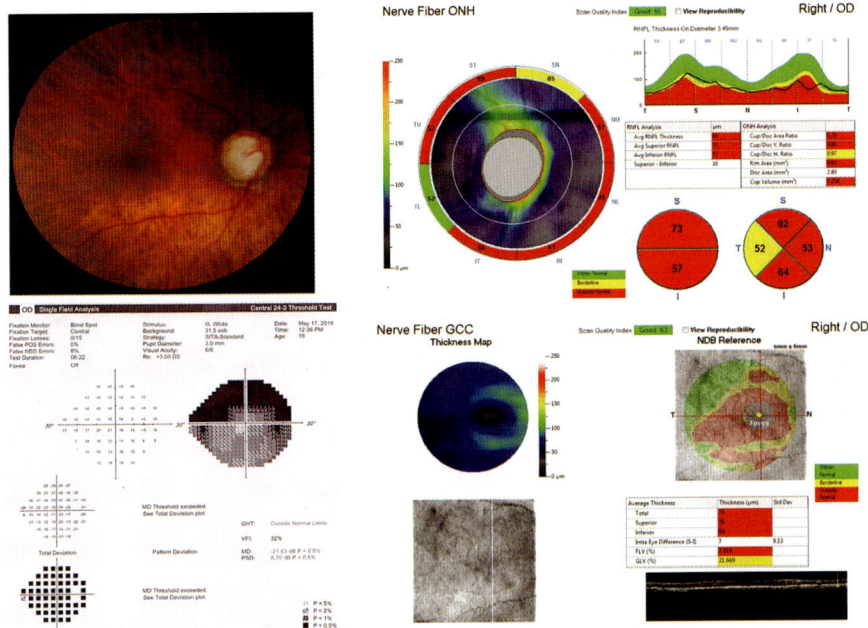

Fig. 7.31: Fundus photo shows enlarged VCD ratio of 0.8 with thinning of superior and inferior neuroretinal rim. Visual field shows severe visual field loss. OCT ONH analysis shows reduction in superior, nasal and inferior RNFL thickness with severely depressed TSNIT graph

Figure 7.31 portrays the details of a patient who underwent glaucoma surgery prior with controlled IOP. Fundus photograph shows enlarged VCDR of 0.8 with thinning of superior and inferior neuroretinal rim. Visual field shows severe visual field loss. OCT-ONH analysis shows reduction in superior, nasal and inferior RNFL thickness with severely depressed TSNIT graph.

FUTURE DEVELOPMENTS IN GLAUCOMA IMAGING

Swept-source OCT (SS-OCT)

Swept-source OCT is the latest milestone in retina, choroid and optic nerve head imaging. It differs from SD-OCT (Table 7.2).

TABLE 7.2: Showing difference between Swept-source OCT and SD-OCT

	Swept-source OCT	Spectral domain OCT
Wavelength	1050 nm	840 nm
Laser source	Short-cavity swept laser	Superluminescent diode laser
Scan speed	100,000 A-scans/sec	50000 A-scans/sec
Field of scan	12 mm	6–9 mm
Field of view	Optic nerve and macula on the same scan	Optic and macula not possible on the same scan
Depth of image	Deeper choroidal layers and lamina cribrosa visible	Only till RPE layer

The widefield scan of SS-OCT enables the view of macula and ONH simultaneously, helping to understand the relationship of macular damage and ONH damage in glaucoma. It displays the RNFL thickness data across 12 × 9 mm grid format. SS-OCT also gives in vivo study of the lamina cribrosa. The histological studies suggest that the lamina cribrosa can undergo morphological changes in glaucomatous eyes. Thinning and the posterior displacement of lamina have been observed and are thought to be a result of raised intraocular pressure.[50] The three-dimensional SS-OCT imaging allows visualization of the lamina cribrosa defects, which may be more prevalent in eyes with longer axial length and related to disc hemorrhages.[51]

Longer Wavelength OCT

Currently, clinical OCT imaging of the retina mainly occurs at wavelengths in the 800–870 nm range, however the melanin contained in the retinal pigment epithelial (RPE) is highly scattering and absorbing in this range of wavelength,[52] making it difficult to image structures below this tissue layer, such as the choroid and choriocapillaris. Additionally, due to the rapid signal drop off, the penetration of light into the optic nerve head is limited. Current research is focused on exploring OCT imaging at wavelengths of 1000 to 1100 nm to achieve deeper imaging capabilities, and allow penetration below the RPE. Long-wavelength imaging may also improve OCT signal quality in patients with media opacity.[53,54] High-speed retinal OCT in the 1000–1100 nm wavelength range has been shown to allow the imaging of choroidal layers. Thus, it is helpful in the evaluation of glaucoma and age-related macular degeneration.[55]

Adaptive Optic OCT (AO-OCT)

Early detection of axonal tissue loss is critical for managing diseases that destroy the RNFL such as glaucoma. AO–OCT systems have been used to capture volume images of retinal structures that were previously visible only with histology. Examples include the bundles within the RNFL; retinal microvasculature such as the capillaries that form the rim of the foveal avascular zone (FAZ); microstructures in the ganglion cell layer and Henle's fiber layer; the 3D photoreceptor mosaic; retinal pigment epithelium; and the tiny pores of the lamina cribrosa of the optical nerve. AO–OCT represents a potential means to measure cross-sectional retinal nerve fiber bundles (RNFB) dimensions, owing to its micron-level 3D resolution.[56] The technical benefits of adding AO to OCT are increased lateral resolution, smaller speckle, and enhanced sensitivity there by increasing the imaging capability of the OCT.

The volume of retinal tissue visualized by AO-OCT is shown as a composite that is made by re-imaging the same retinal patch, with focus systematically shifted to different depths. In this way it preserves the high image quality provided by AO for the retinal layer of interest. Extracted en face slices are shown of individual RNFBs, microstructures in the ganglion cell layer, retinal capillaries, and outer segments of cone photoreceptors.

Polarization Sensitive OCT (PS-OCT)

Polarization sensitive OCT extends the concept of OCT and utilizes the information that is carried by polarized light to obtain additional information on the tissue. Several structures in the eye like cornea, retinal nerve fiber layer and retinal pigment epithelium alter the polarization state of the light and therefore show a tissue specific contrast in PS-OCT images. In PS-OCT images of the eye, birefringent structures like the retinal nerve fiber layer, depolarizing tissues like the retinal pigment epithelium and polarization preserving structures like the photoreceptor layer, can be distinguished.[57]

OCT Angiography: ANGIOVUE

It is a non-invasive technique that acquires volumetric angiographic information without the use of dye. The en-face images (OCT angiograms) images are obtained and they can be analyzed layer wise from internal limiting membrane to the choroid along with the vascular plexus. It employs motion contrast imaging to high-resolution volumetric blood flow information generating angiographic images.

In glaucoma it is useful in evaluating the optic disc perfusion which shows attenuation in both superficial disc vasculature as well as the microvascular network along the lamina cribrosa. In eyes with glaucoma, the flow index is reduced, which is obtained by averaging the de correlation signal and the area of microvasculature. The flow index has been shown to have both a very high sensitivity and specificity in differentiating glaucomatous eyes from normal eyes.[58,59]

REFERENCES

1. Steven T Simmons. American Academy of ophthalmology. Basic and clinical science course, Glaucoma Section 10, 2005-2006.
2. Vizzeri G, Kjaergaard SM, Rao HL, Zangwill LM. Role of imaging in glaucoma diagnosis and follow-up. Indian J Ophthalmol. 2011;59,Suppl S1:59-68.
3. Medeiros FA, Bowd C, Zangwill LM, Patel C, Weinreb RN. Detection of glaucoma using scanning laser polarimetry with enhanced corneal compensation. Invest Ophthalmol Vis Sci. 2007;48(7):3146-53.
4. Reus NJ, Zhou Q, Lemij HG. Enhanced imaging algorithm for scanning laser polarimetry with variable corneal compensation. Invest Ophthalmol Vis Sci. 2006; 47(9):3870-7.
5. Bowd C, Zangwill LM, Berry CC, et al. Detecting early glaucoma by assessment of retinal nerve fiber layer thickness and visual function. Invest Ophthalmol Vis Sci. 2001; 42(9):1993-2003.
6. Da Pozzo S, Fuser M, Vattovani O, et al. GDx-VCC performance in discriminating normal from glaucomatous eyes with early visual field loss. Graefes Arch clin Exp Ophthalmol. 2006;244(6):689-95.
7. Brusini P, Salvetat ML, Parisi L, et al. Discrimination between normal and early glaucomatous eyes with scanning laser polarimeter with fixed and variable corneal compensator settings. Eur J Ophthalmol. 2005;15(4):468-76.
8. Tjon-Fo-Sang MJ, Lemij HG. The sensitivity and specificity of nerve fiber layer measurements in glaucoma as determined with scanning laser polarimetry. Am J Ophthalmol. 1997;123(1):62-69.
9. Ramakrishnan R, Krishnadas SR, Khrana M, Robin AL. Diagnosis and Management of Glaucoma: Interpretation of Visual Fields. 1st edition. Jaypee Highlights Medical Publishers; New Delhi. 2013;182-95.
10. Wollstein G, Garway-Heath DF, Hitchings RA. Identification of early glaucoma cases with the scanning laser ophthalmoscope, Ophthalmology. 1998;105(8):1557-63.

11. Zangwill LM, Weinreb RN, Berry CC, et al. The confocal scanning laser ophthalmoscopy ancillary study to the ocular hypertension treatment study: study design and baseline factors. Am J Ophthalmol. 2004;137(2):219-27.
12. Zangwill LM, Weinreb RN, Berry CC, et al. Racial differences in optic disc topography: baseline results from the confocal scanning laser ophthalmoscopy ancillary study to the ocular hypertension treatment study. Arch Ophthalmol. 2004;122(1):22-8.
13. Mikelberg FS, Parfitt CM, Swindale NV, Graham SL, Drance SM, Gosine R. Ability of the Heidelberg Retina Tomograph to detect early glaucomatous visual field loss. J Glaucoma. 1995;4(4):242-7.
14. Uchida H, Brigatti L, Caprioli J. Detection of structural damage from glaucoma with confocal laser image analysis. Invest Ophthalmol Vis Sci. 1996;37(12):2393-401.
15. Caprioli J, Park HJ, Ugurlu S, Hoffman D. Slope of the peripapillary nerve fiber layer surface in glaucoma. Invest Ophthalmol Vis Sci. 1998;39(12):2321-8.
16. Bathija R, Zangwill L, Berry CC, Sample PA, Weinreb RN. Detection of early glaucomatous structural damage with confocal scanning laser tomography. J Glaucoma. 1998;7(2):121-7.
17. Bowd C , Weinreb RN, Lee b, et al. Optic disk topography after medical treatment to reduce intraocular pressure. Ophthalmol Vis Sci. 2000;41(3);775-82.
18. Swindale NV, Stjepanovic G, Chin A, Mikelberg FS. Automated analysis of normal and glaucomatous optic nerve head topography images. Invest Ophthalmol Vis Sci. 2000;41(7):1730-42.
19. Taibbi G, Fogagnolo P, Orzalesi N, Rossetti L. Reproducibility of the Heidelberg Retina Tomograph III Glaucoma Probability Score. J Glaucoma. 2009;18(3):247-52.
20. Moreno-Montañés J, Antón A, García N, Mendiluce L, Ayala E, Sebastián A. Glaucoma probability score vs Moorfields classification in normal, ocular hypertensive, and glaucomatous eyes. Am J Ophthalmol. 2008;145(2):360-8.
21. Fujimoto JG, Pitris C, Boppart SA, et al. Optical Coherence Tomography: an emerging technology for biomedical imaging and optical biopsy. Neoplasia. 2000;2(1-2):9-25.
22. Nassif N, Cense B, Park BH, et al. In vivo human retinal imaging by ultrahigh-speed spectral domain optical coherence tomography. Opt Lett. 2004;29(5):480-2.
23. Wojtkowski M, Srinivasan V, Ko T, et al. Ultra-high resolution, high speed, Fourier domain optical coherence tomography and methods of dispersion compensation. Opt Express. 2004;12(11):2404-22.
24. Huang D, Swanson EA, Lin CP, et al. Optical coherence tomography. Science. 1991;254(5053):1178-81.
25. Mansoori T, Viswanath K, Balakrishna N, et al. Quantification of retinal nerve fiber layer thickness using spectral domain optical coherence tomography in normal Indian population. Indian J Ophthalmol. 2012;60(6): 555-8.
26. Sowmya V, Venkataramanan VR, Vishnu Prasad KP. Analysis of retinal nerve fiber layer thickness using optical coherence tomography in normal South Indian population. Muller J Med Sci Res. 2014;5:5-10.
27. Appukuttan B, Giridhar A, Gopalakrishnan M, Sivaprasad S. Normative spectral domain optical coherence tomography data on macular and retinal nerve fiber layer thickness in Indians. Indian J Ophthalmol. 2014;62:316-21.
28. Pawar N, Maheshwari D, Ravindran M, Ramakrishnan R. Retinal nerve fiber layer thickness in normal Indian pediatric population measured with optical coherence tomography. Indian J Ophthalmol. 2014;62:412-8.
29. Strouthidis NG, Yang H, Reynaud J, et al. Comparison of clinical and spectral domain optical coherence tomography optic disc margin anatomy. Invest Ophthalmol Vis Sci. 2009;50(10):4709-18.
30. Curcio CA, Allen KA. Topography of ganglion cells in human retina. J Comp Neurol.1990;300(1):5-25.

31. Mwanza JC, Durbin MK, Budenz Dl, et al. Glaucoma diagnostic accuracy of ganglion cell–inner plexiform layer thickness: comparison with nerve fiber layer and optic nerve head. Ophthalmology. 2012;119(6):1151-8.
32. Wu Z, Vazeen M, Varma R, et al. Factors associated with variability in retinal nerve fiber layer thickness measurements obtained by optical coherence tomography. Ophthalmology. 2007;114(8):1505-12.
33. Wu Z, Huang J, Dustin L, Sadda SR. Signal strength is an important determinant of accuracy of nerve fiber layer thickness measurement by optical coherence tomography. J Glaucoma. 2009;18(3):213-16.
34. Lee JY, Hwang YH, Lee SM, Kim YY. Age and Retinal Nerve Fiber Layer Thickness Measured by Spectral Domain Optical Coherence Tomography. Korean J Ophthalmol. 2012;26(3):163-8.
35. Kim YW, Jeoung JW, Yu HG. Vitreopapillary traction in eyes with idiopathic epiretinal membrane: a spectral-domain optical coherence tomography study. Ophthalmology. 2014;121(10):1976-82.
36. Hood DC, Kardon RH. A framework for comparing structural and functional measures of glaucomatous damage. Progress in retinal and eye research. 2007;26(6):688-710.
37. Medeiros FA, Zangwill LM, Alencar LM, et al. Detection of glaucoma progression using stratus OCT retinal nerve fiber layer, optic nerve head and macular thickness measurements. Invest Ophthalmol Vis Sci. 2009;50(12):5741-8.
38. Strouthidis NG, Scott A, Peter NM, Garway-Heath DF. Optic disc and visual field progression in ocular hypertensive subjects: Detection rates, specificity, and agreement. Invest Ophthalmol Vis Sci. 2006;47(7):2904-10.
39. Balasubramanian CM, Weinreb RN, et al. Performance of Confocal Scanning Laser Tomograph Topographic Change Analysis (TCA) for Assessing Glaucomatous Progression. Invest. Ophthalmol. Vis. Sci. 2009;50(2):691-701.
40. Garas A, Vargha P, Hollo G. Reproducibility of retinal nerve fiber layer and macular thickness measurement with the RTVue-100 optical coherence tomograph. Ophthalmology. 2010;117(4):738-46.
41. Gonzalez-Garcia AO, Vizzeri G, Bowd C, et al. Reproducibility of RTVue retinal nerve fiber layer thickness and optic disc measurements and agreement with Stratus optical coherence tomography measurements. Am J Ophthalmol. 2009;147(6): 1067-74.
42. Lee SH, Kim SH, Kim TW, Park KH, Kim DM. Reproducibility of retinal nerve fiber thickness measurements using the test-retest function of spectral OCT/SLO in normal and glaucomatous eyes. J Glaucoma. 2010;19(9):637-42.
43. Li JP, Wang XZ, Fu J, Li SN, Wang NL. Reproducibility of RTVue retinal nerve fiber layer thickness and optic nerve head measurements in normal and glaucoma eyes. Chin Med J (Engl). 2010;123:1898-1903.
44. Mwanza JC, Chang RT, Budenz DL, et al. Reproducibility of peripapillary retinal nerve fiber layer thickness and optic nerve head parameters measured with CirrusTM HD-OCT in glaucomatous eyes. Invest Ophthalmol Vis Sci. 2010;51(11):5724-30.
45. Menke MN, Knecht P, Sturm V, Dabov S, Funk J. Reproducibility of nerve fiber layer thickness measurements using 3D Fourier-domain OCT. Invest Ophthalmol Vis Sci. 2008;49:5386-91.
46. Schuman JS. Spectral domain optical coherence tomography for glaucoma (an AOS thesis) Trans Am Ophthalmol Soc. 2008;106:426-58.
47. Leung CK, Chiu V, Weinreb RN, et al. Evaluation of retinal nerve fiber layer progression in glaucoma: a comparison between spectral-domain and time-domain optical coherence tomography. Ophthalmology. 2011;118(8):1558-62.
48. Leung CK, Cheung CY, Weinreb RN, et al. Retinal nerve fiber layer imaging with spectral-domain optical coherence tomography: a variability and diagnostic performance study. Ophthalmology.2009;116(7):1257-63.

49. Kim JS, Ishikawa H, Sung KR, et al. Retinal nerve fibre layer thickness measurement reproducibility improved with spectral domain optical coherence tomography. Br J Ophthalmol. 2009;93(8):1057-63.
50. Bellezza AJ, Rintalan CJ, Thompson HW, et al. Deformation of the lamina cribrosa and anterior scleral canal wall in early experimental glaucoma. Invest Ophthalmol Vis Sci. 2003;44(2):623-37.
51. Takayama K, Hangai M, Kimura Y, et al. Three-dimensional imaging of lamina cribrosa defects in glaucoma using swept-source optical coherence tomography. Invest Optom Vis Sci. 2013;54(7):4799.
52. Wolbarsht ML, Walsh AW, George G. Melanin, a unique biological absorber. Appl Opt. 1981;20:2184-6.
53. Povazay B, Hermann B, Unterhuber A, Hofer B, Sattmann H, Zeiler F, et al. Three-dimensional optical coherence tomography at 1050 nm versus 800 nm in retinal pathologies: enhanced performance and choroidal penetration in cataract patients. J Biomed Opt. 2007;12:041211.
54. Esmaeelpour M, Povazay B, Hermann B, et al. Three-dimensional 1060-nm OCT: choroidal thickness maps in normal subjects and improved posterior segment visualization in cataract patients. Invest Ophthalmol Vis Sci. 2010;51:5260-6.
55. Povazay B, Hofer B, Torti C, et al. Impact of enhanced resolution, speed and penetration on three-dimensional retinal optical coherence tomography. Opt Express. 2009;17:4134-50.
56. Miller DT, Kocaoglu OP, Wang Q, Lee S. Adaptive optics and the eye (super resolution OCT). Eye. 2011;25(3):321-30.
57. Pircher M, Götzinger E, Leitgeb R, Sattmann H, Findl O, Hitzenberger CK. Imaging of polarization properties of human retina in vivo with phase resolved transversal PS-OCT. Opt Express. 2004;12(24):5940-51.
58. Jia Y, Morrison JC, Tokayer J, Tran O, Lombardi L, Baumann B, et al. Quantitative OCT Angiography of Optic Nerve Head Blood Flow. Biomed Opt Express. 2012;3(12):3127-37.
59. Jia Y, Wei E, Wang X, Zhang X, Morrison JC, Parikh M, et al. Optical Coherence Tomography Angiography of Optic Disc Perfusion in Glaucoma. Ophthalmology. 2014;7(121):1322-32.

Chapter 8

Postoperative Endophthalmitis

Lalit Verma, Arindam Chakravarti

INTRODUCTION

Postoperative endophthalmitis is the most devastating complication after intraocular surgery, which is commonly associated with a poor prognosis.[1] Postoperative endophthalmitis can occur following any ocular surgery in which the globe is penetrated. However, 90% of postoperative endophthalmitis occurs following cataract surgery, because cataract surgery is one of the most frequently performed intraocular surgeries in the world.[2] Fortunately, postoperative endophthalmitis after intraocular surgery is a rare clinical occurrence, but it often causes severe visual impairment or even the loss of an eye.[3]

Worldwide, the reported incidence of postoperative endophthalmitis is 0.04–4%. Post-cataract surgery incidence is 0.265% (more with clear corneal incision), post-keratoplasty 0.382% and post-vitrectomy 0.05%. The incidence of bleb associated infection is 0.2–9.6%. This range in the incidence of infection appears to be consistent across numerous patient populations from all over the world.[4,5] In a study of ten-year incidence of endophthalmitis rate at Bascom Palmer Eye Institute (1984–1994),[6] the incidence of post-cataract surgery endophthalmitis was 0.09%. In a meta-analysis of and Taban et al.[7] the overall incidence rate of postoperative endophthalmitis was 0.128% from 1963 to 2003. However, the incidence of postoperative endophthalmitis has changed over time and has increased to 0.265% per year over the last few decades, which coincides temporally with the development of self-sealing clear corneal incisions. Several retrospective, comparative, case-controlled studies found a significantly higher endophthalmitis rate associated with clear corneal incisions compared to sclera tunnel incisions.[8-11] Recently, Nagaki et al.[12] reported a statistically increased risk with clear corneal incisions (0.29%) compared to sclerocorneal incisions (0.05%).

Though rare, it is potentially the most feared and devastating complication of intraocular procedures and can lead to a permanent, complete loss of vision. Endophthalmitis has been associated with severe visual loss in 20% of patients. A series of endophthalmitis cases may force a temporary shutdown of the operation theater.

Infectious endophthalmitis is classified by the events leading to the infection and by the timing of the clinical diagnosis. The broad categories include postoperative endophthalmitis (acute-onset, chronic or delayed-onset, conjunctival filtering-bleb associated), post-traumatic endophthalmitis, and endogenous endophthalmitis.

Miscellaneous categories include cases associated with microbial keratitis, intravitreal injections, or suture removal. These categories are important in predicting the most frequent causative organisms and in guiding therapeutic decisions before microbiologic confirmation of the clinical diagnosis (Table 8.1).

Patient symptoms indicative of endophthalmitis include ocular pain, diminished vision and headache. Although pain is an important symptom, it is not universal.

It is important to differentiate infective endophthalmitis from sterile postoperative inflammation (Table 8.2).

Toxic anterior segment syndrome (TASS) is an acute postoperative inflammatory reaction in which a noninfectious substance enters the anterior segment and induces toxic damage to the intraocular tissues. Almost all cases occurred after uneventful cataract surgery.

In TASS most develop symptoms within 12–24 hours, there is decrease in visual acuity, corneal edema is from limbus to limbus, there is moderate to severe AC reaction with cells, flare, hypopyon and fibrin, pupil may be dilated and non-reactive and IOP may be normal or raised.

BACTERIAL ENDOPHTHALMITIS

Postoperative endophthalmitis may be early or delayed. Most common causative agents are Gram-positive coagulase negative organisms. However in India, Gram-negative organisms and fungi are important in etiology.[16-21]

Differentiation is important as the management and prognosis of TASS is significantly different. Delay in diagnosis leads to delay in initiating appropriate treatment.

Endophthalmitis should be suspected when there is pain and increased in AC reaction on slit lamp examination on first postoperative day. However, pain may

TABLE 8.1: Classification of endophthalmitis (most frequent organisms in various clinical settings)

- Postoperative
  - Acute-onset postoperative endophthalmitis: Coagulase-negative staphylococci, *Staphylococcus aureus*, *Streptococcus* species, Gram-negative bacteria
  - Delayed-onset (chronic) pseudophakic endophthalmitis (>6 weeks postoperative): *Propionibacterium acnes*, coagulase-negative staphylococci, fungi
  - Conjunctival filtering bleb-associated endophthalmitis: *Streptococcus*, *Haemophilus influenzae*, *Staphylococcus* species
- Post-traumatic (open globe): *Bacillus* species, staphylococci
- Endogenous: *Candida* species, *S. aureus*, Gram-negative bacteria
- Miscellaneous:
  - Keratitis: *Staphylococcus* and *Pseudomonas* species
  - Intravitreal injection (intravitreal triamcinolone, intravitreal ganciclovir, pneumatic retinopexy, etc.): Coagulase negative staphylococci
  - Suture removal: Both bacteria and fungi

Source: Results in the ESCRS postoperative endophthalmitis study, the Endophthalmitis Vitrectomy Study (EVS),[4] and other studies assessing the causative organism demonstrate that Gram-positive organisms account for 90% or more of pathogens isolated in culture-positive cases of postoperative endophthalmitis following cataract surgery, with coagulase-negative staphylococci (i.e. *Staphylococcus epidermidis*) and *Staphylococcus aureus* representing the leading causes.[12-18, 6, 14-16,19-21]

TABLE 8.2: Differences between TASS and infective endophthalmitis

	TASS	Endophthalmitis
Cause	Noninfectious reaction to toxic agent present in: • BSS solution • Antibiotic injection • Endotoxin • Residue	Bacterial, fungal, or viral infection
Onset	12–24 hours	4–7 days
Signs/Symptoms *distinguishing feature	• Blurry vision • Pain: None, or mild to moderate • Corneal edema: diffuse, limbus to limbus* • Pupil: Dilated, irregular, nonreactive* • Increased IOP* • Anterior chamber: Mild to severe reaction with cells, flare, hypopyon, fibrin • Signs and symptoms are limited to anterior chamber* • Gram stain and culture negative • Ultrasound is anechoic	• Decreased VA • Pain (25% have no pain) • Lid swelling with edema • Conjunctival injection • Hyperemia • Anterior chamber: Marked inflammatory response with hypopyon • Vitreous involvement • Inflammation in entire ocular cavity* • Ultrasound shows vitreous echoes
Treatment	• Rule out infection • Culture anterior chamber • Intensive corticosteroids • Monitor IOP closely for signs of damage to trabecular meshwork and side effects of steroids • Watch closely over next few hours for signs of bacterial infection	• Culture anterior chamber and vitreous • Intravitreal and topical antibiotics • Vitrectomy

be absent in 25% cases. Decreased glow on distant direct ophthalmoscopy has high sensitivity but low specificity on first postoperative day.

On subsequent postoperative days, decrease in vision following initial improvement along with pain should immediately raise the index of suspicion. Presence of exudates in vitreous on indirect ophthalmoscopy is 100% specific.

Presence of hypopyon and vitreous exudates is usually diagnostic of endophthalmitis.

If there is no hypopyon, role of distant direct ophthalmoscopy, slit lamp examination, indirect ophthalmoscopy and ultrasound B scan is very important in deciding surgical intervention, rule out other causes like masquerade.

Slit lamp examination helps to see dilatability of pupil, wound margin (many cases related to suture removal). In cases with poorly dilating pupils and significant AC reaction (+++) and best corrected visual acuity better than 6/60, sterile reaction should be considered and treatment started with intravenous bolus steroids and topical steroids and antibiotics. However, if best corrected visual acuity (BCVA) is <6/60, endophthalmitis should be considered and patient should be administered intravitreal antibiotics. An USG B scan may aid in the diagnosis with non-dilating pupils and severe AC reaction by demonstrating vitreous echoes.

Presence of vitreous exudates clinches the diagnosis of endophthalmitis.

Case Situations and Studies

CASE 1: Postoperative day 1: Good glow, AC reaction 2–3 +, no hypopyon (Fig. 8.1).

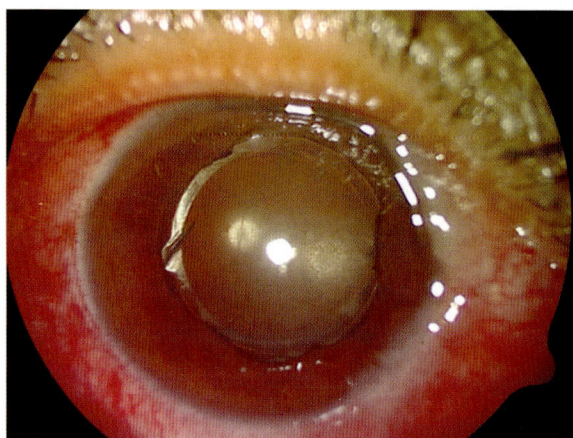

Fig. 8.1: Whether to give intravitreal antibiotics or topical + S/C + IV steroids

Can be treated as TASS with topical and IV steroids but requires close follow-up.

CASE 2: Postoperative day 1: BCVA 6/24, unusual postoperative reaction, good glow after treatment with steroid (Figs 8.2A and B). Gradual improvement in vision was noted on day 2 (Figs 8.3A and B) and day 14 (Figs 8.4A and B).

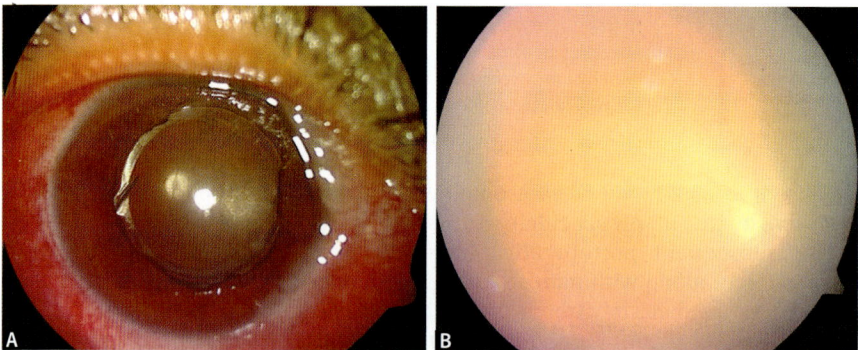

Figs 8.2A and B: Treated with intensive steroids

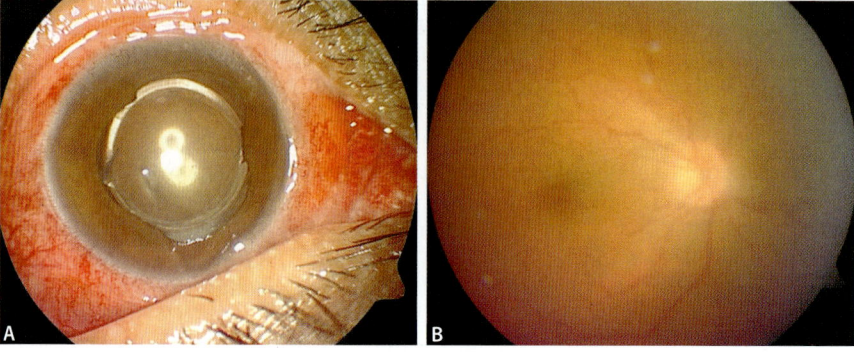

Figs 8.3A and B: DAY 2: BCVA 6/18, reaction significantly less, fundus details much clearer

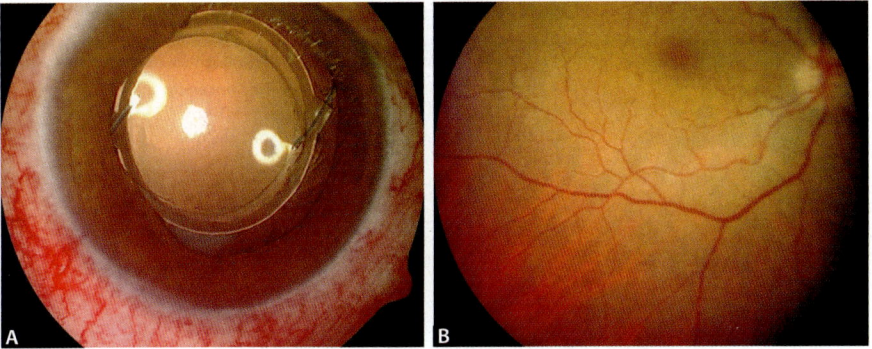

Figs 8.4A and B: Day 14: BCVA 6/6, quiet AC, normal appearance of fundus

Case situation of definite endophthalmitis: Vision of at least HM, has not received intravitreal antibiotics (Fig. 8.5).

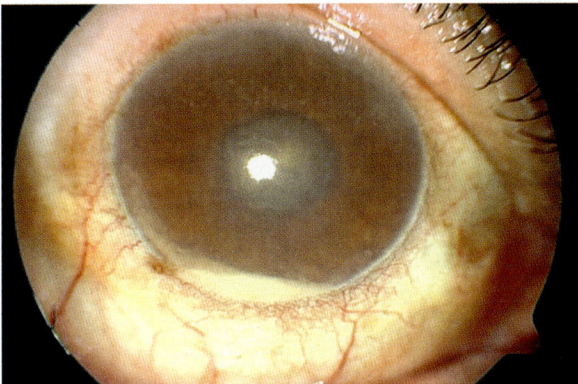

Fig. 8.5: At present, best choice of intravitreal antibiotics is vancomycin (1 mg in 0.1 mL) combined with ceftazidime (2.25 mg in 0.1 mL) in separate syringes

Alternatively, vancomycin may be combined with amikacin (400 μg in 0.1 mL). Topical treatment comprises ciprofloxacin/gatifloxacin/moxifloxacin 1 hourly or fortified cefazolin + tobramycin 1 hourly along with cycloplegics in the form of atropine every six hourly. The topical drug dosage is tailored according to response. Topical steroids are added 1–2 days later intravenous ciprofloxacin 200 mg twice daily is required in very severe cases.

Oral steroids administered as 1–1.5 mg/kg single dose along with oral antibiotics. Ciprofloxacin 750 mg twice daily for 7–10 days usually preferred although currently many clinicians prefer oral gatifloxacin or moxifloxacin. After intravitreal antibiotics, patient is monitored for 24–36 hours. If there is worsening, patient has to be taken up for surgical intervention in the form of pars plana vitrectomy. If there is no worsening, medical treatment can be continued for 48 hours following which decision regarding additional intravitreal antibiotics or surgical intervention is to be taken. Improvement in fundus glow with decrease in hypopyon is indicative of clinical improvement. Medical treatment should be continued.

TABLE 8.3: Commonly used intravitreal drugs in endophthalmitis

Intravitreal drugs in postoperative bacterial endophthalmitis				Anti-fungal drugs in endophthalmitis	
Vancomycin (1 mg in 0.1 mL) 500 mg powder		**Amikacin** (400 µg in 0.1 mL) 100 mg in 2 mL vial/50 mg in 1.0 mL/10 mg in 0.2 mL		**Amphotericin B** (5 µg in 0.1 mL) 50 mg powder	
Add 10 mL	500 mg in 10 mL			Add 10 mL 5% dextrose	50 mg in 10 mL
	50 mg in 1.0 mL	Take 0.2 mL	10 mg		0.5 mg in 0.1 mL
	10 mg in 0.2 mL	Add 2.3 mL	10 mg in 2.5 mL	Take 0.1 mL	0.5 mg
Take 0.2 mL	has 10 mg	Take 0.1 mL	0.4 mg in 0.1 mL	Add 9.9 mL of 5% dextrose	0.5 mg/10 mL
Make it 1.0 mL	10 mg in 1 mL	**Gentamicin** (200 µg in 0.1 mL) 80 mg in 2 mL vial/40 mg in 1.0 mL			0.05 mg/1.0 mL
Take 0.1 mL	1 mg in 0.1 mL			Take 0.1 mL	0.005 mg
Ceftazidime/cefazoline (2.25 mg in 0.1 mL) 500 mg powder		Take 0.1 mL	4 mg	**Voriconazole** (50–100 µg in 0.1 mL) 200 mg powder	
		Add 1.9 mL	4 mg in 2 mL		
Add 2.0 mL	500 mg in 2 mL	Take 0.1 mL	0.2 mg	Add 19 of d/w	200 mg in 20 mL
	250 mg in 1.0 mL	• Diluent used (Water for injection/Ringer lactate) • All preparations done by surgeon himself, under strict aspetic conditions • Recommended (for bacterial endophthalmitis) Vancomycin + ceftazidime or Vancomycin + amikacin • For fungal endophthalmitis voriconazole or amphotericin B			10 mg in 1.0 mL
Take 0.1 mL	22.5 mg in 0.1 mL			Take 1.0 mL	
Make it to 1.0 mL	22.5 mg in 1.0 mL			Add 9.0 mL of d/w	10 mg in 10 mL
Take 0.1 mL	2.25 mg in 0.1 mL				1.0 mg in 1.0 mL
Dexamethasone (0.4 mg in 0.1 mL) 8 mg in 2 mL vial/4 mg in 1.0 mL				Take 0.05 mL/ 0.1 mL	50/100 µg
Take 0.1 mL directly	0.4 mg				

CASE 3: Post cataract surgery (phaco) day 4: BCVA: HM+, no glow (Fig. 8.6).

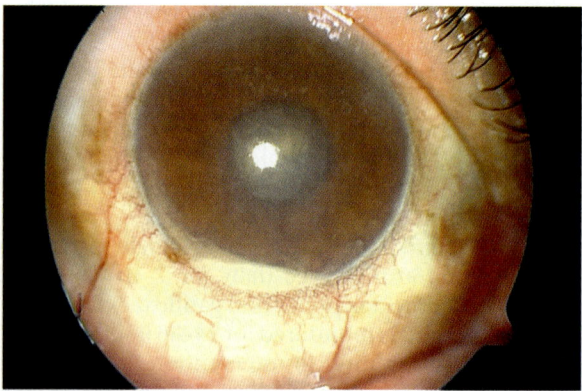

Fig. 8.6: Patient treated with intravitreal vancomycin + ceftazidime and medical management

Some improvement was noted on postoperative day 3: BCVA FC ½ meters (Fig. 8.7).

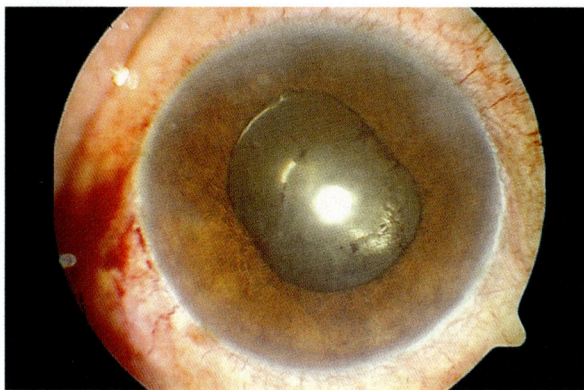

Fig. 8.7: Postoperative day 3: BCVA FC ½ meters

Postoperative day 6: FC 3 meters (Fig. 8.8).

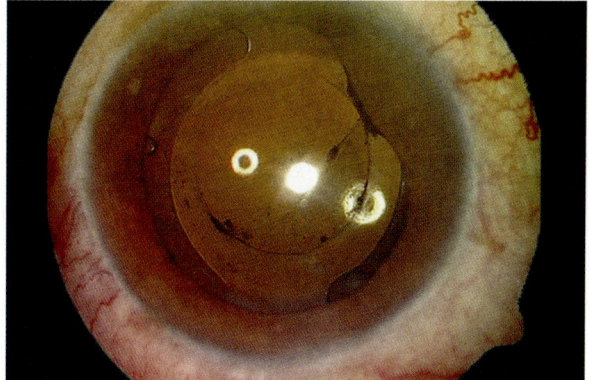

Fig. 8.8: Postoperative day 6: FC 3 meters

Postoperative 2 weeks: BCVA 6/24 (Figs 8.9A and B).

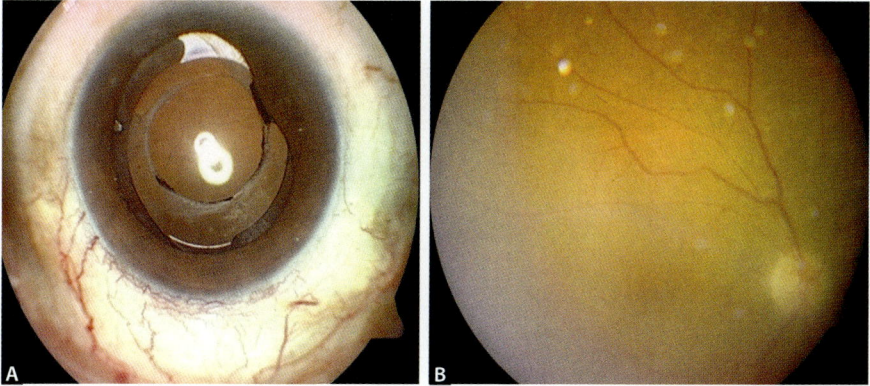

Figs 8.9A and B: Postoperative 2 weeks: BCVA 6/24

Postoperative 3 weeks: BCVA 6/6 (Fig. 8.10).

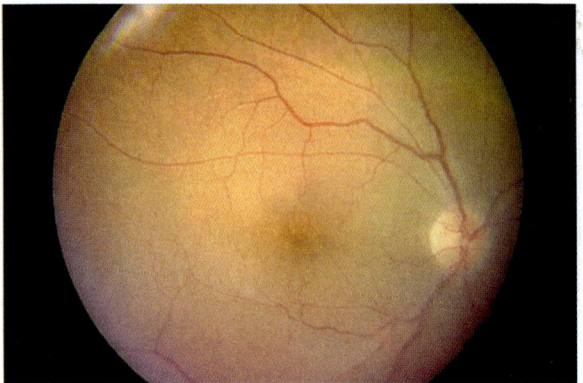

Fig. 8.10: Postoperative 3 weeks: BCVA 6/6

However in situations where there is a partial response to intravitreal antibiotics with resolution of hypopyon but persisting AC reaction (3–4+), further intravitreal antibiotics are not preferred, conservative medical management is continued and patient is readied for surgical intervention.

In situations where there is no response to intravitreal antibiotics or in very severe infection, radical pars plana vitrectomy with peeling of hyaloid and base dissection is required. There is no role for core vitrectomy in this situation.

CASE 4: Post pars plana vitrectomy (PPV) 4 days, VA: PL +, no glow (Fig. 8.11).

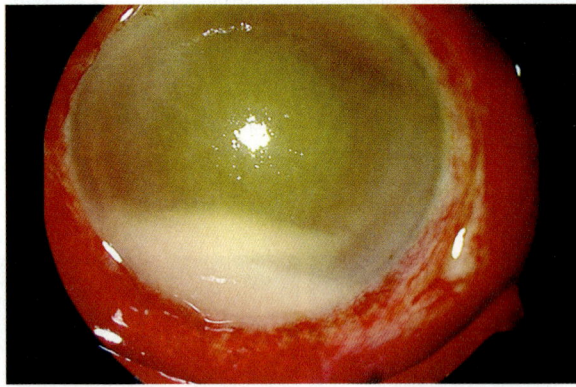

Fig. 8.11: Post PPV 4 days, VA: PL +, no glow

Post radical PPV + IOL removal, day 9, VA: FCCF (Figs 8.12A and B).

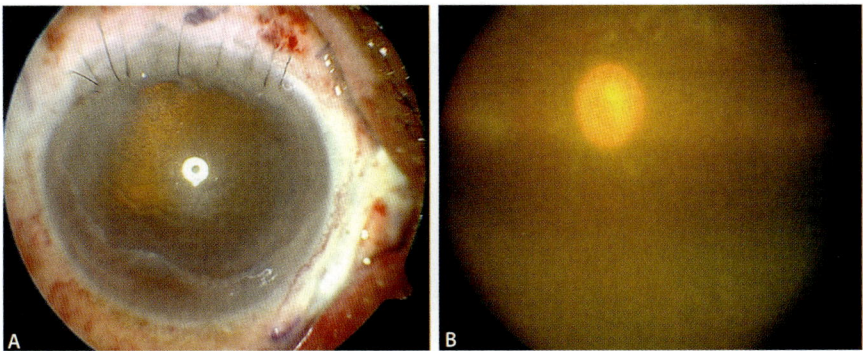

Figs 8.12A and B: Post radical PPV + IOL removal, day 9, VA: FCCF

IOL removal during vitrectomy for endophthalmitis may be indicated in severe endophthalmitis, P acne endophthalmitis, fungal endophthalmitis and recurrent endophthalmitis.

CASE 5: Endophthalmitis with corneal abscess, VA: PL+ at presentation (Figs 8.13A and B).

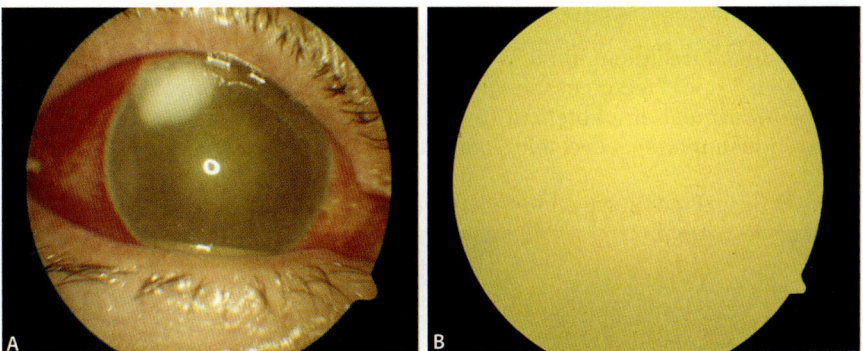

Figs 8.13A and B: Endophthalmitis with corneal abscess, VA: PL+ at presentation

Situation improved 4 weeks after radical vitrectomy with silicone oil, BCVA 6/24 (Figs 8.14A and B).

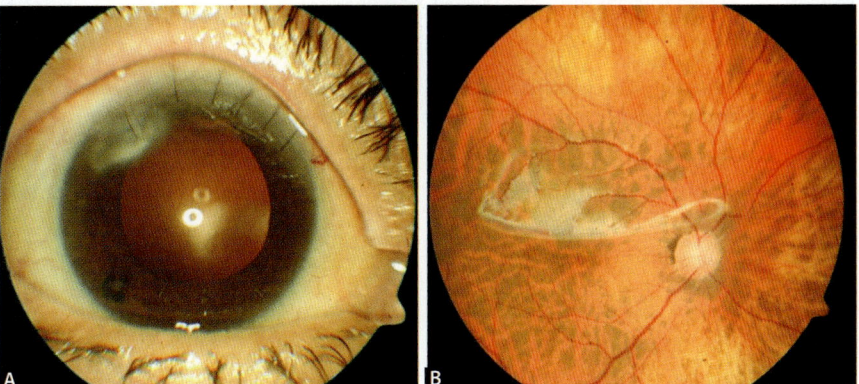

Figs 8.14A and B: Four weeks after radical vitrectomy with silicone oil, BCVA 6/24

FUNGAL ENDOPHTHALMITIS

Predisposing history may include diabetes mellitus, immunocompromised patient, injury with vegetable matter and in patients on intravenous line.

Usually, a quite eye is encountered where signs are more prominent than symptoms. Vitreous balls, fungal granuloma may be seen (Fig. 8.15). Smears, cultures may help.

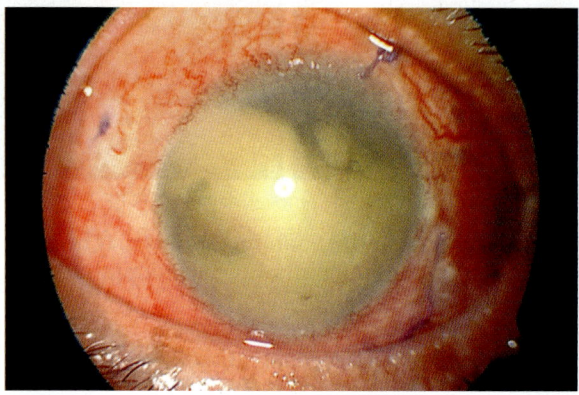

Fig. 8.15: Fungal endophthalmitis

If on initial treatment, there is no/partial response or worsening, vitrectomy is the only hope. Treatment includes oral and intravitreal voriconazole (50–100 µg) or intravitreal amphotericin (5–10 µg). Steroids should be stopped. Oral/intravenous antibiotics, cycloplegics and topical antibiotics are usually continued.

CASE 6: Suspected fungal endophthalmitis with VA: HM + (Figs 8.16A and B).

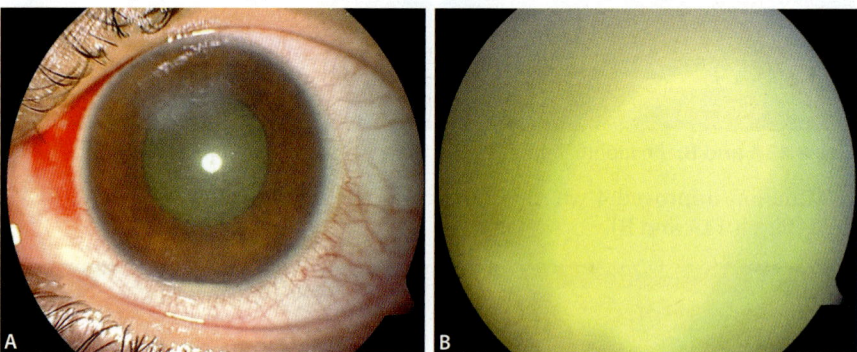

Figs 8.16A and B: Suspected fungal endophthalmitis with VA: HM +

Patient underwent radical vitrectomy with posterior hyaloid peeling and removal of subhyaloid pus pockets. Postoperative improvement is documented in Figure 8.17A and B.

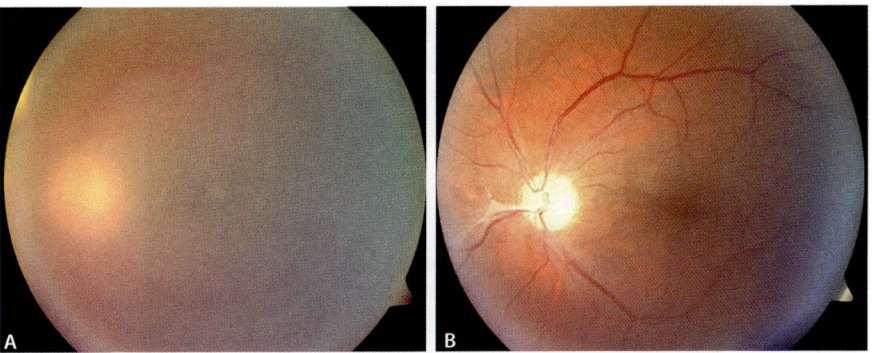

Figs 8.17A and B: Postoperative improvement. Postoperative day 1: Postoperative day 21

CHRONIC ENDOPHTHALMITIS

Typical is *Propionibacterium acnes* related endophthalmitis. It runs a chronic course with multiple recurrences.

Usual intravitreal antibiotic injections are not of much help.

Treatment options:
- 'In the bag' vancomycin 1 mg/0.1 mL
- PPV + Partial capsulectomy
- PPV + Total capsulectomy + IOL explantation.

CASE 7: Patient with recurrent attacks of uveitis with PC plaque and improvement with steroids (Figs 8.18A and B) underwent PPV + Partial capsulectomy + In-the-bag vancomycin. Postoperative improvement is documented in Figures 8.19 to 8.21A and B.

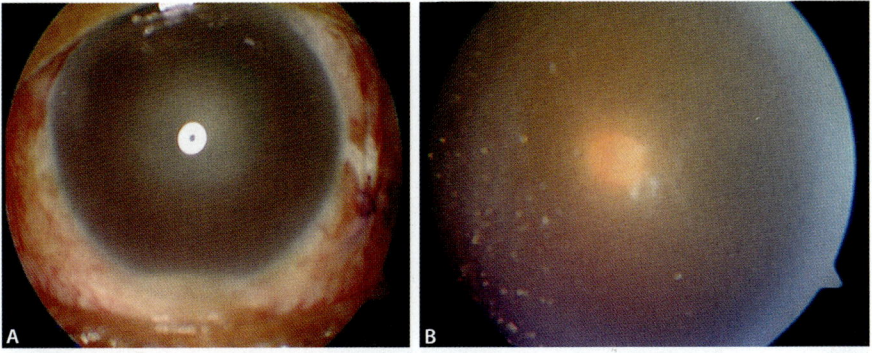

Figs 8.18A and B: Preoperative: BCVA FC

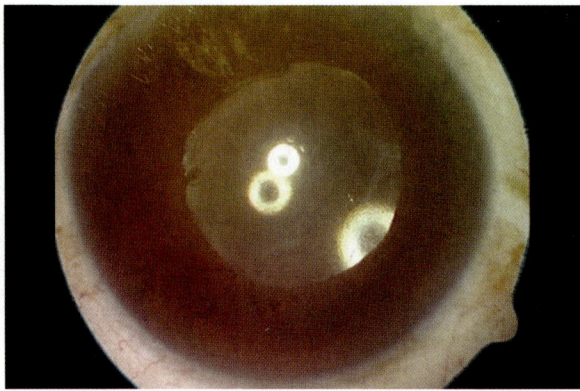

Fig. 8.19: Postoperative day 27: BCVA 6/18

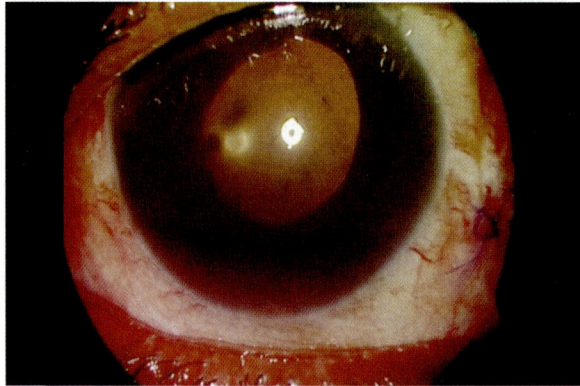

Fig. 8.20: Postoperative day 49: BCVA 6/9

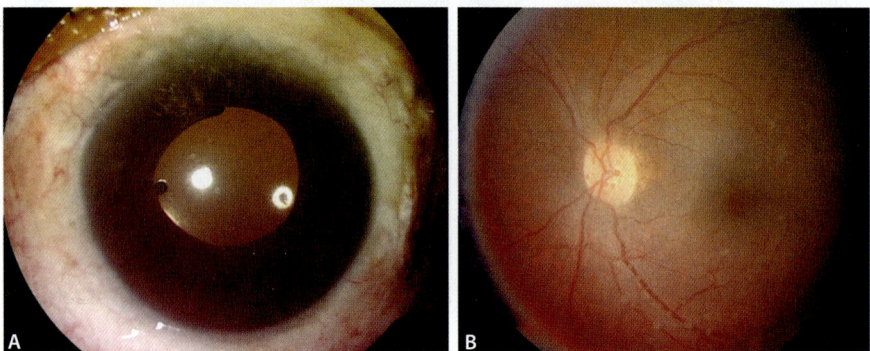

Figs 8.21A and B: Postoperative follow-up

CASE 8:

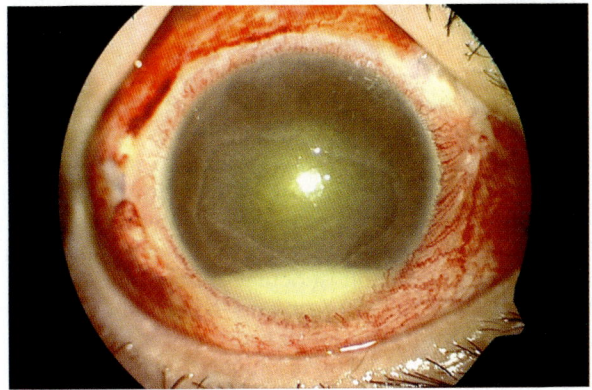

Fig. 8.22: Endophthalmitis after intravitreal Avastin

It is extremely severe due to direct inoculation of organism in vitreous (Fig. 8.22). Prognosis is very poor and vitrectomy is the only answer.

Lucentis scores over Avastin because of its efficacy and safety. Safety with regard to preparation of Avastin is always a source of concern as there is no uniform method; muliple pricks are involved during aliquoting.

There have been incidents of cluster endophthalmitis with Avastin. And even cornea is severely involved (Fig. 8.23).

CASE 9:

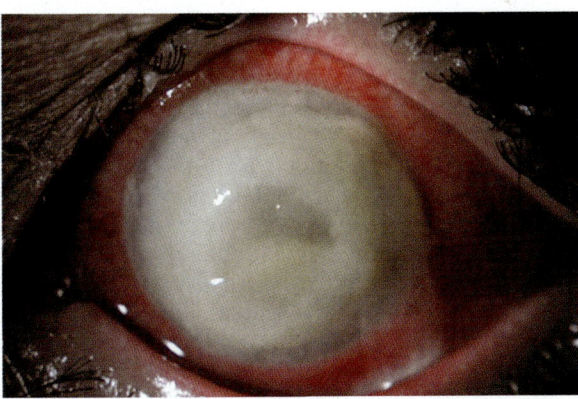

Fig. 8.23: Endophthalmitis with corneal involvement

Prognosis is generally poor. Management requires the help of a cornea specialist.

Clinician has to depend upon intravitreal antibiotic injections + intensive topical treatment. Definitive vitreous surgery is difficult.
- If no response: Can try core vitrectomy—if possible
- Keratoprosthesis: Vitrectomy + PK
- Endoscopic vitrectomy.

PREVENTION AND PROPHYLAXIS

Eyelid and ocular surface microflora have been implicated as the source of infection in most cases of postoperative endophthalmitis.[19-21] Because bacteria can be cultured from the ocular surface of almost any person, certain risk factors may make patients more susceptible to infection by their ocular surface microflora. Risk factors for endophthalmitis include chronic bacterial blepharitis, active conjunctivitis, infections of the lacrimal drainage system, tear drainage obstruction, contaminated eye drops, contact lens wear, prosthesis in the fellow eye, and active nonocular infections. These conditions may lead to an abnormally elevated population of ocular surface microbes or colonization of the ocular surface by atypical organisms with greater virulence than the normal microflora. Host factors that lower resistance to infection such as chronic immunosuppressive therapy and diabetes mellitus have also been reported to be significant risk factors for postoperative endophthalmitis.

To reduce the incidence of postoperative endophthalmitis, each of the factors implicated in the pathogenesis should be addressed. First, an attempt should be made to decrease or eliminate eyelid and conjunctival microflora both preoperatively and intraoperatively. This goal may be accomplished by using preoperative topical antibiotics and topical antiseptic agents. Second, administering subconjunctival antibiotic at the time of surgery should be considered.

Studies evaluating the effectiveness of preoperative administration of antibiotics and povidone-iodine19-21 have reported a significant decrease in conjunctival bacterial colony counts. Topical antibiotics were reported to be most effective in decreasing conjunctival bacterial colony counts when administered 2 hours before surgery rather than one or more days before surgery. The combination of topical antibiotics and povidone-iodine was found to sterilize the conjunctiva in more than 80% of treated patients.

Subconjunctival antibiotics are commonly administered after intraocular surgery. The rationale for subconjunctival antibiotic administration at the completion of the ocular procedure is to inhibit growth of bacteria that may gain entry into the eye during the operative procedure. Studies performed evaluating the effectiveness of prophylactic subconjunctival antibiotics in reducing the incidence of postoperative endophthalmitis reported conflicting results.

Administering antibiotics in the irrigating fluid for cataract surgery has become a common technique for infection prophylaxis. This technique carries the risks of antibiotic toxicity, cost, and the possibility of emergence of resistant bacteria. The various strategies to prevent postoperative endophthalmitis are based on current knowledge regarding the pathogenic mechanisms of postoperative endophthalmitis. Perhaps of greatest importance, the preoperative ocular examination will help to identify the high-risk patient as previously described. In these patients, eyelid and conjunctival cultures can be performed before performing intraocular surgery. Based on the culture results and the overall clinical evaluation, preoperative topical antibiotic treatment may be considered. In patients with eye diseases requiring chronic administration of topical medications, new sterile medications should be provided to the patient before and after intraocular surgery.

On the day of cataract surgery, treating patients with prophylactic topical antibiotics that have activity against organisms commonly causing endophthalmitis can be considered. A thorough surgical prep, which includes lid margins, is performed. Instillation of 5% povidone-iodine on the conjunctiva followed by irrigation with saline is part of the surgical prep. The eyelids and eyelashes can be draped out of the surgical field with a plastic eye drape. A dry surgical field can be maintained when instruments are passed in and out of the eye. Attention to water-tight wound closure is a priority, particularly in complicated surgical procedures or in reoperations that tend to have a higher incidence of postoperative wound leak. Vitreous incarceration in the wound should be eliminated by anterior vitrectomy techniques. At the conclusion of surgery, subconjunctival antibiotic injection using a combination of agents effective against the majority of causative Gram-positive and Gram-negative organisms can be considered.

NEWER INTRAVITREAL ANTIBIOTICS

Intravitreal injection of piperacillin and tazobactam could be effective in the management of multidrug-resistant endophthalmitis caused by Gram-negative bacteria. *Enterobacter* species develop resistance rapidly to antibiotics due to their capacity to produce extended spectrum beta-lactamases. Piperacillin and tazobactam complement in their mechanism of action against beta-lactamase-producing organisms. Due to the production of high levels of beta-lactamase, combination therapy with piperacillin and tazobactam is a safe and effective alternative in the management of multidrug-resistant Gram-negative infections. Combination of tazobactam and piperacillin is given in dosage of 225 μg/0.1 mL intravitreally based on available experimental data.

Intravitreal injection of colistin could be an option effective in the management of multidrug-resistant endophthalmitis caused by Gram-negative bacteria. Colistin belongs to polymyxins, a group of polypeptide antibiotics which includes five different chemical compounds (polymyxins A, B, C, D and E). Colistin binds to Gram-negative bacterial cell membrane phospholipids, producing a disruptive physiochemical effect, which leads to the cell membrane permeability changes and ultimately cell death. Most Gram-negative microorganisms are susceptible to colistin, including multidrug-resistant *Acinetobacter baumannii* and *P. aeruginosa* strains. Two forms of colistin are commercially available, colistin sulfate and colistimethate sodium (also called colistin methanesulfate, pentasodium colistimethate sulfate and colistin sulfonylmethate). The target of antimicrobial activity of colistin is a bacterial cell membrane. The initial association of colistin with bacterial membrane occurs through electrostatic interactions between the cationic polypeptide (colistin) and anionic lipopolysaccharide (LPS) molecules in the outer membrane of the Gram-negative bacteria, leading to derangement of the cell membrane. The endotoxin of Gram-negative bacteria is the lipid A portion of LPS molecules and colistin binds and neutralizes LPS. Polymyxin E (colistin), only polymyxin B has been used in clinical practice in several countries. Polymyxin B has the same mechanism of action and resistance as does colistin.

Colistin sulfate has greater activity than polymyxin B against *P. aeruginosa*. Intravitreal dose was—0.1 mg/0.1 mL (1000 IU/0.1 mL) and IV dose was 2.5–5 mg/kg daily in 2–4 doses.

Imipenem has a broad spectrum of activity against both aerobic and anaerobic and Gram-positive and Gram-negative bacteria including *Pseudomonas* and *Enterococcus* species. It acts by inhibiting cell wall synthesis of various Gram-positive and Gram-negative bacteria. It is stable to hydrolysis by the common plasmid-mediated beta-lactamases produced by various bacteria and lacks cross resistance with penicillins and third-generation cephalosporins. Intravitreal imipenem may limit intraocular inflammation and retinal tissue damage when given early in the course of *Pseudomonas* endophthalmitis. It is generally nontoxic in animal models at concentrations that are far higher than the MIC 90 of 3.6 to 12.5 μg/mL against *Pseudomonas* infection and may offer promise in the treatment of endophthalmitis after intraocular surgery or perforating eye injuries.

When to refer? (After giving first intravitreal injection)
- Severe infection
  - Very poor vision ±
  - Post-trabeculectomy infection
  - After intravitreal injections
  - Suspected fungal
  - Endophthalmitis panophthalmitis
- Non-response to first intravitreal injection
- Associated CD/RD
- Associated corneal abscess
- Unsatisfied patient
- Cluster infection.

Early, prompt and appropriate treatment with (intravitreal antibiotics/vitrectomy/re-vitrectomy) may show gratifying results.

WHAT TO DO, IN CASE OF INFECTION?

- Dialogue with patient and relatives
- Clearly explain the possible causes and pathophysiology of infection and further management. Need for co-operation and referral should be emphasized
- All findings should be documented
- Review all sterility factors
- Have a peer review
- Referral to higher center
- Treat energetically with intravitreal antibiotics and supportive therapy
- OT should be sealed and cultures for microbiological evaluation should be taken
- Batch numbers of all solutions used should be noted and samples sent for culture
- All solutions used should be sealed and kept in safe custody
- Seek help from legal cell of All India Ophthalmological Society (AIOS).

WHAT TO DO IN CLUSTER INFECTIONS OR OUTBREAK?

- Cluster infection is defined as occurrence of two or more than two infections at a time, or the occurrence of repeated postoperative infection
- Inform authorities (CMO, Medical Superintendent, Senior Authority)
- Institute Infection Control Committees
- Inform AIOS and seek help of legal cell
- Engage and seek help of lawyer
- Press has to be handled carefully to prevent Pandemonium from spreading
- It is desirable that medical superintendent/hospital committee does press briefing.

LEGAL ISSUES RELATED TO ENDOPHTHALMITIS

Legal issues related to endophthalmitis are multifold and can be patient-related, surgeon-related, institution-related, media-related or government-related.

Handling of the media is of particular importance and one must ensure that the surgeon involved does not speak to the press. The institutional head or some other institutional representative should handle the press. One wrong quote by the surgeon may be misquoted and made a huge issue. The surgeon should however ensure that he/she has completely documented each and every clinical record of every patient to protect one-self from such eventualities.

There have been certain landmark court rulings in the recent past on the issue of medical negligence. Some of the rulings are not favorable to medical professionals. One approach towards a more objective measure in determining the legal standard of care could be the use of clinical guidelines decided upon by an expert medical body. This is where the printed guidelines on prevention of intraocular infections assume vital importance.

REFERENCES

1. Maguire JI. Postoperative endophthalmitis: optimal management and the role and timing of vitrectomy surgery. Eye. 2008;22(10):1290-300.
2. Verbraeken H. Treatment of postoperative endophthalmitis. Ophthalmologica. 1995;209(3):165-71.
3. Kresloff MS, Castellarin AA, Zarbin MA. Endophthalmitis. Survey of Ophthalmology. 1998;43(3):193-224.
4. Results of the endophthalmitis vitrectomy study: a randomized trial of immediate vitrectomy and of intravenous antibiotics for the treatment of postoperative bacterial endophthalmitis. Archives of Ophthalmology. 1995;113(12):1479-96.
5. Fintelmann RE, Naseri A. Prophylaxis of postoperative endophthalmitis following cataract surgery: current status and future directions. Drugs. 2010;70(11):1395-409.
6. Endophthalmitis Study Group and European Society of Cataract and Refractive Surgeons. Prophylaxis of postoperative endophthalmitis following cataract surgery: results of the ESCRS multicenter study and identification of risk factors. Journal of Cataract and Refractive Surgery. 2007;33: 978-88.
7. Taban M, Behrens A, Newcomb RL. Acute endophthalmitis following cataract surgery: a systematic review of the literature. Archives of Ophthalmology. 2005;123(5):613-20.
8. Aaberg TM, Flynn HW, Schiffman J, Newton J. Nosocomial acute-onset postoperative endophthalmitis survey: a 10-year review of incidence and outcomes. Ophthalmology. 1998;105(6):1004-10.
9. Cooper BA, Holekamp NM, Bohigian G, Thompson PA. Case-control study of endophthalmitis after cataract surgery comparing scleral tunnel and clear corneal wounds. American Journal of Ophthalmology. 2003;136(2):300-5.
10. Lertsumitkul S, Myers PC, O'Rourke MT, Chandra J. Endophthalmitis in the western Sydney region: a case-control study. Clinical and Experimental Ophthalmology. 2001;29(6):400-5.
11. McDonnell PJ, Donnenfeld ED, Perry HD. New horizons in fluoroquinolone therapy. Ophthalmology Times. 2002;27(1):1-15.
12. Barrow D, McDermott M, Elliot D, Frank R. Acute postoperative endophthalmitis and modern cataract surgery technique [ARVO abstract 1340]. Investigative Ophthalmology and Visual Science. 2001;42:S24.

13. Nagaki Y, Hayasaka S, Kadoi C. Bacterial endophthalmitis after small-incision cataract surgery: effect of incision placement and intraocular lens type. Journal of Cataract and Refractive Surgery. 2003;29(1):20-6.
14. Han DP, Wisniewski SR, Wilson LA. Spectrum and susceptibilities of microbiologic isolates in the Endophthalmitis Vitrectomy Study: the Endophthalmitis Vitrectomy Study Group. American Journal of Ophthalmology. 1996;122:1-17.
15. Benz MS, Scott IU, Flynn Jr HW, Unonius N, Miller D. Endophthalmitis isolates and antibiotic sensitivities: a 6-year review of culture-proven cases. American Journal of Ophthalmology. 2004;137(1):38-42.
16. Recchia FM, Busbee BG, Pearlman RB, Carvalho-Recchia CA, Ho CA. Changing trends in the microbiologic aspects of postcataract endophthalmitis. Archives of Ophthalmology. 2005;123(3):341-6.
17. Barry P, Cordovés L, Gardner S. ESCRS guidelines for prevention and treatment of endophthalmitis following cataract surgery: data, dilemmas and conclusions. Paper presented at: the European Society of Cataract and Refractive Surgeons; 2013; Dublin, Ireland.
18. Speaker MG, Menikoff JA. Prophylaxis of endophthalmitis with topical povidone-iodine. Ophthalmology. 1991;98:1769-75.
19. Verma L, Venkatesh P, Tewari HK. AIOS CME Series.2000; 4.
20. Das TP, Dogra MR, Gopal L, Jalali S, Kumar A, Malpani A, et al. Postsurgical endophthalmitis: diagnosis and management. Current Ophthalmology. 1995; 43(3):103-16.
21. Anand AR, Therese KL, Madhavan HN. Spectrum of aetiological agents of postoperative endophthalmitis and antibiotic susceptibility of bacterial isolates. Indian J Ophthalmol. 2000;48(2):123-8.

Chapter 9

Toxic Anterior Segment Syndrome

Kamaljeet Singh, Arshi Misbah

INTRODUCTION

Toxic anterior segment syndrome (TASS) is an acute, noninfectious inflammation of the anterior segment of the eye occurring 12–48 hours following the anterior segment surgery. It is an uncommon, potentially devastating complication that occurs when a noninfectious toxic agent enters the anterior segment of the eye causing an inflammatory reaction and resulting in toxic damage to the intraocular tissues. Cataract extraction is the most common form of surgery associated with TASS, but it can occur after any kind of anterior segment surgery. It was initially referred to as *sterile postoperative endophthalmitis.* It was termed TASS by Monson et al.[1] in 1992. TASS became a subject of clinical interest over the last so many years.[2-5] Gopal and Vijaya wrote an editorial in the British Journal of Ophthalmology and elaborated on its causes and investigations.[6] When the damage is restricted to corneal endothelial cells, TASS is classified as toxic endothelial cell destruction syndrome (TECDS); a rare complication of intraocular operations.

EPIDEMIOLOGY

Frequency

Data on the incidence of TASS are lacking. Clusters ranging from a few cases to up to 20 cases occur several times each year in United States of America.

Aravind Eye Hospital, Pondicherry, India determined the incidence of long-term outcomes of TASS at a single institution. The records of all eyes developing TASS during a 1-year period after cataract surgery were retrospectively reviewed. TASS occurred in 60 eyes (0.22%) in 26408 consecutive cataract surgeries.[7] There were two identifiable clusters of TASS sporadic and epidemic outbreak.[8]

Incidence

The TASS can present as sporadic cases (52%) or in outbreaks. Many cases are never diagnosed and many cases are not reported because they are not severe and represent a very low percentage of the total cataract surgeries performed, thus the real incidence rate of TASS remains unknown.

ETIOLOGY

The etiology of TASS is not infectious. It has been associated with many factors. They can be divided into extraocular substances which penetrate in the anterior chamber during or after surgery. Often the cause cannot be found, even after thorough investigations. Common causes of TASS are discussed below.[9-12]

Bacterial Endotoxin Residues

Many think that since it is sterile it cannot be toxic. Sterile does not mean nontoxic. Bacteria produce heat stable endotoxins that are not destroyed during the sterilization process. These endotoxins even in small amount can cause an outbreak of TASS. Instruments, which are cleaned using ultrasonic bath in same unchanged tap water, have accumulation of debris which encourages the growth of gram-negative bacteria. These bacteria with passage of time produce heat-stable endotoxins causing TASS.

In Indian set up where the disposable instruments are used in selected hospitals and institutes, the chances of TASS episodes are high.

Viscoelastic Residues

Viscoelastic solutions are used in majority of intraocular surgeries. Usually, viscoelastic residues are nontoxic. However, if reusable irrigation and aspiration cannulas are not cleaned properly after surgery, the viscoelastic residues are denatured during the sterilization process. These denatured viscoelastic residues are toxic to eye and act as carrier for detergents and enzymatic cleaners used in processing of instruments before sterilizing them. These sterilized cannulas, when used during subsequent procedures, may introduce these toxic materials into the eye causing TASS.[13]

Other Residues

Detergents, enzymes and tiny particulate matter can contaminate instruments and tubing. They can get trapped inside irrigating cannulas, which when introduced into the eye can cause TASS. Most of the enzymatic detergents contain subtilisin, an exotoxin that causes corneal edema, marked inflammation, and corneal decompensation.

Phacoemulsification hand pieces: Phacoemulsification hand pieces that are sterilized with ethylene oxide gas may have gas residue left on them when they are not aerated completely. This gas residue can cause TASS.[13]

Other particulate contaminants like talc from gloves, clothing cotton fibers, rubber stopper pieces, metallic flakes, introduced unknowingly in the eye can lead to TASS. Residual lens cortex can also induce reaction. TASS may be associated with sulfate, copper or zinc residues found in autoclave steam used for sterilization.

Solutions and Intraocular Fluids

Any solution injected in or around the eye during or after surgery can potentially cause TASS. Balanced salt solution (BSS) is a sterile physiological solution that contains sodium chloride, potassium chloride, calcium chloride, magnesium chloride, sodium acetate and sodium citrate dehydrate. BSS is isotonic and is used for irrigation during eye surgery. BSS can be a major contributing factor in

TASS as it can act as a carrier for toxic material in several ways. The solution may have an abnormal ionic composition or pH. Refrigerated BSS has been associated with TASS outbreaks. Earlier, it was thought that cold temperature reduces postoperative inflammation and endothelial cell loss. However, cold BSS reduces corneal swelling, leading to improper sealing of incision and thereby allowing potentially toxic subconjunctival fluids to enter the eye causing TASS.

Preservatives

Preservatives used in ophthalmic solutions like benzalkonium chloride can damage corneal endothelium and can cause TASS. Other toxic preservatives include edetic acid, 0.1% sodium bisulfite and 0.01% thimerosal. Anesthetics used intracamerally may also contain preservative which can cause TASS.

Medications

Medications like antimetabolites used during glaucoma surgery, postoperative subconjunctival antibiotic injections or postoperative application of antibiotic drops or ointments may penetrate through the surgical wounds into the eye and can cause TASS. Toxicity may also occur while irrigating solutions containing antibiotic agents like gentamycin sulfate, moxifloxacin or when antibiotics are injected directly in the anterior chamber at the end of procedure for prevention of endophthalmitis.

Intraocular Lenses

Ethylene oxide is used for sterilizing the IOL, where residue may be left on IOL when it is not aerated completely. This IOL, when introduced into the eye causes TASS.[8,9] IOL polishing compound aluminum oxide is also associated with chronic inflammation. Although low level of aluminium does not cause ocular inflammation, the higher level may cause late onset TASS (Taka).[8] Therefore, it should be thoroughly washed with BSS before implanting. It has also been demonstrated that most common risk factors for TASS arise from problems with the instrument cleaning process. Inadequate flushing of the hand pieces, the use of enzymatic detergents, and the use of ultrasound baths are the most prevalent factors responsible for TASS.

CLINICAL FEATURES

Most patients with TASS develop symptoms within 12–24 hours of the surgery. Patients have decreased visual acuity, corneal edema, a nonreactive dilated pupil and moderate to severe anterior chamber reaction with cells, flare, hypopyon and especially fibrin with eventual increased intraocular pressure. Pain is mild to moderate.

There is significant overlap between the clinical presentation of TASS and that of infectious endophthalmitis. Differentiating TASS from endophthalmitis may be difficult at times. The onset of signs and symptoms and response to therapy are all very important factors in differentiating TASS from infectious endophthalmitis (Table 9.1). To differentiate between the two complete evaluation should be done including.
- Slit lamp examination
- Fundus examination

TABLE 9.1: Showing differences between TASS and postoperative endophthalmitis

	Toxic anterior segment syndrome	Endophthalmitis
Onset	12–48 hours after surgery	4–7 days after surgery
Pain	Often painless or mild pain	Often present and severe
Vision	Impaied early	Impaired late
Corneal edema	Marked limbus to limbus	Near the surgical incision
IOP	Increased	Decreased
Vitreous	Clear	Hazy with exudates
Smear and culture	Negative	Positive large percentage
Response to steroids	Very good	Poor
Prognosis	Very good	Poor

- Gonioscopy
- IOP measurement
- Aqueous and vitreous tap and
- B-Scan.

Following points are helpful in differentiating TASS from endophthalmitis:

Onset: Usually, TASS occurs within 12 to 24 hours after surgery whereas usual onset of infectious endophthalmitis is within 4–7 days postoperatively.

Pain: Mild to moderate pain occurs in TASS whereas in infectious endophthalmitis, pain is more severe and regarded as diagnostic. But approximately 25% of patients diagnosed with infectious endophthalmitis however, do not complain of pain.

Corneal edema: Although corneal edema exists in both conditions, the edema in TASS is more profound and characteristically described as diffuse, from "limbus to limbus". The corneal edema in infectious endophthalmitis is more marked near or opposite the wound.

Inflammation: Toxic anterior segment syndrome is characterized by immediate and marked anterior segment inflammation, with increased presence of cells as a result of the marked breakdown of the blood-aqueous barrier, causes hyopyon (Fig. 9.1) and significant fibrin formation. Sometimes, the hypopyon may be out of proportion with the quantity of cells and amount of flare observed (Fig. 9.2). In infectious endophthalmitis, there is an increased cellular reaction in the anterior chamber, which occurs over a longer period of time than the inflammation in TASS.

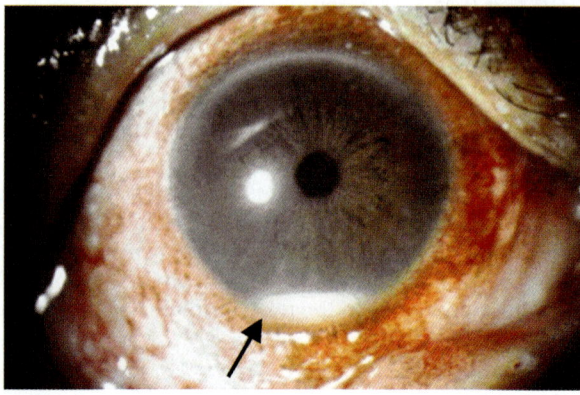

Fig. 9.1: Anterior chamber reaction with hypopyon

Pupil: Iris atrophy may occur early and significantly in TASS. The damaged iris sphincter causes pupillary distortion. As a result, it reacts poorly to light. A fixed, dilated pupil, therefore, is more commonly found in TASS than in infectious endophthalmitis.

Intraocular pressure (IOP): A marked inflammation is often associated with lowering of IOP but gradually the pressure rises postoperatively. The pressure may be as high as 40–70 mm Hg. Permanent damage to the trabecular meshwork can occur. Usually, the IOP of a patient with infectious endophthalmitis is usually subnormal.

Cultures: Cultures can determine whether the inflammation is sterile or infectious. With TASS, cultures of the anterior chamber and vitreous aspirates are negative. Usually cultures are positive with infectious endophthalmitis.

B-scan: Vitreous is not involved in TASS (Fig. 9.3). B-scan is anechoic in TASS whereas in infectious endophthalmitis, vitreous echoes are present (Fig. 9.4).

These are only guidelines for differentiating TASS from endophthalimits. There are reports indicating that *Bacillus cereus* endophthalmitis can occur within 12–24 hours after operation (Rishi et al.).[14] On the other hand, a mild toxic anterior segment syndrome can mimic a delayed onset toxic anterior segment syndrome after cataract surgery.[15]

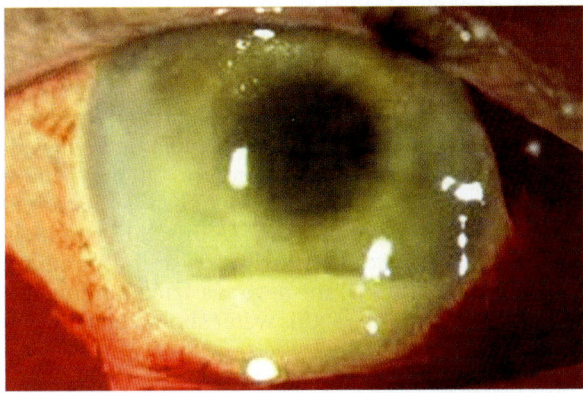

Fig. 9.2: Corneal edema with marked hypopyon

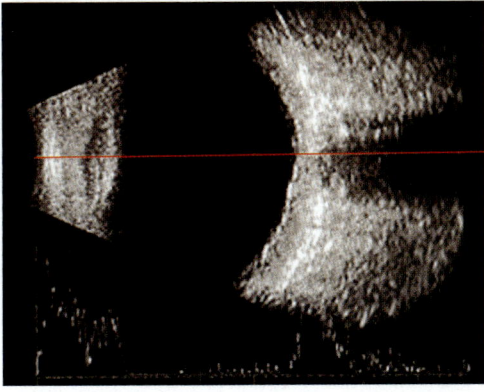

Fig. 9.3: B-scan in TASS

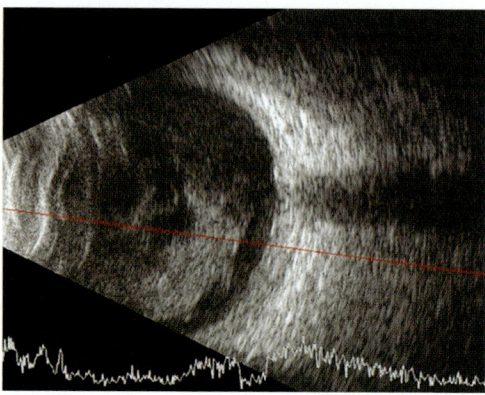

Fig. 9.4: B-scan in endophthalmitis

PREVENTION

To prevent TASS a team should be created including of surgeon, nurses, sterilization area staff, pharmacists, and ideally preventive medicine or public health doctors. The medical records of the TASS patient should be presented to the team for the documentation of surgical procedure, clinical presentation, the first time the inflammatory process was diagnosed, therapeutic approach and follow up. Data including names of surgical team, anesthetics, intraocular drugs or viscoelastic devices, intraocular lenses and surgical incidences should be registered and reviewed. Practice protocols must be reviewed to detect any error during application. This is very important for those members of the staff responsible for cleaning and sterilization. The reusable instruments should be replaced regularly, especially cannulas and I/A tips. It is extremely important to rinse with sterile deionized water both irrigation and aspiration ports and I/A tips of the phacoemulsification. Gram-negative bacteria growth is frequent in ultrasound water baths and therefore this water should be replaced daily.[4,16,17]

TREATMENT

Hourly topical prednisolone acetate must be started immediately. Cycloplegics should be frequently instilled. Oral steroids (1 mg/kg body weight) should be prescribed. Antibiotics must be continued till the diagnosis is clear.

Toxic anterior segment syndrome may cause trabecular meshwork damage, so the patient's IOP should be monitored daily for the several days after the onset of symptoms. After beginning intensive topical steroid therapy, anything that could worse inflammation, such as prostaglandin analogues, usually is avoided. Prostaglandin analogues, medications similar to naturally produced prostaglandins, play a part in causing and increasing inflammation and can adversely increase the inflammatory reaction in TASS.

Close monitoring for several days is necessary to ensure that the inflammation does not worsen and to rule out an infectious etiology. If infectious endophthalmitis is suspected, treatment includes vitreous taps, cultures, and antibiotics.

CLINICAL OUTCOME AND PROGNOSIS

If the reaction is mild, there is rapid improvement in signs and symptoms of inflammation. Hypopyon resolves very fast. Within 24–48 hours there is improvement in visual acuity. From hand movement to counting fingers within a day is seen. Patient's vision improves remarkably thereafter. The inflammation usually clears within one to three weeks.[6,9] Moderate cases take between three to six weeks to resolve. In severe cases, TASS can cause permanent damage. If severe symptoms are still present after six weeks, the eye is less likely to recover. Glaucoma may be resistant to treatment and may require multiple surgical procedures. In patients with very high IOP, the risk of chronic glaucoma is 50%. The corneal edema produced by TASS can permanently damage the corneal endothelium, causing permanent and irreversible corneal decompensation. Such cases may improve by keratoplasty.[17]

TASS may also cause profound cystoid macular edema. If a fixed, dilated pupil is observed on the first postoperative day it is less likely that it will come back to its original size.

The follow up should include frequent IOP measurements, visual acuity, slit lamp examination, corneal endothelial functions and iritis. Gonioscopy and dilated fundus examination should be done in each follow up.

Our experience[18] on ten patients (six females; four males) with mean age of 63.5 year, developed TASS after uneventful cataract surgeries on 12th June 2009. Their symptoms on the second postoperative day were pain, blurry vision, and red eye. Visual acuity was 20/200 to counting fingers, diffuse limbal to limbal corneal edema (ten patients), hypopyon (six patients), marked aqueous flare (ten patients), dilated nonreactive pupil (seven patients), faint fundal glow in all patients, and high intraocular pressure (in three patients). B-scan revealed a clear vitreous in all patients. Culture of vitreous tap was negative from all cases.

After diagnosing TASS, topical and systemic steroids and cycloplegics were started. Improvement in pain was noted within 24 hours of initiation of treatment. Corneal edema started decreasing on third day and cleared in 15 days in eight patients. Visual acuity gain started on third day. Vision improved to 20/30 in nine cases within two weeks. Hypopyon started disappearing on third day and resolved completely in one week in all the patients. Improvement in fundal glow was seen on third day. IOP remained high in only one patient.

Outcome was good within a fortnight. Only one patient developed secondary glaucoma.

CONCLUSION

Toxic anterior segment syndrome is a serious and potentially devastating complication of anterior segment surgery. When it occurs, the patient requires timely and appropriate management. TASS can be prevented by using standard surgical protocol. A proper pH of BSS, and preservative free ocular medicines should be used. Meticulous precautions should be taken in cleaning, sterilization and irrigation of surgical instruments.

REFERENCES

1. Monson MC, Mamalis N, Olson RJ. Toxic anterior segment inflammation following cataract surgery. J Cataract Refract Surg. 1992;18:184-9.
2. Meltzer DW. Sterile hypopyon following intraocular lens surgery. Arch Ophthalmol. 1980;98:100-4.
3. Apple DJ, Mamalis N, Steinmetz RL, Loftfield K, Crandall AS, Olson RJ. Phacoanaphylactic endophthalmitis associated with extracapsular cataract extraction and posterior chamber intraocular lens. Arch Ophthalmol. 1984;102: 1528-32.

4. Richburg FA, Reidy JJ, Apple DJ, Olson RJ. Sterile hypopyon secondary to ultrasonic cleaning solution. J Cataract Refract Surg. 1986;12:248-51.
5. Nelson DB, Donnenfeld ED, Perry HD. Sterile endophthalmitis after sutureless cataract surgery. Ophthalmology. 1992;99:1655-7.
6. Lingam Golpal, Vijaya L. Toxic anterior segment syndrome Br J. Ophthalmology. 2013;97:953.
7. Sen Gupta S, Chang DF, Gandhi R, et al. Incidence and long-term outcomes of toxic anterior segment syndrome. J Cataract Refract Surgery. 2011;37:1673-8.
8. Takashi et al. Outbreak of late onset toxic anterior segment syndrome after implantation of one-piece intraocular lens. American Journal of Ophthalmology. 2015;159:934-9.
9. Jehan FS, Mamalis N, Spencer TS, Fry LL, Kerstine RS, Olson RJ. Postoperative sterile endophthalmitis (TASS) associated with the memory lens. J Cataract Refract Surg. 2000;26:1773-7.
10. Cutler Peck CM, Brubaker J, Clouser S, Danford C, Edelhauser HE, Mamalis N. Toxic anterior segment syndrome: Common causes. J Cataract Refract Surg. 2010; 36:1073-80.
11. Bodnar Z, Clouser S, Mamalis N. Toxic anterior segment syndrome: Update on the most common causes. J Cataract Refract Surg. 2012;38:1902-10.
12. Carolee M. Cutler Peck, Jacob Brubaker, Sue Clouser, Chris Danford, Henry E Edelhauser, et al. Toxic anterior segment syndrome: Common causes Journal of Cataract & Refractive Surgery. 2010;36:1073-80.
13. Kreisler KR, Martin SS, Young CW, Anderson CW, Mamalis N. Postoperative inflammation following cataract extraction caused by bacterial contamination of the cleaning bath detergent. J Cataract Refract Surg.1992;18:106-10.
14. Rishi E, Rishi P, Sengupta S, et al. Acute postoperative Bacillus cereus endophthalmitis mimicking toxic anterior segment syndrome. Ophthalmology. 2013; 120:181-5.
15. Lee Su. Mild toxic anterior segment syndrome mimicking delayed onset toxic anterior segment syndrome after cataract surgery. Ind J Ophthalmol. 2014;62:890-92.
16. ASCRS Toxic anterior segment syndrome task force guidelines. Recommended practices for cleaning and sterilizing intraocular surgical instruments Available online at http://www.ascrs.org/TASS/upload /TASS_guidelines.pdf.
17. Mamalis N, Edelhauser HF, Dawson DG. Toxic anterior segment syndrome. J Cataract and Refractive Surgery. 2006;32:324-33.
18. Singh Kamaljeet, Suman Santosh. Clinical outcome of toxic anterior segment syndrome in an outbreak. Paper presented at XXVII ESCRS, Barcelona, 2009.

Chapter 10

Control of Infection in Ocular Surgery

Vaibhavi Subhedar

INTRODUCTION

Eye infection may be bacterial, viral, chlamydial, fungal or Acanthamoebic, and these infections account for a large proportion of the workload in ophthalmic centers.[1] Cross-infection may occur through contaminated instruments, hands, communal towels and droplets. Patients with dry eye or inadequate lid closure are more susceptible. Other risk factors are low immunity, malnutrition, general disease and extremes of age.[2] The incidence of endophthalmitis has been reported to be between 0.13% and 0.7%.[3] The primary source of this intraocular infection is considered to be bacteria from the patient's ocular surface (cornea, conjunctiva) or adnexa lacrimal glands, eyelids, and extraocular muscles).[4]

Multiple factors can lead to endophthalmitis. The source of the bacteria is considered to be from the patient's own ocular surface or adnexa. For this reason, simple measures in the preparation of the patient have a dramatic effect on the reduction of endophthalmitis rates, in particular the instillation of povidone-iodine and careful draping to isolate the lid and lashes. The use of antibiotics at the conclusion of surgery, especially intracameral or subconjunctival cefuroxime, is also recommended.[5,6]

PROGRESS IN INTRAOCULAR CATARACT SURGERY

In the past 4 decades, cataract surgery has undergone remarkable technical refinement, with simplified postoperative care and faster visual recovery as consequences.[7,8] With improved instrumentation, small-incision phacoemulsification became possible in the late 1980s, leading to the current state of the art of sutureless phacoemulsification surgery with foldable intraocular lens implantation.[9,10]

Removal of the lens through a corneal incision was reported as early as 1668;[11] however, the current self-sealing clear corneal incision was first introduced in 1992 by Fine.[12] Since then, increasing popularity of clear corneal incisions over limbal and scleral tunnel incisions among cataract surgeons across the United States and Europe has resulted in greater intraoperative control, decreased surgical time, simplified postoperative care, less induction of astigmatism, and faster visual recovery.[12] In the most recent survey of American Society of Cataract and Refractive Surgery members (2003), Leaming[3] reported that clear corneal incision was preferred by 72% of US surgeons and the no-suture closure was preferred by 92%. This acceptance is part of a gradual uptrend from 1.5%, 12.4%, 30%, 40%, and 47% in 1992, 1995, 1997, 1999, and 2000, respectively.[4] Among European surgeons, 51.4% prefer clear corneal incisions,[13] while a 1999 French survey reported a more than 86% preference for clear corneal incisions.[14] Furthermore, sutureless cataract incisions are reportedly preferred among 92%, 94%, and 58% of cataract surgeons in the United States, New Zealand, and Japan, respectively.[9,12]

EPIDEMIOLOGY OF POSTOPERATIVE ENDOPHTHALMITIS

The reported incidence of postoperative endophthalmitis varies by the specific surgical procedure and across studies, but the overall incidence has been declining since the late 19th to late 20th century. The incidence of endophthalmitis after cataract surgery was approximately 5% to 10% in the late 1800s and early 1900s,[15,16] 1.5% to 2% during the 1930s,[16,17] 0.5% to 0.7% in the mid 1900s,[17-19] and 0.06% to 0.09% according to nationwide patient registries in the early 1990s.[2] Improvements in microsurgical and aseptic techniques, advancements in surgical materials, and use of prophylactic broad-spectrum antibiotics, in combination with a better understanding of causes of the infection, may explain this favorable trend. In a meta-analysis of studies published from 1979 to 1991, a period that predates the use of self-sealing clear corneal incisions, Powe et al[20] reported a 0.13% incidence of acute postoperative endophthalmitis following cataract extraction. However, recent reports suggest that the postcataract endophthalmitis rate may be substantially higher, suggesting a greater risk of endophthalmitis coincident with the increase in self-sealing clear corneal incisions.[21,22] Colleaux and Hamilton,[22] reported 0.129% and 0.05% incidences of endophthalmitis following cataract extraction with sutureless clear corneal and scleral tunnel incisions, respectively. Similarly, 3 retrospective, comparative, case-controlled studies found a significantly higher endophthalmitis rate associated with clear corneal incisions compared with scleral tunnel incisions.[23,24] In a study from the Massachusetts Eye and Ear Infirmary (Boston), the incidence of endophthalmitis was 0.68% for clear corneal incisions vs 0.18% for scleral tunnel incisions.[25] More recently, Nakagi et al.[26] reported a statistically increased risk with clear corneal incisions (0.29%) compared with sclerocorneal incisions (0.05%). Various other anecdotal reports by cataract surgeons and retinal specialists have also claimed a higher incidence of endophthalmitis with clear corneal incisions.[25] These studies indicate an apparently increased occurrence of endophthalmitis in the last decade and a several-fold increase in endophthalmitis risk associated with self-sealing clear corneal incisions compared with scleral tunnel and sclerocorneal wounds. However, the relative rarity of endophthalmitis following intraocular surgery poses significant difficulty in ascertaining accurate incidence rates or in analyzing effects of multiple risk factors. Most reports regarding the rates of endophthalmitis are based on the experience of individual institutions or groups of surgeons and are limited by the small sample sizes, thereby making comparisons and statistical validity of data difficult. Only more appropriate methods such as extensive reviews or multicenter, prospective studies can help reveal clinical and statistical trends for this adverse outcome.[27]

Endophthalmitis is a rare but devastating complication of ocular surgery. Despite the advances in surgical techniques, the use of antibiotics and the improvement in surgical environment endophthalmitis still occurs after different types of ocular surgery at different rates worldwide.[28]

A postoperative endophthalmitis is an uncommon complication of any ocular surgery. The reported incidence of postoperative endophthalmitis ranges from 0.01% to 0.367%, with incidence varying among different surgical procedures and across studies and different countries.[28] The analysis showed an increase in the incidence of postsurgical endophthalmitis from 0.087% in the 1990s to 0.265% in the 2000s, and this was attributed to the change in surgical technique towards clear corneal sutureless wounds that allow exogenous microorganisms for easy access into the intraocular space. Apart from identification of the causative infectious agent, investigations are necessary not only to determine the incidence of this condition but also to identify the sources of such infections. It is necessary to understand its epidemiology in the given ophthalmic hospital to develop a plan for the prevention of its occurrence. Often, the identity of the infective agent can be presumed with reasonable accuracy depending on the clinical presentation such as acute, delayed and chronic endophthalmitis, depending on the time of onset of symptoms, may be grouped according to the onset of symptoms as acute, which occurs within 6 weeks of surgery, delayed if it is more than 6 weeks and less than 1 year of time and chronic if it is beyond 1 year.[29,30]

Nearly 70% of postoperative infectious endophthalmitis follow cataract surgery.[31] Varying incidence of postoperative infectious endophthalmitis has been reported from different parts of the world, but data of value from India are sparsely available in the literature. There are two reports from south India: one on its incidence following cataract surgery[32] and another with a description of the relationship between the visual outcome and clinical presentations of postcataract endophthalmitis.[33]

Endogenous endophthalmitis is even rarer than exogenous endophthalmitis (approximately 2–15% of all endophthalmitis cases). An American study reported an average annual incidence of 5 in 10,000 hospitalized patients.[34]

RISK FACTORS FOR ENDOPHTHALMITIS[6,22,27]

- Surgical
    - Previous presence of infection (e. g. bacterial conjunctivitis)
    - Poor surgical technique
    - Contaminated intraocular lens.
- Accidental injury
    - Retained infected foreign material, particularly if this is organic.
- Ophthalmic risk factors
    - Contact lens wearer (where there is poor hygiene)
    - Chronic corneal ulceration.
- Non-ophthalmic risk factors
    - Debility
    - Distant infection (e. g. indwelling catheter)
    - Immunosuppression
    - Intravenous drug use
    - AIDS.

The Endophthalmitis Vitrectomy Study (EVS) demonstrated that most isolates causing clinical endophthalmitis are introduced into the eye from the patient's conjunctival flora.[35,36] However, contamination of sterilized instruments, disposable supplies, prepared solutions, surgical field, or the intraocular lens, has been reported. Epidemic clusters of endophthalmitis have resulted from these types of external contaminations.[37,38]

Normally, the blood-ocular barrier prevents invasion from infective organisms but if this is breached (directly through trauma or indirectly due to a change in its permeability secondary to inflammation), infection can occur. Endophthalmitis may be the result of:
- Associated with surgery: early or delayed postoperative
- Traumatic: bacterial or fungal endophthalmitis
- Endogenous: bacterial or fungal endophthalmitis
- Associated with corneal infection (microbial keratitis)
- Associated with intravitreal injection
- Bleb-associated endophthalmitis.

PATHOGENS

The most common pathogens in endophthalmitis vary by cause.[35,36]
- Staphylococci coagulase-negative are the most common causes of post-cataract endophthalmitis (Fig. 10.1)
- Coagulase-negative staphylococcal bacteria and streptococci viridans viridans cause most cases of postintravitreal anti-VEGF injection endophthalmitis
- *Bacillus cereus* is a major cause of post-traumatic endophthalmitis
- *Staphylococcus aureus* and *Streptococcus* species are important causes of endogenous endophthalmitis associated with endocarditis
- *Klebsiella pneumoniae* causes most cases of endogenous endophthalmitis, in association with liver abscess in Southeast Asia

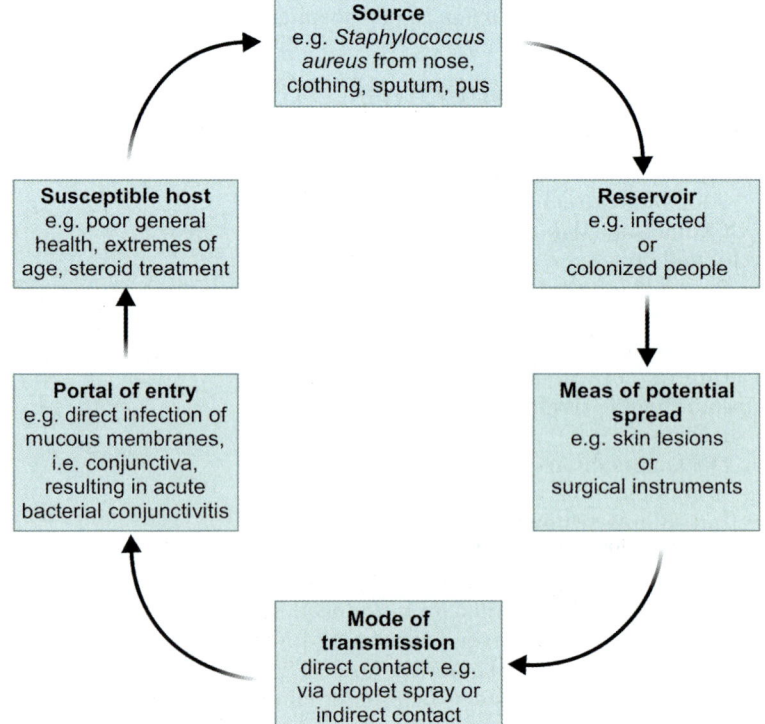

Fig. 10.1: Cycle of *Staphylococcus* infection

- Endogenous fungal endophthalmitis in hospitalized patients is usually caused by *Candida* species, particularly *Candida albicans*, *Fusarium* species and *Aspergillus* species
- Other pathogens which may be seen include:
    - Protozoans: *Acanthamoeba, Toxoplasma gondii, Toxocara* species
    - Viruses: Herpes simplex
    - Bacteria: *Pseudomonas aeruginosa*.

The bacteria most frequently isolated are gram-positive coagulase-negative cocci (mainly *Staphylococcus epidermidis*) which account for 70% of culture-positive cases.[31] *Staphylococcus aureus* is isolated in 10% of culture-positive cases, *Streptococcus* species in 9%, *Enterococcus* species in 2%, and other gram-positive species in 3% of cases.[30] Gram-negative bacteria account for just 6% of culture-positive cases; however, an infection with these bacteria, particularly with *Pseudomonas aeruginosa*, can lead to a devastating visual outcome.[30]

PROPHYLAXIS

Prevention of infection has to be done at all levels.[39,40]

Staff	• Consider all patients and staff a potential infection risk. • Staff should wash hands with soap before commencing any examination. • Wash hands with soap before and after every clinical procedure, even if gloves are worn. • Staff and patients with any broken skin, however small, must wear an occlusive dressing. • Staff with any known or suspected infection should not have direct patient contact.
Environment	• Wear heavy duty gloves for any cleaning procedures. • Clear up any spillages of blood or other body fluids immediately. Cover with bleach and leave for 15 minutes, wipe with disposable paper tissue or cloth. Wash the surface with a clean cloth, detergent and water. Burn all cleaning tissue and cloths. • Burn or bury soiled materials and other waste. • Soiled linen—soak first, dispose of the water carefully, and boil the linen before (gloved) hand-washing.
Equipment	• Used needles and other sharps—dispose of immediately into a puncture-resistant container. Make sure plenty are available in all areas where needles are used. • Never re-sheath a disposable needle! One-third of needle stick injuries are reported to occur during re-sheathing. • If a needle stick injury occurs—remove the glove and instrument from the surgical field. (See below the procedure following a needle stick injury). • Applanation tonometer prisms (tips only), diagnostic contact lenses, A-scan probes, occluders and pin-holes should be wiped with disposable paper tissue after each use. Store in sodium hypochlorite 1%, in a non-metallic pot, for 10 minutes, rinse in sterile water and dry before re-use. • Slit lamp—chin rest, head rim, handgrips and table top should be washed with detergent and water between each patient examination.
Surgical Instruments and deconta-mination procedures	• Loaded needle holders—lie point down on trolley and table tops. • Pass sharp instruments to colleagues with verbal warning and eye contact communication. • Sharp instruments should not project beyond the surface edge.

Contd...

Contd...

	• Ensure surgical instruments are thoroughly cleaned before being passed for sterilization or disinfection. • Choose the appropriate sterilization or disinfection method for the specific instrument. • Emphasize care of instruments and sterilization and disinfection procedures in training programs.
Clinical practice and safety issues	• Critically review work practices regularly. • Include control of infection policies in training programs. • Implement and emphasize strict adherence to universal control of infection policies. • Teach correct hand-washing technique and display a written procedure in all relevant areas (Fig. 10.2). • Eye drops and ointments—provide individual containers for each patient. • Eye dressings—following removal, dispose of immediately, by burning. • Eye shields—if removed from a knowingly infected patient, never re-use. • Pathological specimens—dispose of needles and blades used to obtain corneal and conjunctival material into 'sharps' container. • Wear rubber boots to protect feet in the operating theatre. Feet are particularly at risk of injury from puncture wounds caused by dropped instruments. Never allow sandals to be worn in the operating theatre. • Wear a plastic or rubber apron under sterile gowns in case a large amounts of blood spillage is expected. • Wear eye protection and face masks in the operating theater. • Wear gloves on both hands for all invasive procedures and when in contact with broken skin, mucous membranes, blood and body fluids.

The event of a needle-stick injury	Hand-washing technique
• Allow the wound to bleed freely for a few minutes. • Wash with soap and water. • Cover with a sterile dressing. • If known, note the details of the person on whom the needle was used and, if possible, check their HIV status. • Report the incident to the person-in-charge. • The injured person should be examined by a medical practitioner and referred for treatment if HIV transmission is a confirmed risk. • Hepatitis B vaccination. • Employers shall make available hepatitis B vaccinations to all employees who have occupational exposure. • These must be provided at no cost to the employee. • The vaccination must be started within 10 working days of the employee's initial assignment. • Should an employee refuse the vaccine? A declination form using specific language requested by OSHA must be signed.	• Wet hands with clean, preferably running, water. • Apply soap or cleanser. • Rub palm to palm. • Rub back of left hand over right palm. • Rub back of right hand over left palm. • Rub palm to palm with fingers interlaced (Fig. 10.2). • Rub backs of fingers on opposing palms with fingers interlocked. • Rub around right thumb with left palm. • Rub around left thumb with right palm. • Rub around fingers of right hand with palm of left hand. • Rub around fingers of left hand with palm of right hand. • Rub around the wrists. • Rinse off soap with clean, preferably running water and dry well.

Instruments[35,36]

All instruments used in the surgery should be thoroughly washed, cleaned and sterilized (Table 10.1).

Control of Infection in Ocular Surgery

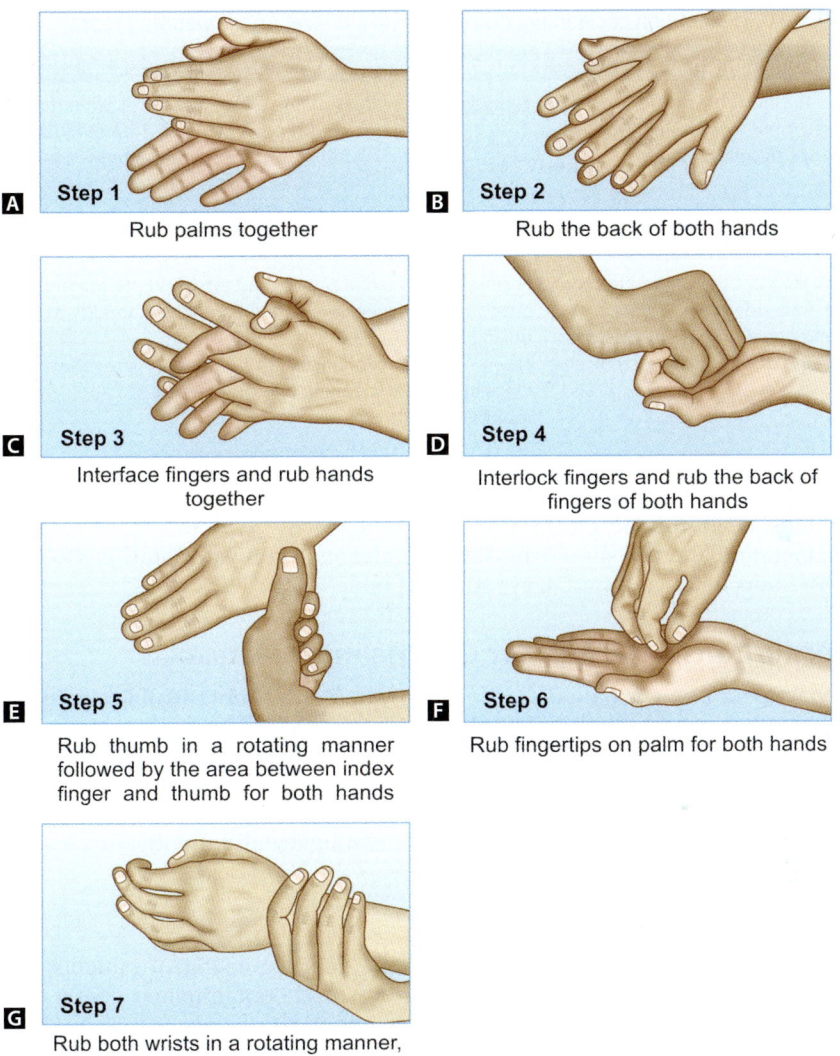

Figs 10.2A to G: Technique of washing hands (WHO guidelines)

TABLE 10.1: Cleaning and sterilization procedure for commonly used surgical instruments

Step	Procedure
• Cleaning and washing of is instruments after use • Ultrasonic cleaning • Drying of instruments • Autoclaving	• Clean the tips of the instruments preferably using distilled water, remove blood and debris from the using a sponge of instrument wipe and wash the instruments in detergent solution • It is better to clean surgical instruments in ultrasonic cleaner except sharp blades and delicate items like phaco or IA handpiecew • Dry the instruments after ultrasonic cleaning and pack in instrument trays • Most of the instruments are sterilized in steam autoclave. Temperature sensitive detectors must always be used to ensure adequate autoclaving

TABLE 10.2: Regimen of cleaning, disinfection of sterilization of operating room

Procedure and agents	Routine	Efficacy
Carbolization of or floor, walls, tables, trolleys with Phenol, Lysol, clearsol, hycolin or Stericol	Everyday	Reasonably effective against wide range of gram-positive and gram-negative bacteria but have little activity against endospores, viruses and hepatitis-B virus
Washing of or walls, floor, tables and trolleys, etc. with detergent	Once a week	Enhances the effect of daily cleaning and disinfection
Fumigation of the operating room with formaldehyde Maintenance, repair of breaches, cleaning of ventilation system, etc.	Fortnightly or after surgery on an infected case Once in six months	Efficacy is uncertain at temperatures below 200°C and relative humidity below 70% Enhances and improves the effect of cleaning and disinfection

Operation room
It must be thoroughly cleaned and sterilized.[39,40]
- Operation theater should be washed, cleaned, fumigated and carbolised 24 hours before the start of eye surgery (Table 10.2).

Specific Considerations for Ophthalmic Practice

A separate unit for eye patients is ideal, but where this is not possible care must be taken that patients with open infected wounds, ulcers or bed-sores are not accommodated in the same area as eye patients. Patients with eye infections should be separated from other ophthalmic patients in the ward, especially those who have had eye surgery. If surgery is performed on an infected eye the operation must be scheduled last on the operating list and the theatre cleaned thoroughly afterwards.

Hands of the Examiner and Patient

Eye infection can be spread through simple social greeting of patients, i.e. shaking of hands. Patients often rub their eyes and contaminated hands may transfer the organism to the examiner. It is important that hands are washed immediately before performing an eye examination and after the patient has left before greeting another patient.

Slit Lamp Biomicroscopy

The areas which come into contact with the patient must be washed with soap solution between patient examinations—chin rest, head rim, not forgetting the hand grips!

Tonometer Prisms

These should be wiped after use on disposable paper tissue and then placed (tip only) in a small pot of sodium hypochlorite 1% for at least 10 minutes between patients.
(NOTE: The prism must be rinsed in sterile water and dried before use). If there is suspected adenoviral infection the soaking must be extended to 30 minutes before re-using the same tonometer prism. A fresh sterile pot and new solution of sodium hypochlorite must be provided for every clinic session.

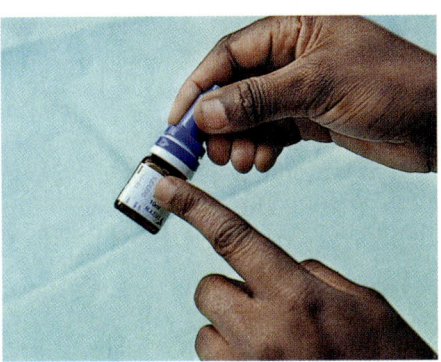

Fig. 10.3: Check the expiry dates

Occluder and Pinhole
This should be stored in a container of sodium hypochlorite 1% for at least 10 minutes between patients, rinsed in sterile water or saline and wiped dry before use. A fresh solution must be provided before each clinic session.
NB: Sodium hypochlorite causes corrosion—do not use stainless steel containers for the above.

Eye Drops
Ideally, each patient should have his or her own bottle of drops and, where there is known infection, separate bottles for each eye. However, in many situations this may be economically impossible. Care should therefore be taken to avoid eye dropper contact with eyelids, lashes, eyebrows and facial skin. Where possible a single-use dispenser should be used in out-patient examinations. Expiry dates must be checked, as out-of-date drops can be a source of infection (Fig. 10.3).

Pathological Specimens
Scrapings of the cornea and conjunctiva may be taken using a disposable sterile surgical needle or blade. If a spatula or loop is used it must be sterilized before and after each procedure by flaming, and allowed to cool. Alternatively, it may be sterilized by chemical soaking.

Eye Dressings
An infected eye must never be covered with a pad and/or bandage. Used eye dressings must be disposed of immediately and burned. Eye shields must be washed before being re-applied and, in known infected cases, must not be used on other patients. Cotton wool, gauze swabs or tissues, used when instilling drops or ointment, must be disposed of immediately.

Spectacles
Spectacles wearers should be encouraged to wash their spectacles daily.

POLICY

Eye infesction can happen anywhere as eyes are particularly susceptible to many organisms including gram-negative bacilli, adenoviruses, herpes simplex virus and fungi.

Cross-infection is a costly and continuing concern. Multi-resistant *Staphylococcus aureus* (MRSA) has made alarming news worldwide as treatment is very difficult. Lives, as well as sight, have tragically been lost.

Health workers must aim to limit hospital-acquired infection. Lack of motivation and poor microbiological knowledge will result in non-compliance. Eye staff is advised to develop and teach an appropriate infection control policy with regular reinforcement and review. Preoperative, intraoperative and postoperative precautions are shown in Table 10.3 and Table 10.4, respectively.

TABLE 10.3: Showing preoperative measures

1. Preoperative antibiotic drops for 24 hours
2. Bath for patients/headwash/facewash
3. Special note of eyebrow, medial canthus area and nasal area
4. Eyebrow to be washed with BSS and Betadine 5%
5. Keratomes, blades, needles not be reused unless sterilization process undertaken
6. Intraocular instruments as canulas not to be reused if possible unless properly sterilized—disposables should be used
7. All doctors and staff (medical and paramedical) should receive a formal training on Biomedical Waste Management
8. OT to be washed/and scrubbed before use, surfaces should be carbolized
9. A drop of Betadine should be instilled before starting the surgery

TABLE 10.4: Showing intraoperative measures

1. A drop of Betadine before starting the surgery
2. Minimal handling of tissues
3. Instruments used for extraocular manipulation not to be used inside the eye
4. No wick left into the anterior chamber-uvea/capsule/vitreous and complete removal and formation of anterior chamber with irrigation fluid/air
5. No foreign material to be left in the surgical area

Besides preoperative and intraoperative measures, postoperative precations are equally or rather more important. They are mentioned in Table 10.5.

TABLE 10.5: Postoperative measures

1. Subconjunctival antibiotics, single drop of Betadine in the conjunctival sac after completion of the surgery
2. Systemic antibiotics only if adnexal infections present
3. Topical antibiotics to be given after the post operatively with steroidal/nonsteroidal agents
4. Personal hygiene to be emphasized
5. Avoid dust, smoke and sunlight
6. Wear protective dark glasses outdoors
7. Routine weekly or if necessary more frequent postoperative visits to be ensured
8. Frequent instillation of eye drops to be ensured
9. Dilatation drops once weekly to keep pupil mobile

Tips for Preventing Endophthalmitis[39-41]
- Instill povidone-iodine 5% eye drops prior to surgery
- Carefully drape the eyelid and lashes prior to surgery
- Use sterile gloves, gowns, and face masks
- Construct watertight incisions, preferably three-plane
- Manage complications (e.g., capsular rupture) effectively
- Acrylic IOLs are better than silicone
- Inject intracameral cefuroxime postoperatively (1 mg in 0.1 mL normal saline).

Protocol for Treating Endophthalmitis
- Admit the patient, stop antibiotics, and prepare for theater
- Perform a vitreous tap with or without capsulectomy
- Give an intravitreal injection (Table 10.6) of vancomycin 2 mg and cefuroxime (or ceftazidime) 2 mg (or 0.5 mg amikacin if the patient is allergic to penicillin)
- Give a subconjunctival injection of vancomycin 50 mg and cefuroxime (or ceftazidime) 125 mg (or amikacin 50 mg if the patient is allergic to penicillin)
- Send the vitreous sample for microscopy and culture
- Monitor the pain experienced by the patient. A reduction in pain suggests bactericidal effect
- Start instilling vancomycin 5% and ceftazidime 5% eye drops hourly
- If you cannot see the posterior segment, do an ultrasound B-scan
- If there is no improvement within 24 hours, consider repeating the vitreous sample and the antibiotic injections
- Consider topical or systemic steroids if you are confident the infection is under control (i.e. pain is diminishing, fibrin is contracting, hypopyon is decreasing).

TABLE 10.6: Types of endophthalmitis, common pathogens, and treatment[35-37]

Type	Most common pathogens	Intial intravitreal treatment[a]	Vitrectomy necessary[c]	Need to remove artificial intraocular lens?	Initial systemic antibiotics[b]
Acute post-cataract	Coagulase-negative staphylococci (70% of cases), other gram-positive cocci (25%)	Intravitreal vancomycin plus ceftazidime	Yes, if severe infection or fungal etiology	No, unless fungal etiology	Value unknown, rarely given
Chronic Post-cataract	*Propionibacterium acnes*	Intravitreal vancomycin	Varies	Yes	No
Post-injection	Coagulase-negative staphylococci, viridans streptococci	Intravitreal vancomycin plus ceftazidime	Yes, if severe infection	No	Moxifloxacin or similar?

Contd...

Contd...

Bleb-related	Streptococci, Haemophilus influenzae	Intravitreal vancomycin plus ceftazidime	Most cases	No	Moxifloxacin or similar?
Post-traumatic	Bacillus cereus, coagulase-negative staphylococci (fungi in some cases)	Intravitreal vancomycin plus ceftazidime (plus amphotericin if fungi suspected)	Most cases	Varies (always if fungal)	Intravenous vancomycin plus either ceftazidime or ciprofloxacin
Endogenous bacterial	Staphylococcus aureus, streptococci, gram-negative bacilli (e.g. Klebsiella)	Intravitreal vancomycin plus ceftazidime (or amikacin)	Yes, nearly all cases	No	Intravenous antibiotics tailored to systemic infection
Candida	Candida species	Intravitreal amphotericin (or voriconazole)	Yes, if vitritis	Often	Yes
Mould	Aspergillus, Fusarium	Intravitreal amphotericin	Yes	Yes	Yes

Note: Vancomycin and cefuroxime (or ceftazidime) must not be mixed in the same syringe—draw up in separate syringes.

- Taper the treatment according to the patient's response and culture results.
- Keep the patient informed of progress.
- Intravitreal antibiotics are given at the end of a vitrectomy in the operating room, or as an office procedure without a vitrectomy. Whereas initial therapy is empirical, subsequent injections may be tailored to culture results.
- Systemic antibiotics alone are not effective in treating endophthalmitis.
- *Candida chorioretinitis* endogenous endophthalmitis is treated with systemic antifungal as well as intravitreal amphotericin or voricanazole.

REFERENCES

1. Seewoodhary M. Effectiveness of sodium hypochlorite solution as a disinfectant in ophthalmic practice. Ophthalmic Nursing. 1998;2(3):4-12.
2. Ayliffe G. Infection control, nosocomial infection, problems and organisation. Africa Health. 1996;18:9-10.
3. Mamalis N, Kearsley L, Brinton E. Postoperative endophthalmitis. Curr Opin Ophthalmol. 2002;13:14-18.
4. Buzard K, Liapis S. Prevention of endophthalmitis. J Cataract Refract Surg. 2004;30:1953-9.
5. Eifrig CWG, Scott IU, Flynn HW, Jr, Miller D. Endophthalmitis caused by *Pseudomonas aeruginosa*. Ophthalmology. 2003;110:1714-7.
6. Tyhurst KN, Hettler DL. Infection control guidelines—an update for the optometric practice. Optometry. 2009;80(11):613-20.
7. Jaffe NS. History of cataract surgery. Ophthalmology. 1996;103S5-16.

8. Olson RJ, Mamalis N, Werner L, Apple DJ. Cataract treatment in the beginning of the 21st Century. Am J Ophthalmol. 2003;136:146-54.
9. Leaming DV. Practice styles and preferences of ASCRS members—2003 survey. J Cataract Refract Surg. 2004;30:892-900.
10. Oshika T, Amano S, Araie M, Majima Y, Leaming DV. Current trends in cataract and refractive surgery in Japan: 1999 survey. Jpn J Ophthalmol. 2001;45:383-7.
11. Kirby DB. Surgery of Cataract. Philadelphia, Pa JB Lippincott Co.1950;3-24.
12. Fine IH. Clear corneal incisions. Int Ophthalmol Clin. 1994;3459-72.
13. O'h Eineachain R. ESCRS survey shows acrylic IOLs and LASIK now dominant features of European ophthalmic practice. Eye World. 2001;626.
14. Hidalgo-Simon. A Changing trends in cataract/refractive surgery reflected in new French survey. Eye World. 2001;622-23.
15. Axenfeld T. *The* Bacteriology of the Eye. London, England Bailliere Tindall and Cox.1908;77-107.
16. Abel R Jr, Binder PS, Bellows R. Postoperative bacterial endophthalmitis: section I. Ann Ophthalmol. 1976;8:731-44.
17. Starr MB. Prophylactic antibiotics for ophthalmic surgery. Surv Ophthalmol. 1983;27:353-73.
18. Javitt JC, Vitale S, Canner JK, et al. National outcomes of cataract extraction: endophthalmitis following inpatient surgery. Arch Ophthalmol. 1991;109:1085-9.
19. Callahan A. Effect of sulfonamides and antibiotics on panophthalmitis complicating cataract extraction. Arch Ophthalmol. 1953;49:212-9.
20. Powe NR, Schein OD, Gieser SC, et al. Synthesis of the literature on visual acuity and complications following cataract extraction with intraocular lens implantation: Cataract Patient Outcome Research Team. Arch Ophthalmol. 1994;112:239-52.
21. Colleaux KM, Hamilton WK. Effect of prophylactic antibiotics and incision type on the incidence of endophthalmitis after cataract surgery. Can J Ophthalmol. 2000;35:373-8.
22. Barrow D, McDermott M, Elliot D, Frank R. Acute postoperative endophthalmitis and modern cataract surgery technique [ARVO abstract 1340]. Invest Ophthalmol Vis Sci. 2001;42:S24.
23. Cooper BA, Holekamp NM, Bohigian G, Thompson PA. Case-control study of endophthalmitis after cataract surgery comparing scleral tunnel and clear corneal wounds. Am J Ophthalmol. 2003;136:300-5.
24. Lertsumitkul S, Myers PC, O'Rourke MT, Chandra J. Endophthalmitis in the western Sydney region: a case-control study. Clin Experiment Ophthalmol. 2001;29:400-5.
25. McDonnell PJ, Donnenfeld ED, Perry HD, et al. New horizons in fluoroquinolone therapy. Ophthalmol Times. 2002;27(suppl 1)1-15.
26. Nagaki Y, Hayasaka S, Kadoi C, et al. Bacterial endophthalmitis after small-incision cataract surgery: effect of incision placement and intraocular lens type. J Cataract Refract Surg. 2003;29:20-26.
27. Niyadurupola N, Astbury N. Endophthalmitis: controlling infection before and after cataract surgery. Community Eye Health. 2008;21(65):9-10.
28. Alshihry AM. Epidemiology of Postoperative Endophthalmitis (POE) in a Specialized Eye Hospital. Epidemiology. 2014;4:145.
29. Busin M, Cusumano A, Spitznas M. Intraocular lens removal from eyes with chronic low-grade endophthalmitis. J Cataract Refract Surg. 1995;21:679-84.
30. Allen G. Gentamicin-loaded sponges; multimodal rehabilitation; nocardial endophthalmitis; acute-onset endophthalmitis. AORN. 2005;5:863-7.
31. Forster RK, Abbott RL, Gelender H. Management of infectious endophthalmitis. Opthalmology. 1980;87:313-9.

32. Lalitha P, Rajagopalan J, Prakash K, Ramasamy K, Prajna NV, Srinivasan M. Post-cataract endophthalmitis in South India Incidence and Outcome. Ophthalmology. 2005;112:1884-9.
33. Das T, Kunimoto DY, Sharma S, Jalali S, Majji AB, Nagaraja Rao T, et al. Relationship between clinical presentation and visual outcome in postoperative and post-traumatic endophthalmitis in South Central India. Indian J Opthalmol. 2005;53: 5-16.
34. Durand ML. Endophthalmitis. Clin Microbiol Infect. 2013;19(3):227-34. doi: 10.1111/1469-0691.12118.
35. Subhedar V, Bharihoke N, Singh P, Gupta P, Jain SK, Chaturvedi K. Microbial endopthalmitis: Incidence spectrum and antibiotic sensitivity pattern of bacterial isolates. J of Evidence Based Med and Health care. 2014;1(12):1534-41.
36. Endophthalmitis Vitrectomy Study Group. Microbiologic factors and visual outcome in the endophthalmitis vitrectomy study. Am J Ophthalmol. 1996;122(6):830-46.
37. Gibb AP, Fleck BW, Kempton-Smith L. A cluster of deep bacterial infections following eye surgery associated with construction dust. J Hosp Infect. 2006;63(2):197-200.
38. Cruciani M, Malena M, Amalfitano G, et al. Molecular epidemiology in a cluster of cases of postoperative *Pseudomonas aeruginosa* endophthalmitis. Clin Infect Dis. 1998;26(2):330-3.
39. Cox I, Stevens S. Ophthalmic Operating Theatre Practice: A Manual for Developing Countries, London: International Centre for Eye Health, 2002.
40. Guidelines for Preoperative, Operative and Postoperative precautions for eye surgery. National Programme for Control of Blindness. Directorate of Health Services Ministry of Health Family Welfare Governement of India in Collaboration with WHO under National Rural health mission. 2009.
41. Fintelmann RE, Naseri A. "Prophylaxis of postoperative endophthalmitis following cataract surgery: current status and future directions," Drugs. 2010;70(11):1395-1409.

Chapter 11

Diabetic Macular Edema

Neha Mohan, Chetan Videkar, Umesh C Behera, Krushna Gopal Panda, TP Das

INTRODUCTION

Diabetic macular edema (DME) is one of the leading causes of visual impairment in the working age population affected by diabetic retinopathy (DR). The 10-year rate of developing macular edema is reported to vary from 14–25% depending on the type of diabetes and the dependence on insulin (The Wisconsin Epidemiologic Study of Diabetic Retinopathy-WESDR).[1] Diabetic retinopathy occurs in 1 in 3 diabetics and DME develops in 1 in 13 diabetics.[2] The relative risk for DME is 6.2 times greater in patients with very severe non-proliferative diabetic retinopathy (NPDR) and 7.7 times greater in patients with proliferative diabetic retinopathy (PDR).[3] With an increasing prevalence of diabetes suspected to reach epidemic proportions in India in the coming years, blindness secondary to DME is poised as a major cause of preventable blindness.[4]

The Early Treatment Diabetic Retinopathy Study (ETDRS) defined macular edema as thickening of the retina and/or hard exudates within 1 disc diameter of the center of the macula while clinically significant macular edema (CSME) was defined as 1 or more of the following (Figs 11.1 A to C):
1. Retinal thickening at or within 500 μm of the center of the macula
2. Hard exudates at or within 500 μm of the center of the macula if associated with adjacent retinal thickening.
3. Zone or zones of retinal thickening 1 disc area in size, at least part of which is within 1 disc diameter of the center of the macula.[3]

RISK FACTORS

Besides chronic hyperglycemia and duration of diabetes, hypertension, nephropathy and hyperlipidemia are major factors that contribute to macular edema.

PATHOGENESIS

Elevated glucose levels lead to osmotic damage to vascular cells due to increased concentration of intracellular sorbitol through aldose reductase pathway.[5] Binding of aldoses to protein side chains on free amine [NH(2)] groups, during the Maillard reaction result in formation of subfunctional and non-functional products, referred to as advanced glycation end-products (AGEs) and reactive oxygen species (ROS).[6] Binding of AGEs to their receptors (RAGE) activates monocytes and endothelial cells, resulting in release of cytokines, adhesion

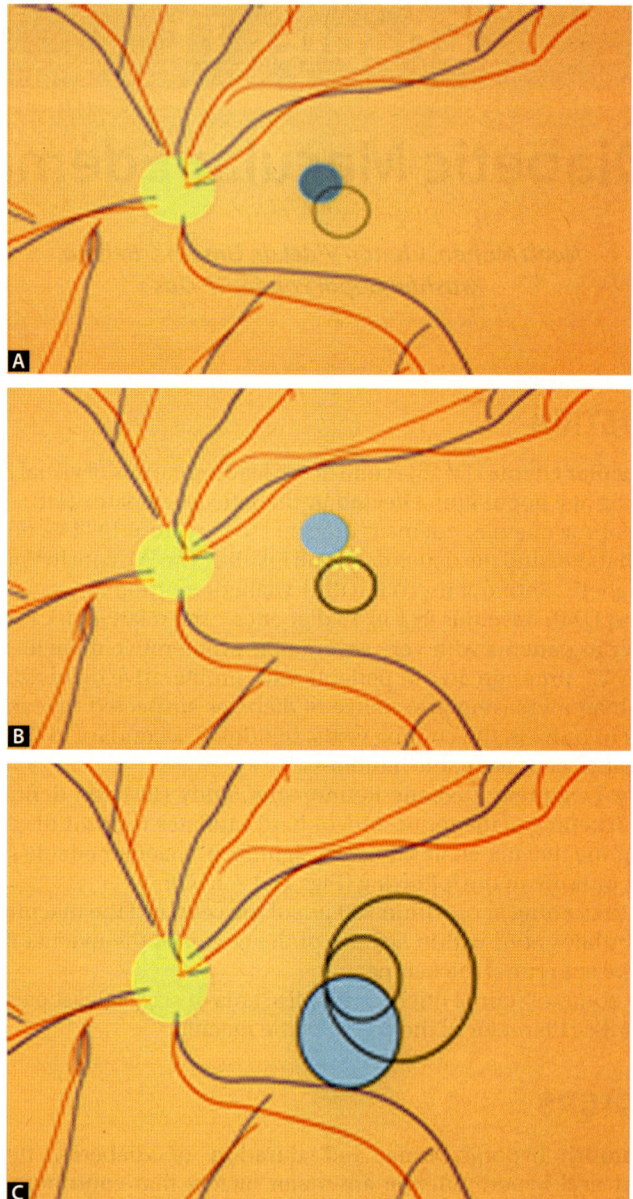

Figs 11.1A to C: Diagrammatic illustration of DME by ETDRS. (*With permission from:* Das T, Rani A (eds). Diabetic Eye Disease. Jaypee Brothers. 2006).

molecules and tissue factors. Enhanced generation of diacylglycerol, causes physiologic activation of protein kinase C (PKC) pathway. PKC causes numerous cellular changes including increased expression of matrix proteins, such as collagen and fibronectin resulting in thickening of basement membrane. PKC also causes increased expression of vasoactive mediators like endothelin which causes loss of pericytes and alters the vascular permeability (Fig. 11.2).

There are many isoforms of PKC but studies suggest that PKC β_2 is preferentially activated in the causation of diabetic retinopathy.[7]

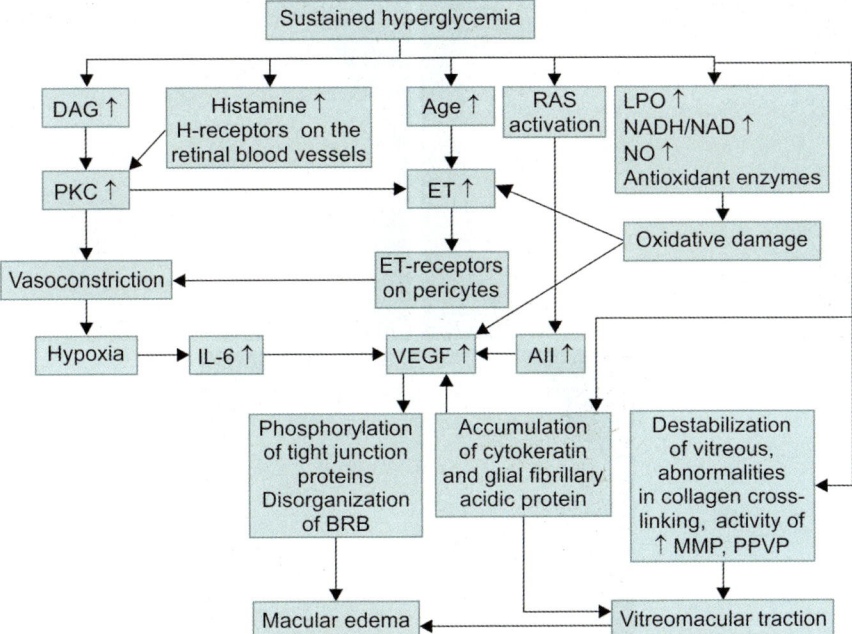

Fig. 11.2: Pathogenesis of diabetic macular edema. AII- angiotensin II: AGE, advanced glycation end products
Abbreviations: DAG, diacylglycerol; ET, endothelin; LPO, lypoxygenase; NO, nitric oxide, PKC, protein kinase C; RAS, rennin angiotensin system; VEGF, vascular endothelial growth factor.[9]

Vascular endothelial growth factor (VEGF) is a potent cytokine that causes angiogenesis and induces changes in the structure of tight junctions. The breakdown of BRB leads to accumulation of plasma proteins such as albumin, which exerts high oncotic pressure in the neural interstitium, leading to interstitial edema.

Vitreoretinal interface also plays an important role in the pathogenesis of DME. A diabetic retina compromised due to microvascular abnormalities may be vulnerable to increased exudation in presence of macular traction. The accumulated AGEs lead to increased cross linkage of collagen fibrils along with structural alteration of posterior hyaloid, that lead to vitreomacular adhesion. The hyaloid often gets infiltrated and thickened with glial and inflammatory cells. Cellular contraction of hyalocytes is enhanced by PKC pathways leading to taut thickened posterior hyaloid that exerts anteroposterior and horizontal traction on fovea. Fibrovascular proliferation on disc or along the arcades also leads to traction on fovea at times. Besides, the preretinal space or the vitreous act as a reservoir for all inflammatory mediators. This explains how even in absence of taut hyaloid or ERM, vitrectomy alone improves DME.[8,9]

More recently, use of troglitazone, a thiazolidinediones (TZDs), has been associated with worsening of macular edema.

CLASSIFICATION

International Clinical Diabetic Retinopathy Disease Severity Scale[10] has classified diabetic retinopathy into five stages: (1) No apparent retinopathy;

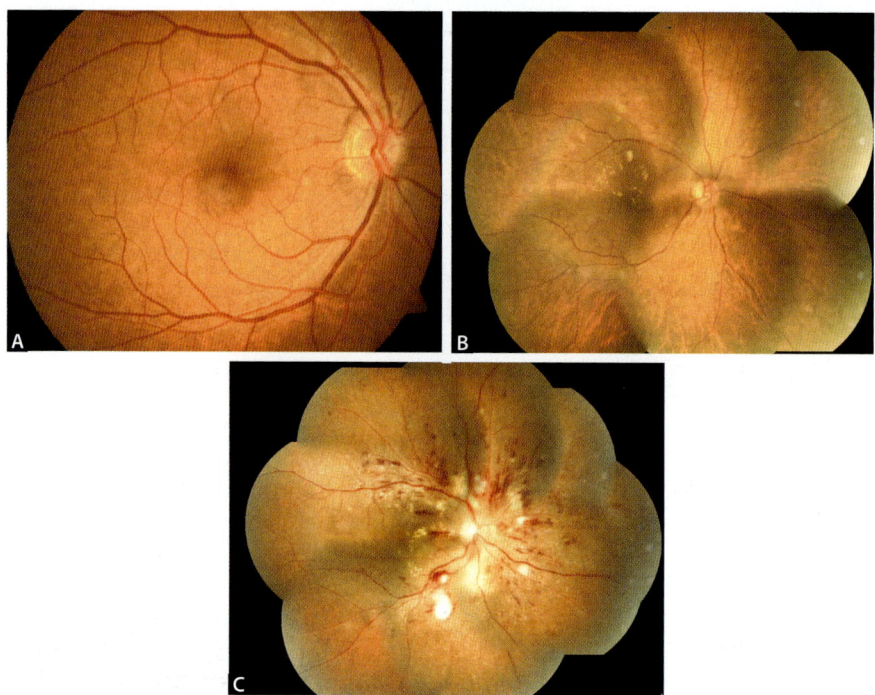

Figs 11.3A to C: (A) Colored fundus photograph showing few microaneurysms suggestive of mild non-proliferative diabetic retinopathy (NPDR); (B) Colored fundus montage showing moderate NPDR with hemorrhages and exudates and (C) Severe NPDR with hemorrhages, hard exudates and macular edema

(2) Mild non-proliferative diabetic retinopathy (NPDR); (3) Moderate NPDR; (4) Severe NPDR and (5) Proliferative diabetic retinopathy (PDR). (Figs 11.3A to C).

Mild NPDR is characterized by presence of a few microaneurysms. Moderate NPDR is characterized by presence of more than just microaneurysms but less than severe NPDR. It also includes the presence of cotton wool spots, hemorrhages and hard exudates. Severe NPDR also known as pre-PDR, is characterized by presence of one or more of the following, in the absence of PDR—the 4:2:1 rule.
- More than 20 intraretinal hemorrhages in each of 4 quadrants
- Definite venous beading in at least 2 quadrants
- Prominent intraretinal microvascular abnormality (IRMA) in at least 1 quadrant

The ETDRS data has shown that the type 2 DM patients with severe NPDR have a 50% probability of developing high-risk characteristics if laser treatment is not instituted.

Clinical Classification of Diabetic Macular Edema

Clinically, the DME is could be classified as—mild, moderate and severe DME.

Mild DME is characterized by some retinal thickening or hard exudates in the posterior pole, distant from the center of the macula; moderate DME is characterized by retinal thickening or hard exudates near the center of the macula but not involving the center, and the severe DME is characterized by retinal thickening or hard exudates involving the center of the macula (Figs 11.4A to C).

Diabetic Macular Edema

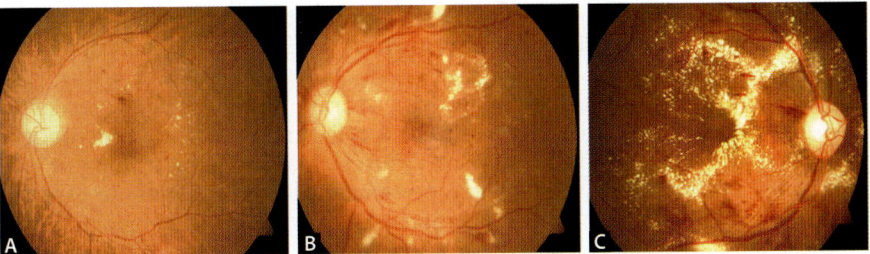

Figs 11.4A to C: Colored fundus photographs showing diabetic macular edema; (A) Mild (hard exudates in posterior pole, but distant from macula); (B) Moderate (hard exudates in macula, center not involved) and (C) Severe (hard exudates and retinal thickening involving macula center)

Pathological Classification of Diabetic Macular Edema

- **Retinovascular**: The pathology is primarily in the vascular system. Depending on whether it is perfused or ischemic it is further divided into:
  - **Focal macular edema** is centred around few microaneurysms that leak on fundus fluorescein angiography (FFA). A ring of hard exudates may be seen surrounding it partly or in a circinate pattern. (Figs 11.5A to D).
  - **Diffuse macular edema** is due to breakdown of blood retinal barrier; in this situation arterioles and retinal capillaries leak besides the microaneurysms. FFA shows leakage from diffusely dilated capillary bed with

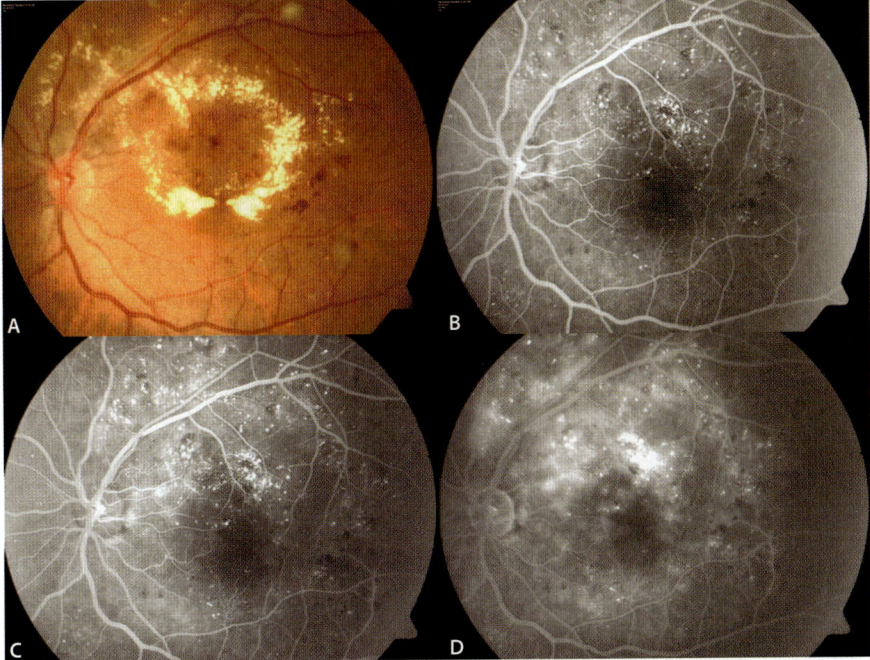

Figs 11.5A to D: Focal macular edema. (A) Color fundus photograph showing a ring of hard exudates surrounding microaneurysms; (B) FFA shows multiple microaneurysms in early phase; (C) that leak profusely in mid; and (D) late phases of angiogram

widened intercapillary spaces that corresponds histologically to dilated hypercellular capillaries and numerous acellular occluded capillaries. (Fig. 11.6A to C).
- **Macular ischemia**: Some amount of ischemia is usually present in edematous diabetic macula either focally in relation to a microaneurysm/ a cotton wool spot or more diffusely. Macular ischemia may or may not be associated with edema; presence of ischemia points to guarded visual prognosis. It could be demonstrated on fluorescein angiography as enlarged foveal avascular zone (FAZ), irregular FAZ margin, widened intercapillary space and baring of the precapillary arterioles. (Figs 11.7A and B).

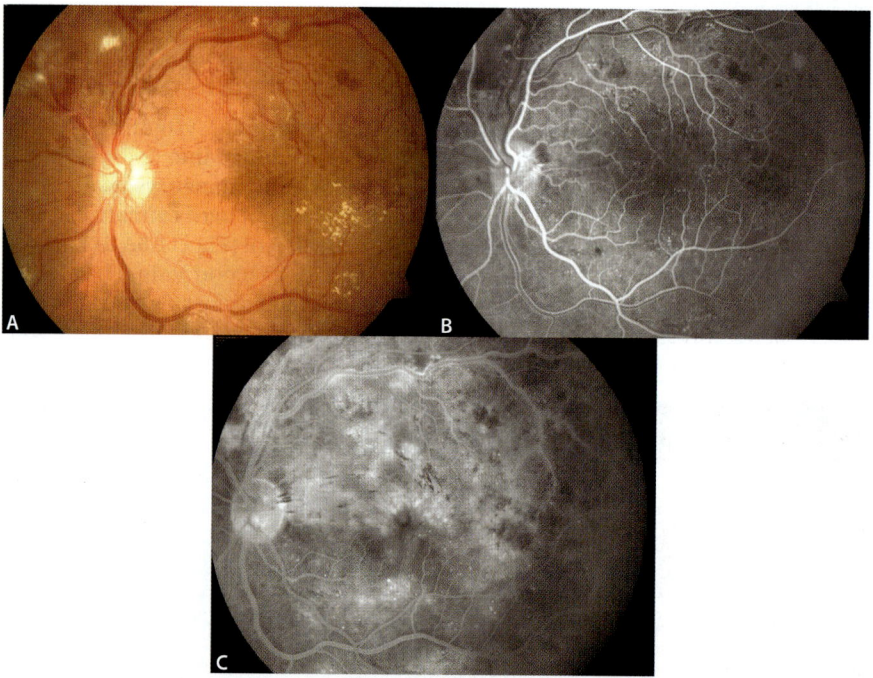

Figs 11.6A to C: Diffuse diabetic macular edema. (A) Color fundus photo showing diabetic macular edema; (B) FFA shows microaneurysms in early phase; and (C) diffuse leakage from capillary bed leading to cystoid edema

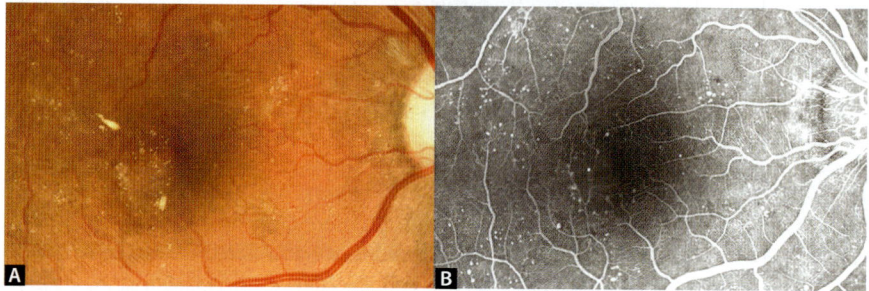

Figs 11.7A and B: Macular ischemia. Color fundus photograph showing (A) diabetic macular edema; (B) FFA shows enlarged, broken foveal avascular zone suggestive of ischemic maculopathy

- **Taut attached posterior hyaloid:** The role of vitreomacular interface contributing to macular edema is now well-established. It has been postulated that the tangential traction by the attached posterior hyaloid leads to macular edema. Hence, posterior vitreous detachment spontaneously, pharmacologically (with plasmin), or surgically (by vitrectomy) has been shown to improve DME.[11-13]
- **Tractional:** Evident traction on macula by a vitreous strand or a fibrovascular proliferation leads to macular edema. OCT demonstrates the traction well, and FFA may show late leakage.

SYMPTOMS AND SIGNS

Reduction of vision is the most common symptom in patients with CSME. Metamorphopsia is not uncommon and may be a significant feature. One may not complain reduction of vision in unilateral CSME. The diagnosis of CSME is basically clinical, done by slit lamp biomicroscopy (with 90D/78D lens) and stereo fundus photography. Further confirmation is made with FFA and OCT. With the increasing indications to treat DME with anti-VEFGs, it is imperative to scan all diabetic macular edemas by OCT to document or rule out the involvement of macular center.

Fundus fluorescein angiography (FFA): It qualifies diabetic macular edema. Its role in DME is to identify areas of increased vasopermeability, like leaking microaneurysms or decompensated capillary beds and to evaluate retinal ischemia. However, leakage on FFA is not synonymous with edema or thickening because extracellular fluid is accumulated only when ingress of fluid exceeds the egress by the retinal pigment epithelium (RPE pump. Based on leakage pattern on FFA, the DME is categorized into three different groups:[14] focal leak, diffuse leak, and cystoid leak (Table 11.1).

TABLE 11.1: Role of fundus fluorescein angiography in DME

Situation	Usually	Occasionally	Never
• Guide laser treatment of CSME	✓		
• Evaluate unexplained visual loss	✓		
• Rule out other causes of macular swelling		✓	
• Evaluate patients with questionable DME		✓	
• Screen a patient with no/minimal DR			✓
• Monitor treatment outcome			

Optical coherence tomography (OCT): It quantifies macular edema. Clinically, accurate detection of macular edema less than 300 µ is difficult.[15] Four types of macular edema have been described on OCT:
- Diffuse retinal thickening (spongiform edema),
- Cystoid macular edema,
- Neurosensory detachment, and
- Vitreomacular traction. (Figs 11.8A to C).

OCT is an indispensable tool in the management of patients with DME though it cannot replace traditional FFA. Both FFA and OCT are complementary in diagnosis and management of DME. The FFA qualifies and OCT quantifies the macular edema. Because the OCT is noninvasive, it is often used to monitor the treatment outcome (Table 11.2).[16]

TABLE 11.2: Role of optical coherence tomography in DME

Situation	Usually	Occasionally	Never
• Evaluate unexplained vision loss	✓		
• Identify extent and type of macular edema	✓		
• Identify areas of vitreo macular traction	✓		
• Evaluate patients with questionable DME		✓	
• Monitor treatment outcome	✓		

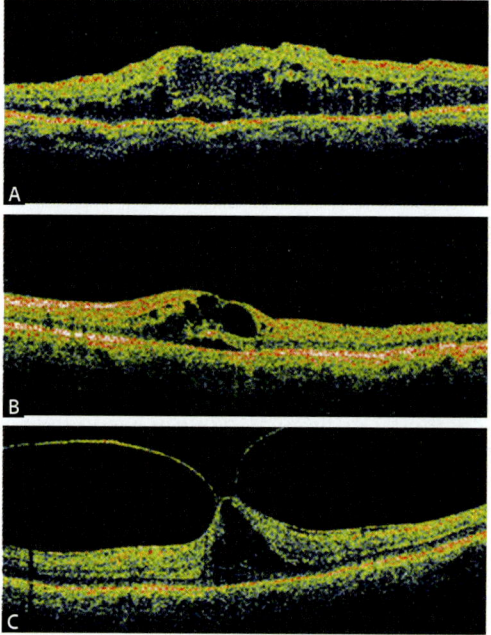

Figs 11.8A to C: Types of macular edema in OCT. (A) Spongiform retinal edema; (B) Cystoid macular edema with serous retinal detachment; and (C) Tractional macular edema

OCT angiography (OCT-A) is a noninvasive diagnostic method, and its reliability makes it an interesting potential diagnostic tool for disease detection and follow-up in retinal pathologies involving foveal microcirculation.

Microperimetry: The visual change may not always be parallel with macular thickness change following treatment, meaning the macular thickness may decrease but vision may not increase correspondingly and vice versa. Visual acuity though is considered the gold standard, does not entirely reflect functional vision. Microperimetry gives a functional assessment and fundus-related quantification of retinal sensitivity. It helps to follow patients on treatment and prognosticate the disease (Figs 11.9A and B).

TREATMENT

Diabetic macular edema can be the most challenging clinical scenario to treat at times. It must be understood that DME is a consequence of diabetes mellitus and the associated diseases. Hence, for DME treatment to be successful, a

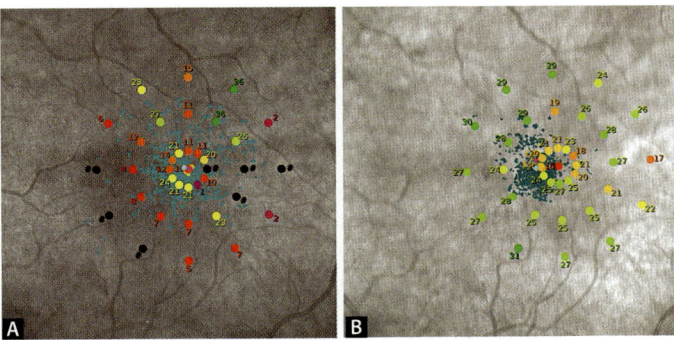

Figs 11.9A and B: Microperimetry in a 62- year type 2 diabetic with left eye macular edema—before (A) and after (B) intravitreal bevacizumab treatment. Sensitivity improved after treatment (black in left panel to green in right panel). Visual acuity improved from 20/50 to 20/40. (*Courtesy:* Jay Chablani, MD)

comprehensive treatment of diabetes and the allied diseases like hypertension, nephropathy, hyperlipidemia and anemia is essential. The systemic investigations include tests for anemia (Hb), blood sugar (HbA1c, fasting and postprandial) renal profile (24 hours urine albumin, serum urea, serum creatinine), serum lipid (low and high density lipid) and blood pressure. A number of studies such as the Diabetes Complication and Control Trial (DCCT), Action to Control Cardiovascular Risk in Diabetes (ACCORD), United Kingdom Prospective Diabetes Study (UKPDS), and Epidemiology of Diabetes Intervention and Complications (EDIC) have reported the importance of systemic control for effective treatment of DME (Table 11.3).

TABLE 11.3: Major studies on impact of systemic control in DME management

Study	Design	Systemic control	Impact on DR care
DCCT[17] (1983–1993) n = 1441, type 1 DM	Standard vs intensive control of blood glucose	HbA1C around 6%	• 76% reduced risk for developing DR • 50% reduction in kidney disease • 60% reduction in nerve disease • 54% reduced DR progression
EDIC[20]	90% of DCCT patients after 1993		• 42% reduced risk of any cardio-vascular disease (CVD) event • 57% reduced risk of nonfatal heart attack, stroke, or death from CVD
ACCORD[21] 1999–2009 ACCORD-Eye (n = 4,065)	Intensive glycemia control, intensive BP control and multiple lipid management	HbA1C <6 Systolic BP<120 mm Hg Fenofibrate to all and open label simvastatin	DR rate decreased with intensive glycemic and lipid control but not intensive BP control
UKPDS[18] 1981–1998 n = 3867 type 2 DM	Tight diastolic BP control v/s less tight BP control	Tight control BP <150/85 mm Hg; less tight control BP <185/105 mm Hg	• 37% reduced microvascular complications • 35% reduced need for retinal photocoagulation

Systemic Factors

Glycemic Control

The DCCT in Type 1 DM[17] and the UKPDS trial in Type 2 DM[18] demonstrated that a good glycemic control (intensive control) reduced the development and progression of diabetic retinopathy. However, intensive therapy seemed to apparently increase the progression of retinopathy probably because of drastic and rapid reduction of glucose and alteration of retinal perfusion or by increased intravascular coagulation or aggregation of platelets.[19] Hence, it is suggested that in patients with bad glycemic control, the therapy should be targeted to achieve a more gradual control. Severe hypoglycemic episodes however, remain a limitation of intensive glycemic control.

Blood Pressure Control

The WESDR study reported an association of higher blood pressure, especially diastolic, with the progression of retinopathy.[1] UKPDS found that a tight blood pressure control with angiotensin converting enzyme (ACE) inhibitors or with β-blockers caused 34% reduction in progression of retinopathy and 47% reduction in deterioration of visual acuity by 3 lines.[18]

Lipid Control

Elevated serum cholesterol has been shown to be associated with higher incidence of hard exudates in DME.[1,3] Poor visual outcomes are often related to increased accumulation of hard exudates, either due to subfoveal deposition or associated subretinal fibrosis. Atrovastatin and Fenofibate are the two main drugs advised to control lipid.

Once the metabolic parameters are well under control, treatment options include pharmacologic therapy, retinal laser and vitreoretinal surgery.

Therapy

Oral Medication

Antioxidants directed against the reactive oxygen species, and high doses of Vitamin E, have been reported to reverse microvascular abnormalities.[22] Other antioxidants such as berry extracts and Gingko biloba leaf extract (vasoprotector) have been studied for their effect on diabetic retinopathy.[23] PKC inhibitors such as Ruboxistaurin has not shown any promising results.[24,25] Aminoguanidine, an AGE inhibitor reduces the progression of retinopathy but has been associated with increase in anemia.[26]

Laser Therapy

Conventional focal laser (direct/grid) has been the gold standard treatment for DME (Figs 11.10A and B). ETDRS reported that at 3 years, treatment with focal laser reduced the risk of moderate visual loss (15 letters) by approximately 50% (from 24% to 12%) in eyes with CSME while visual acuity improved in only 3%.[27] Laser photocoagulation was prescribed for all cases with edema within two disc diameters of macular center. Initially treatment was not planned closer to 500 μm from center but if vision was less than 20/40 and if retinal edema and leakage persisted, treatment of lesions up to 300 μm was recommended. The various mechanisms proposed by which laser seems to act are (Table 11.4):

Diabetic Macular Edema

TABLE 11.4: Recommended laser techniques in CSME

Wavelength 532 nm	Spot (μm)	Duration (msec)	Power (mW)	Intensity	Number	Location
Focal	50–100	50–100	50–100	Whiten or darken MA	To all leaking MA	500 μm away from fovea
Grid	50–200	50–100	50–100	Faint white burns 1.5 to 2 burns apart	Area of diffuse DME	500 μm away from fovea

Abbreviations: DME: diabetic macular edema; MA: microaneurysm (*Modified from:* Das T, Rani A (eds). Diabetic Eye Disease. Jaypee Brothers. 2006)

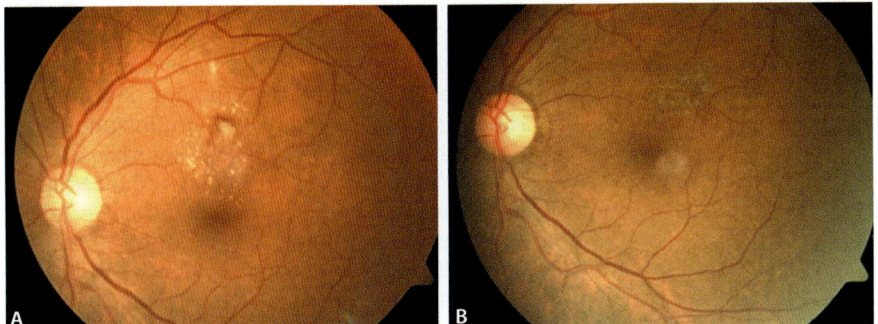

Figs 11.10A and B: Laser treatment in DME—before (A) and after (B) laser. Following laser there was complete disappearance of macular exudates. Vision improved from 20/25;N8 to 20/20;N6.

- Thrombosis of leaking microaneurysms, either directly by absorption of light by hemoglobin or indirectly by heat conducted by RPE.[28]
- Atrophy of RPE and outer retina and autoregulation leads to increased oxygenation of inner retina. This causes vessel constriction and lower intravascular pressure, which reduces edema formation.[29]
- Repair and restoration of blood retinal barrier as a result of enhanced proliferation of endothelial cells and RPE.[30]
- Release of antiangiogenic factors like pigment epithelial derived factors (PEDF) from RPE.[31]

Conventional laser therapy aims at a visible end point referred to as threshold lesion and has been reported to be associated with complications like paracentral scotomas, accidental foveal photocoagulation, choroidal neovascularization, juxtafoveal laser creep into the fovea and subfoveal fibrosis. A less visible clinical end point (subthreshold) was recommended and modified laser protocol was suggested to avoid these complications.[32] Two newer lasers, the subthreshold micropulse laser and selective retinal therapy laser are currently explored with promising results.

Subthreshold micropulse laser energy is delivered via short repetitive pulses (each is typically 100–300 ms) within an "envelope', the width of which is typically **0.1–0.15s.** A duty cycle needs to be set, which determines the frequencies of micropulse train. A 5% of duty cycle is considered safe in limiting the tissue damage[33] caused by heat conduction to RPE with minimal spread to choriocapillaris and inner neural retina. Many commercial micropulse lasers are available at wavelengths of 532 nm, 577 nm, 586 nm, 660 nm, and 810 nm.[34]

Selective retinal laser therapy (SRT) aims at selective damage of RPE that stimulates RPE cell migration and proliferation into the irradiated areas to improve metabolism at diseased sites.[35] A burst of microsecond laser pulses in green spectral range is applied, which is primarily absorbed by the melanosomes of RPE cells. Microvaporization around these intracellular melanosomes forms short-lived microbubbles that mechanically disrupt RPE cells. Since, there is clinically no end point to determine the dose adequacy, optoacoustic method and reflectometric methods are used for dosimetry.

Intravitreal Therapy

It is the current standard of care. Two kinds of molecules—anti-VEGF and corticosteroid are currently used, either alone or in combination with retinal laser.

- **Anti-VEGF therapy:** The available molecules include ranibizumab, aflibercept and bevacizumab. Pegaptanib sodium, an apatamer with specific binding affinity to VEGF 165 isoform is not in vogue. Both ranibizumab and aflibercept are FDA approved and are backed by robust clinical trials.
  - **Bevacizumab** *(Avastin, Genetech, San Francisco, CA)* is used for treating colorectal cancer and its use in eye is off-label. Its usual intravitreal dose is 1.25 mg in 0.05 mL. BOLT study[36] compared the use of bevacizumab (BVZ) for center involving DME to macular laser therapy (MLT) and found that at 2 years, mean ETDRS best corrected visual acuity (BCVA) was 64.4 (Snellen: 20/50) in the BVZ arm and 54.8 (Snellen: 20/80) in the MLT arm (p = .005). The median number of treatments over 24 months was 13 for BVZ and 4 for MLT.
  - **Ranibizumab** *(Lucentis, Genetech, San Francisco, CA)* is a recombinant humanized monoclonal antibody fragment specific for all isoforms of human VEGF-A and has been FDA approved for intravitreal injections. Its dose is 0.5 mg in 0.05 mL, although higher and lower doses have been used in various clinical trials.

  The RESTORE study showed that ranibizumab (RBZ) alone or in combination with laser was superior to laser alone in improving BCVA and causing reduction in the mean central macular thickness (-118.7 µm in RBZ group, -128.3 µm in RBZ+laser group and -61.3 µm in the laser alone group). Eyes originally receiving laser monotherapy for 12 months, then ranibizumab for 24 months achieved similar gains by 36 months to eyes receiving RBZ monotherapy for 36 months.[38] The DRCR.net Protocol I compared the relative efficacy of intravitreal ranibizumab with prompt or deferred laser treatment, the combination of intravitreal triamcinolone (IVTA) with prompt laser, and laser alone treatment. This study demonstrated that deferred focal/grid laser with intravitreal RBZ had a higher chance of relatively larger improvement in visual acuity through 5 years.[39] The RISE and RIDE trials randomized DME patients to 3 groups sham injection, 0.3 mg RBZ and 0.5 mg RBZ. At 24 months, 18.1% of the sham group of eyes gained ≥ 15 letters vs 44.8% of the 0.3 mg and 39.2% of the 0.5 mg treated eyes in the RISE study; it was 12.3% of sham group vs 33.6% of the 0.3 mg and 45.7% of the 0.5 mg RBZ patients in the RIDE study.[40] RBZ treated eyes received significantly fewer macular laser treatments.
  - **Aflibercept** *(VEGF Trap-Eye, Regeneron Pharmaceutical, Inc, Tarrytown, NY)* is a recombinant fusion protein consisting of VEGF-binding portions from the extracellular domains of human VEGF receptors 1 and 2, fused to the Fc portion of the human IgG1 immunoglobulin. As a result, it binds

the circulating VEGF and acts as a VEGF-trap. It inhibits VEGF-A, VEGF-B as well as placental growth factor (PGF). The DA VINCI study[41] compared different doses and dosing regimens of aflibercept with laser photocoagulation in patients with DME: aflibercept 0.5 or 2 mg every 4 weeks, 2 mg every 8 weeks, or 2 mg as needed after 3 initial monthly injections or macular laser treatment. At 52 weeks, the mean improvement ranged from 9.7 to 12 letters in the aflibercept groups and 1.3 for laser group. The mean reduction in central retinal thickness in the aflibercept groups ranged from 165.4 µm to 227.4 µm and it was 58.4 µm for the laser group. VISTA and VIVID study, compared two regimen of intravitreal aflibercept injection (IAI)—2 mg every 4 weeks (2q4); and 2 mg every 8 weeks after 5 initial monthly doses (2q8) with macular laser photocoagulation.[42] The mean vision gain from baseline to week 52 in the IAI 2q4 and IAI 2q8 groups versus the laser group were 12.5 and 10.7 versus 0.2 letters ($P < 0.0001$) in VISTA; and 10.5 and 10.7 versus 1.2 letters ($P < 0.0001$) in VIVID.

DRCR.net protocol T compared the relative efficacy and safety of aflibercept, bevacizumab and ranibizumab in DME. From baseline to 1 year, the mean visual-acuity improved by 13.3 letters with aflibercept, by 9.7 letters with bevacizumab, and by 11.2 letters with ranibizumab. The study showed that while both ranibizumab and aflibercept had a similar improvement when the vision was relatively good ($\geq 20/40$) at the start of the treatment, there was better improvement with aflibercept than ranibizumab when the presenting vision was worse ($\leq 20/50$). Vision improvement was less in bevacizumab in all situations.[43]

Table 11.5 summarizes selected randomized control trials (RCT) in DME.

- **Intravitreal steroids**
  - **Intravitreal injections** (triamcinolone acetonide—IVTA) **or sustained release implants** (flucinolone/dexamethasone). Steroid inhibits phospholipase A-2 and subsequent release of arachidonic acid, which is precursor of prostaglandins and leukotrienes. It also down regulates the VEGF production and modulates the ICAM-1 expression. In addition to the anti-inflammatory effect, it increases the levels of tight-junctions in endothelial cells.[48]
  - **Triamcinolone acetonide (TA):** Intravitreal TA (IVTA) has been reported to improve vision and reduce macular thickness in eyes with macular edema, especially refractory, although the results are not well-sustained. In non-vitrectomized eye, the mean elimination half-life of TA is 18.6 days, and in vitrectomized eyes it is 3.2 days.[49] Its use in DME is off-label. Both 2 mg and 4 mg dosages are used frequently. The DRCR.net protocol B compared IVTA (1- and 4-mg doses) with modified ETDRS focal/grid photocoagulation for the treatment of DME. Although at 4 months, mean visual acuity was better in the 4 mg TA group than both laser and the 1 mg TA group, the IVTA effect was not sustained at 2-years. The focal/grid photocoagulation was more effective with fewer side effects than 1 mg or 4 mg doses of TA for most patients with DME.[50]

  DRCR.net Protocol I demonstrated that in the subset of pseudophakic eyes (n = 273) the degree of improvement with IVTA appeared comparable to that of the pseudophakic eyes in the ranibizumab groups and superior to the pseudophakic eyes in the sham + prompt laser group at year 1 and 2.[51] Besides cataract, increase in IOP of at least 5 mm Hg has been observed in 68% of eyes receiving IVTA of which 44% required antiglaucoma medication and around 6% required trabeculectomy.[52] Endophthalmitis,

TABLE 11.5: Selected anti-VEGF randomized controlled trials in DME

Treatment	Study components	≥10 letter gain	≥10 letter lost	≥15 letter gain	≥15 letter lost
Pegaptanib Phase II/III, 2 year Pegaptanib 0.3 mg Vs Sham[44] n = 207	0.3 mg pegaptanib = 107	38.3%	3%	23.4%	3.8%
	Sham = 100	30.0%	6.3%	15.0 %	9.0%
RESOLVE Phase II, 1 year RBZ Vs Sham n = 151[45]	RBZ =102	60.8 %	4.9 %	32.4 %	2.9 %
	Sham = 49	18.4 %	24.5%	10.2 %	20.4 %
RISE Phase III, 1 year Two doses of RBZ Vs Sham n= 377[40]	0.3 mg RBZ = 125	62.7%	3.2%	44.8%	2.4%
	0.5 mg RBZ = 125	62.4%	4%	39.2%	2.4%
	Sham = 127	29.9%	16.6%	18.1%	10.3%
RIDE Phase III, 1 year Two doses of RBZ Vs Laser n= 382[40]	0.3 mg RBZ = 125	59.2%	3.2%	33.6%	1.6%
	0.5 mg RBZ = 127	64.5%	4%	45.7%	4%
	Laser = 130	25.4%	13.8%	12.3%	8.4%
READ-2 Phase II, multicenter RBZ monotherapy/with laser Vs Laser alone n= 126[46]	RBZ = 28	46 %	NA	24 %	NA
	Laser = 22	23 %		18 %	
	RBZ + Laser = 24	38 %		26 %	
RESTORE Phase III study. RBZ monotherapy/ with laser Vs Laser alone n= 345[37]	RBZ = 116	37.4 %	3.5%	22.6%	0.9%
	RBZ + Laser = 118	43.2%	4.2%	27.9%	3.4%
	Laser = 111	15.5%	12.7%	8.2%	8.2%

Contd...

Contd...

DRCR.net Protocol I. RBZ with prompt laser Vs RBZ with deferred Laser n= 361 (3 years)[47]	RBZ + prompt laser = 144	42%	10%	26%	6%
	RBZ + deferred laser = 147	56%	5%	32%	3%
BOLT Phase II single center study BVZ Vs Laser. 2 year. n = 65[36]	Bevacizumab = 37	49%	NA	32%	NA
	Laser = 28	7%	NA	4%	NA
DA VINCI Phase II study, 1 year Multidose different time Aflibercept Vs Laser[41]	0.5 mg q4. n = 44	57%	NA	40.9%	NA
	2 mg q4. n = 44	71%	NA	45.5%	NA
	2 mg q8. n = 42	45%	NA	23.8%	NA
	2 mg PRN. n = 45	62%	NA	42.2%	NA
VIVID DME; VISTA DME Phase III parallel study 2 doses of Aflibercept Vs Laser n = 872. 1 year[42]	VIVID. Aflibercept 2q4			32.4%	
	Aflibercept 2q8			33.3%	
	LASER			9.1%	
	VISTA Aflibercept 2q4			41.6%	
	Aflibercept 2q8			31.1%	
	LASER			7.8%	
DRCR.net Protocol T. Phase III study 1:1:1 ratio 3 anti-VEGF agents. n = 660. 1 year[43]	Aflibercept 2.0 mg	Aflibercept 77%	Aflibercept 1%	Aflibercept 67%	Aflibercept 1%
	Bevacizumab 1.25 mg	Bevacizumab 60%	Bevacizumab 4%	Bevacizumab 41%	Bevacizumab 2%
	Ranibizumab 0.3 mg	Ranibizumab 69%	Ranibizumab 2%	Ranibizumab 50%	Ranibizumab 2%
	In general, the mean improvement was 13.3 letters with aflibercept, 9.7 letters with bevacizumab and 11.2 letters with ranibizumab. There was more improvement with aflibercept when presenting vision was ≤20/50.				

Adapted from: Das T et al. Evidence based review of diabetic macular edema management: Consensus statement on Indian Treatment Guidelines. Indian J Ophthalmol. 2016;64(1):14-25.

vitreous hemorrhage and retinal detachment are other procedure-related complications.
- **Sustained release intravitreal implants** (fluocinolone/dexamethasone). Long-acting intravitreal drug delivery implants help overcome the need for frequent intravitreal injections or systemic side effects, by providing long-term localized delivery of therapeutic agents to the posterior segment at sufficiently high local dosages necessary to elicit the desired therapeutic effects. The Retisert implant (fluocinolone acetonide(FA) intravitreal implant 0.59 mg; *Bausch and Lomb, Rochester, NY*) is the first-generation FDA approved device for chronic macular edema. It is nonbiodegradable implant, inserted surgically and sutured to the eye wall. However, alarming rates (28%) of patients requiring filtering procedure and 5% of patients requiring explantation, has limited its use in DME.[53]

Iluvien *(Alimera Sciences, Alpharetta)* is an injectable second-generation of the Retisert FA implant that can be delivered without surgery using a 25-gauge injector. The Fluocinolone Acetonide in Diabetic Macular Edema (FAME) study randomized patients of persistent DME, low-dose (0.2 μg/day) insert or high-dose insert (0.5 μg/day) groups and found comparable results in both the implant groups, and was superior to sham group.[48] Glaucoma requiring incisional surgery at 24 months was 3.7%, 7.6% and 0.5% of the low-dose, high-dose and sham groups, respectively.

Ozurdex (dexamethasone), a biodegradable intravitreal implant, is another device recommended for DME treatment. It is placed in the vitreous cavity by a 22-gauge applicator. The implant contains 0.7 mg of dexamethasone and the drug is released in a biphasic fashion, with initial high doses for 6 weeks, followed by low but therapeutic doses for 4 to 6 months. The Macular Edema Assessment of implantable Dexamethasone (MEAD) trial[55] randomized patients to treatment with DEX implant 0.7 mg, DEX implant 0.35 mg, or sham procedure. Percentage of patients with ≥15-letter improvement in BCVA at 36 months was greater with DEX implant 0.7 mg, so also in the mean reduction in central retinal thickness (DEX implant 0.7 mg: 111.6 μm; DEX implant 0.35 mg: 107.9 μm and sham: 41.9 μm; $P < 0.001$).

Table 11.6 summarized the current status of intravitreal corticosteroids.

TABLE 11.6: Overview of selected intravitreal corticosteroid in DME

Treatment	Study components	≥ 10 letter gain	≥10 letter lost	≥15 letter gain	≥15 letter lost
DRCR.net. Phase III. 2 years Triamcinolone 1 and 4 mg Vs Laser [50]	IVTA 1 mg = 256	25%	28%	14%	20%
	IVTA 4 mg = 254	28%	26%	17%	20%
	Laser = 330	31%	19%	18%	14%
DRCR Protocol I. Phase III RBZ + Laser Vs TA + Laser [51]	IVTA 4 mg + Prompt laser = 188	21%	33%	14%	8%
	Sham + Prompt Laser = 293	17%	28%	10%	8%
FAME. Phase III. 3 years 2 Fluocinolone acetonide (FA) doses Vs Sham. n= 956 [54]	FA 0.2 μg/day n = 373	NA	3.2%	28.7%	NA
	FA 0.5 μg/day n = 393	NA	4%	27.8%	NA
	Sham = 175	NA	16.6%	18.9%	NA

Contd...

Contd...

Study	Dose (n)			
MEAD. Phase III. 2 parallel studies; 2 doses of dexa implant Vs Sham n = 1048 (Completed 607)[55]	700 µg dexa = 351 (225)	NA	22%	NA
	350 µg dexa = 347 (230)		18.4%	
	Sham = 350 (152)		12%	
Champlain Study Implantable Dexa in vitrectomized eyes n = 55[56]	7,000 µg dexamethasone = 55	30.4%		

Adapted from: Das T, et al. Evidence based review of diabetic macular edema management; Consensus statement on Indian treatment guidelines. Indian J Ophthalmol. 2016;64(1):14-25.

Table 11.7 has tabulated the status and major effects of current intravitreal therapy in DME.

TABLE 11.7: Current intravitreal therapy

Treatment	Landmark study	Approval	Effects
Traimcinolone	DRCR.net (Oph 2008)[50]	Unlicensed	Temporary effect; glaucoma and early cataract are concerns
Dexamethasone	MEAD (Oph 2014)[55]	FDA Sep 2014	Visual acuity improvement corresponds to injection; 36% rise in IOP
Fluocinolone	FAME (Oph 2014)[54]	FDA Sep 2014	Greater benefit in chronic DME; antiglaucoma medicine in 36–42%
Bevacizumab	BOLT (Oph 2010)[36]	Unlicensed	Not inferior to ranibizumab
Ranibizumab	Rise and Ride (Oph 2012)[40]	FDA Aug 2012	After 3 loading doses; monthly injection
Aflibercept	Vivid and Vista (Oph 2014)[42]	FDA Jul 2014	After 5 loading doses; monthly or bimonthly injection

SURGERY: VITRECTOMY

The role of vitrectomy with or without ILM peel has been now studied and it is found to be beneficial not only in cases having traction at macula but also those without any tractional component.[57-59] The comparative results of vitrectomy with lasers have been conflicting, but complications like retinal tears and detachment, vitreous hemorrhage, cataract and glaucoma are likely to occur in vitrectomies.

CONCLUSION

Diabetic Macular Edem a is a complex, chronic clinical entity with variable response. Hence, a single treatment entity may not be enough for the entire course of the disease. Laser therapy has been traditionally used to stabilize the vision. New pharmacotherapeutic agents have replaced it. The current level of evidence is summarized in Table 11.8.

Variable combination of laser with anti-VEGF agents, IVTA and steroid implants may be needed for best visual results. Many randomized clinical trials have helped us understand the dynamic treatment strategy. Essentially, it gears to center involved and center-noninvolved macular edema. In absence of any vitreoretinal traction (as evidenced by OCT) treatment begins with anti-VEGF monotherapy and possibly topped with retinal laser, and the treatment begins with retinal lasers in noncenter involved macular edema. Intravitreal or implantable steroids are reserved for refractory cases and could be considered in pseudophakic eyes. The recommended treatment strategy is illustrated in Flowchart 11.1.

TABLE 11.8: Evidences for DME management

Key points	Evidence
Laser treatment in non-center involved DME	A:I
Anti-VEGF treatment in center involved DME of VA <20/30	A:I
ETDRS Laser for eyes not meeting anti-VEGF threshold	A:III
Loading doses of anti-VEGF, then as needed (PRN)	A:I
Monthly follow-up visits till VA is stable for 3 consecutive visits	A:I
ETDRS laser if anti-VEGF treatment is unsatisfactory, usually after 6 months	A:I
Intravitreal corticosteroid (in pseudophakic eyes)	A:I

Note: A- very important or crucial to good clinical outcome; B- Moderately important to clinical outcome; C- May be relevant, but may not relate to clinical outcome. I- Strong evidence in support of clinical evidence; II- Substantial evidence, but evidence lacks quality; III- Infrequent evidence or against recommendation.

Flowchart 11.1: Recommended treatment strategy in DME

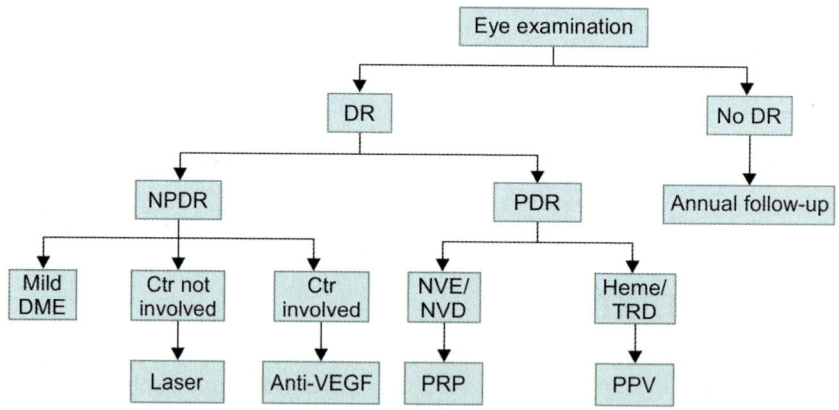

Abbreviations: DR, diabetic retinopathy; NPDR, non-proliferative diabetic retinopathy; PDR, Proliferative diabetic retinopathy; Ctr, center; TRD, tractional retinal detachment; PRP, panretinal photocoagulation; PPV, pars plana vitrectomy.

REFERENCES

1. Klein R, Klein BE, Moss SE, et al. The Wisconsin Epidemiologic Study of Diabetic Retinopathy. XV. The long-term incidence of macular edema. Ophthalmology. 1995;102:7-16.
2. Ding J, Wong TY. Current epidemiology of diabetic retinopathy and diabetic macular edema. Curr Diab Rep. 2012; 12:346-54.
3. Early Treatment Diabetic Retinopathy Study Research Group Report 10. Grading diabetic retinopathy from stereoscopic color fundus photographs—an extension of the modified Airlie house classification. Ophthalmology. 1991;98:786-806.

4. Rema M, Premkumar S, Anitha B, et al. Prevalence of diabetic retinopathy in urban India: the Chennai Urban Rural Epidemiology Study (CURES) Eye Study I. Invest Ophthalmol Vis Sci. 2005;46:2328-33.
5. Gabbay KH. Hyperglycemia, polyol metabolism and complications of diabetes mellitus. Annu Rev Med. 1975;26:521-36.
6. Wautier JL, Guillausseau PJ. Advanced glycation end products, their receptors and diabetic angiopathy. Diabetes Metab. 2001;27: 535-42.
7. Inoguchi T, Battan R, King GL, et al. Preferential elevation of protein kinase C isoform beta II and diacylglycerol levels in the aorta and heart of diabetic rats: differential reversibility of glycemic control by islet cell transplantation. Proc Natl Acad Sci USA. 1992;89:11059-63.
8. Yamamoto T[1], Akabane N, Takeuchi S. Vitrectomy for diabetic macular edema: the role of posterior vitreous detachment and epimacular membrane. Am J Ophthalmol. 2001;132(3):369-77.
9. Bhagat N, Grigorian RA, Tutela A, Zarbin MA. Diabetic Macular Edema: pathogenesis and treatment. Survey Ophthalmol. 2009;54(1):1-32.
10. Wilkinson CP, Ferris FL 3rd, Klein RE, et al. Proposed international clinical diabetic retinopathy and diabetic macular edema disease severity scales. Ophthalmology. 2003;110:1677-82.
11. Nasrallah FP, Jalkh AE, Van Coppenolle F, et al. The role of vitreous in diabetic macular edema. Ophthalmology. 1988;95:1335-9.
12. Diaz-Llopis M, Udaondo P, Millan JM, Arevalo JF. Enzymatic vitrectomy for diabetic retinopathy and diabetic macular edema. World J Diabetes. 2013;4:319-23.
13. Harbour JW, Smiddy WE, Flynn HW Jr, Rubsamen RE. Vitrectomy for diabetic macular edema associated with a thickened and taut posterior hyaloid membrane. Am J Ophthalmol. 1996;121:405-13.
14. Kang SW, Park CY, Ham DI. The correlation between fluorescein angiographic and optical coherence tomographic features in clinically significant diabetic macular edema. Am J Ophthalmol. 2004;137: 313-22.
15. Hee MR, Puliafito CA, Duker JS, et al. Topography of diabetic macular edema with optical coherence tomography. Ophthalmology. 1998;105:360-70.
16. Das T, Simanjuntak G, Sumasri K. Optical coherence tomography titrated photocoagulation in diabetic clinically significant macula edema. In: Binder, (Ed). The Macula. Diagnosis, Treatment, and Future trends. Springer–Verlag, Wein;2004. p:185-94.
17. The Diabetes Control and Complications Trial Research Group. The effect of intensive treatment of diabetes on the development and progression of long-term complications in insulin-dependent diabetes mellitus. N Engl J Med. 1993;329:977-86.
18. UK Prospective Diabetes Study Group (UKPDS) Group. Intensive blood-glucose control with sulphonylureas or insulin compared with conventional treatment and risk of complications in patients with type 2 diabetes (UKPDS 33). Lancet 1998; 352:837-53.
19. Hilsted J, Madsbad S, Nielsen JD, et al. Hypoglycemia and hemostatic parameters in juvenile-onset diabetes. Diabetes Care. 1980;3:675-8.
20. Nathan DM, Cleary PA, Backlund JY, et al. DCCT/EDIC Research Group: Intensive diabetes treatment and cardiovascular disease in patients with type 1 diabetes. N Engl J Med. 2005;353:2643-53.
21. The ACCORD Study Group and ACCORD Eye Study Group. Effects of medical therapies on retinopathy progression in type 2 diabetes. N Engl J Med. 2010; 363:233-44.
22. Kunisaki M, Bursell SE, Clermont AC, et al. Vitamin E prevents diabetes-induced abnormal retinal blood flow via the diacylglycerol-protein kinase C pathway. Am J Physiol.1995; 269: E239-46.

23. Moshetova LK, Vorob'eva IV, Alekseev IB, Mikhaleva LG. Results of the use of antioxidant and angioprotective agents in type 2 diabetes patients with diabetic retinopathy and age related macular degeneration. Vestn Oftalmol. 2015;131:34-40, 42-4.
24. Strom C, Sander B, Klemp K, et al. Effect of ruboxistaurin on blood-retinal barrier permeability in relation to severity of leakage in diabetic macular edema. Invest Ophthalmol Vis Sci. 2005;46:3855-8.
25. PKC-DMES Study Group. Effect of ruboxistaurin in patients with diabetic macular edema: thirty-month results of the randomized PKC-DMES clinical trial. Arch Ophthalmol. 2007;125:318-24.
26. Freedman BI, Wuerth JP, Cartwright K, et al. Design and baseline characteristics for the aminoguanidine Clinical Trial in Overt Type II Diabetic Nephropathy (ACTION II). Control Clin Trials. 1999;20:493-510.
27. Early Treatment Diabetic Retinopathy Study Research Group. Treatment techniques and clinical guidelines for photocoagulation of diabetic macular edema: Early Treatment Diabetic Retinopathy Study Report Number 2. Ophthalmology. 1987; 94:761-74.
28. Royster AJ, Nanda SK, Hatchell DL, et al. Photochemical initiation of thrombosis. Fluorescein angiographic, histologic and ultrastructural alterations in the choroid, retinal pigment epithelium and retina. Arch Ophthalmol. 1988;106:1608-14.
29. Arnarsson A, Stefansson E. Laser treatment and the mechanism of edema reduction in branch retinal vein occlusion. Invest Ophthalmol Vis Sci. 2000; 41:877-9.
30. Wallow IH, Sponsel WE, Stevens TS. Clinicopathologic correlation of diode laser burns in monkeys. Arch Ophthalmol 1991;109:648-53.
31. Ogata N, Tombran-Tink J, Jo N, et al. Upregulation of pigment epithelium-derived factor after laser photocoagulation. Am J Ophthalmol. 2001;132:427-9.
32. Fong DS, Strauber SF, Aiello LP, et al. Comparison of the modified early treatment diabetic retinopathy study and mild macular grid laser photocoagulation strategies for diabetic macular edema. Arch Ophthalmic. 2007;125:469-80.
33. Luttrull JK, Sramek C, Palanker D, et al. Long term safety, high resolution imaging and tissue temperature modeling of subvisible diode micropulse photocoagulation for retinovascular macular edema. Retina. 2012;32:375-86.
34. Park YG, Kim EY, Roh YJ. Laser-based strategies to treat diabetic macular edema: history and new promising therapies. J Ophthalmol. 2014:769213.
35. Roider J, Lieu SH, Klatt C, et al. Selective retina therapy (SRT) for clinically significant diabetic macular edema. Graefe's Arch Clin and Exp Ophthalmol. 2010;248:1263-72.
36. Rajendram R, Fraser-Bell S, Kaines A, et al. A 2-year prospective randomized controlled trial of intravitreal bevacizumab or laser therapy (BOLT) in the management of diabetic macular edema: 24-month data: report 3. Arch Ophthalmol. 2012; 130: 972-9.
37. Mitchell P, Bandello F, Schmidt-Erfurth U, et al. The RESTORE study: ranibizumab monotherapy or combined with laser versus laser monotherapy for diabetic macular edema. Ophthalmology. 2011;118:615-25.
38. Mitchell P, Massin P, Bressler S, et al. Three-year patient-reported visual function outcomes in diabetic macular edema managed with ranibizumab: the RESTORE extension study. Curr Med Res Opin. 2015;1-9.[Epub]
39. Elman MJ, Ayala A, Bressler NM, et al. Diabetic retinopathy clinical research network. Intravitreal Ranibizumab for diabetic macular edema with prompt versus deferred laser treatment: 5-year randomized trial results. Ophthalmology. 2015;122:375-81.
40. Nguyen QD, Brown DM, Marcus DM, et al. Ranibizumab for diabetic macular edema: results from 2 phase III randomized trials: RISE and RIDE. Ophthalmology. 2012;119:789-801.

41. Do DV, Nguyen QD, Boyer D, et al. One-year outcomes of the daVINCI study of VEGF trap-eye in eyes with diabetic macular edema. Ophthalmology. 2012;119:1658-65.
42. Korobelnik JF, Do DV, Schmidt-Erfurth U, et al. Intravitreal aflibercept for diabetic macular edema. Ophthalmology. 2014;121:2247-54.
43. DRCR.net. Aflibercept, bevacizumab, or ranibizumab for diabetic macular edema. N Engl J Med. 2015;372:1193-203.
44. Sultan MB, Zhou D, Loftus J, et al. Macugen 1013 Study group. A phase 2/3, multicenter, randomized, double-masked, 2-year trial of pegaptanib sodium for the treatment of diabetic macular edema. Ophthalmology. 2011;118:1107-18.
45. Massin P, Bandello F, Garweg JG, et al. Safety and efficacy of ranibizumab in diabetic macular edema (RESOLVE Study): a 12-month, randomized, controlled, double-masked, multicenter phase II study. Diabetes Care. 2010;33:2399-405.
46. Nguyen QD[1], Shah SM, Khwaja AA, et al. Two-year outcomes of the ranibizumab for edema of the macula in diabetes (READ-2) study. Ophthalmology. 2010;117:2146-51.
47. DRCR.net. Intravitreal ranibizumab for diabetic macular edema with prompt vs deferred laser treatment: 3-year randomized trial results. Ophthalmology. 2012; 119:2312-8.
48. Sears JE, Hoppe G. Triamcinolone acetonide destabilizes VEGF mRNA in Müller cells under continuous cobalt stimulation. Invest Ophthalmol Vis Sci. 2005;46:4336-41.
49. Beer PM, Bakri SJ, Singh RJ, et al. Intraocular concentration and pharmacokinetics of triamcinolone acetonide after a single intravitreal injection. Ophthalmology. 2003;110:681-6.
50. DRCR.net. A randomized trial comparing intravitreal triamcinolone acetonide and focal/grid photocoagulation for diabetic macular edema. Ophthalmology. 2008;115:1447-79.
51. DRCR.net. Randomized trial evaluating ranibizumab plus prompt or deferred laser or triamcinolone plus prompt laser for diabetic macular edema. Ophthalmology. 2010;117:1064-77.
52. Gillies MC, Sutter FK, Simpson JM, et al. Intravitreal triamcinolone for refractory diabetic macular edema: two-year results of a double-masked, placebo-controlled, randomized clinical trial. Ophthalmology. 2006;113:1533-8.
53. Pearson PA, Comstock TL, Ip M, et al. Fluocinolone Acetonide Implant Study Group. Fluocinolone acetonide intravitreal implant for diabetic macular edema: 3-year multicenter, randomized controlled clinical trial. Ophthalmology. 2011;118;1580-87.
54. Campochiaro PA, Brown DM, Pearson A, et al; FAME Study Group. Sustained delivery fluocinolone acetonide vitreous inserts provide benefit for at least 3 years in patients with diabetic macular edema. Ophthalmology. 2012;119:2125-32.
55. Boyer DS, Yoon YH, Belfort R Jr, et al. Ozurdex MEAD Study Group. Three-year, randomized, sham-controlled trial of dexamethasone intravitreal implant in patients with diabetic macular edema. Ophthalmology. 2014;121:1904-14.
56. Boyer DS, Faber D, Gupta S, et al. Ozurdex CHAMPLAIN Study Group. Dexamethasone intravitreal implant for treatment of diabetic macular edema in vitrectomized patients. Retina. 2011;31:915-23.
57. Lewis H, Abrams GW, Blumenkranz MS, Campo RV. Vitrectomy for diabetic macular traction and edema associated with posterior hyaloidal traction. Ophthalmology. 1992; 99:753-9.
58. La Heij EC, Hendrikse F, Kessels AGH, Derhaag PJ. Vitrectomy results in diabetic macular oedema without evident vitreomacular traction. Graefes Arch Clin Exp Ophthalmol. 2001; 239:264-70.
59. Yanyali A, Nohutcu AF, Horozoglu F, Celik E. Modified grid laser photocoagulation versus pars plana vitrectomy with internal limiting membrane removal in diabetic macular edema. Am J Ophthalmol. 2005;139:795-801.

Chapter 12

New Frontiers in the Treatment of AMD

Suresh R Chandra, Amol D Kulkarni

INTRODUCTION

Age-related macular degeneration (AMD) is one of the leading causes of irreversible blindness in the elderly patients. The current prevalence is 8.7% worldwide and the number is projected to increase to approximately 196 million in 2020.[1] Early stage of AMD is characterized by drusen and pigmentary changes in the macula. The advanced stage of AMD is subdivided in two categories: Atrophic dry form and neovascular form. The atrophic dry AMD is also called geographic atrophy (GA) and is characterized by well-defined areas of RPE loss followed by the degeneration of the corresponding photoreceptors and thinning of the retina (Figs 12.1A and B).[2] Neovascular AMD is also called wet or exudative AMD and is characterized by choroidal neovascular membrane (CNVM).[2] In exudative AMD the subretinal fluid may persit in spite treatment with anti VEGF drugs (Fig. 12.2). Both the GA and wet AMD can lead to severe central visual impairment or legal blindness. This review will focus on the new advances in the management of dry and wet AMD.

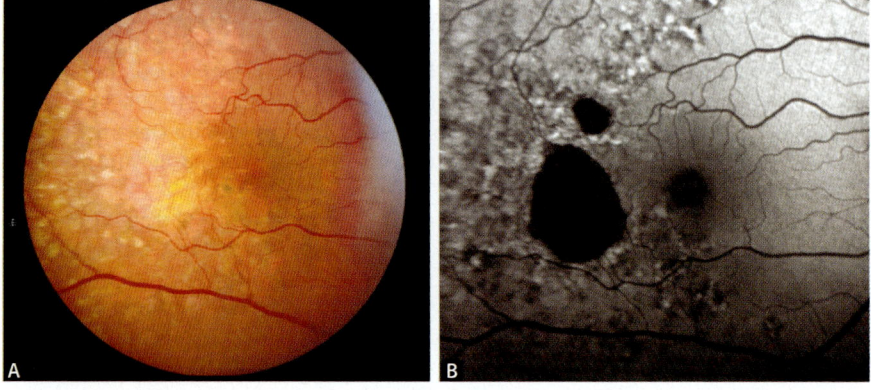

Figs 12.1A and B: (A) Fundus photo of patient with GA showing retinal atrophy; and choroidal vessels; (B) Corresponding hypofluorescence on the autofluorescence image

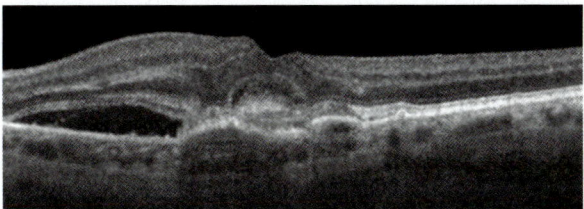

Fig. 12.2: OCT image of patient with wet AMD showing subretinal fluid indicative of persistent activity despite multiple anti-VEGF injections

EMERGING THERAPEUTIC OPTIONS IN DRY AMD

The current standard of care for dry AMD is the Age-related Eye Disease Study (AREDS) formulations, which reduce the risk of AMD progression by 25–30% over a 5-year period. There is no other approved therapy to prevent progression to GA, however there are multiple agents in clinical trials (Fig. 12.1). The current research treatments are focused on modifying the insults from oxidative stress, and chronic inflammation. There is also research directed at minimizing the risks from genetic and environmental factors. These newer treatments can be broadly categorized into:
- Anti-inflammatory therapies
- Anti-oxidative stress therapies
- Visual cycle modifying agents
- Choroidal blood flow enhancing agents
- Regenerative stem cell therapies.

Anti-Inflammatory Therapies

The anti-inflammatory therapies target the complement pathways which has been associated with AMD. Drusen accumulation together with oxidative stress can result in retinal pigment epithelial (RPE) cell damage or death, leading to activation of the complement pathway. This leads to the formation of the membrane attack complex that causes target cell lysis and chronic inflammation. Hence anti-inflammatory agents seem to be a viable option in stopping progression.

The various anti-inflammatory agents in clinical trials include:
- Lampalizumab
- Sirolimus
- Eculizumab
- Zimura.

Lampalizumab

Lampalizumab is an antigen-binding fragment (Fab) of a humanized, monoclonal antibody directed against complement factor D.[3] Complement factor D is a rate-limiting enzyme involved in the activation of the alternative complement pathway which has been implicated in the development of AMD including GA. It is the first complement targeted therapy for GA to enter phase III trials. The MAHALO phase II trial was a multi-center, randomized, single-masked, controlled study of the safety, tolerability and evidence of activity of lampalizumab in patients with GA associated with AMD.[3] Study participants received lampalizumab injections in one eye either monthly or every other month for 18 months. The primary endpoint was change of GA area from baseline to month 18 compared with control, as assessed with fundus autofluorescence (FAF). Lampalizumab showed a reduction rate of 20.4% in the GA area at 18 months in patients with advance dry AMD. Additionally, data from a sub-population of GA patients receiving monthly lampalizumab and positive for the complement factor I (CFI) biomarker, demonstrated a 44% decrease in the rate of disease progression at 18 months. The most frequently reported adverse effects in the MAHALO study were associated with the injection procedure. There were no serious ocular adverse effects or death suspected to be caused by the studied drug.

Sirolimus

Sirolimus (rapamycin), is an immunosuppressive agent that has been approved for preventing organ rejection following renal transplantation and coated stent to prevent coronary artery restenosis. It has been used in oral formulation in refractory uveitis. It acts by inhibiting the mechanistic target of rapamycin (mTOR) pathway, which regulates diverse cell processes, such as growth, metabolism, survival and proliferation.[4] It has been tested at a single center phase II study at the National Eye Institute. This study recruited 11 participants aged 55 years and older to evaluate the safety of sirolimus in patients with GA. The participants received 440 µg subconjunctival injections of sirolimus in the study eye at baseline and every 3 months thereafter. The rate of change in area of GA was evaluated by fundus photography at 24 months and compared with baseline. This study concluded that repeated subconjunctival sirolimus was well-tolerated in patients with GA, although no positive anatomic or functional effects were identified.

Eculizumab

Eculizumab is a humanized IgG antibody that acts by inhibition of terminal complement activation (C5).[5] It is approved by the US Food and Drug Administration for the systemic treatment of paroxysmal nocturnal hemoglobinuria and atypical hemolytic uremic syndrome. The complement inhibition with eculizumab for the treatment of non-exudative age-related macular degeneration (COMPLETE) phase II trial was the first prospective, randomized, placebo-controlled investigation of complement inhibition for the treatment of AMD.[5] A total of 30 patients were enrolled in the study and were randomized 2:1 to receive eculizumab or placebo. All patients underwent fundus photography, fundus autofluorescence (FAF), fluorescein angiography and spectral-domain (SD) optical coherence tomography (OCT) imaging with both the Cirrus (Carl Zeiss Meditec, Inc., Dublin, CA) and Spectralis (Heidelberg Engineering) instruments. The first 10 patients who received eculizumab received the low-dose regimen (600 mg weekly for 4 weeks followed by 900 mg for every 2 weeks until week 24), and the next 10 patients received the high-dose regimen (900 mg weekly for every 4 weeks followed by 1200 mg for every 2 weeks until week 24). Eighteen fellow eyes met inclusion criteria and were analyzed as a secondary endpoint. The primary outcome measured change in GA area at 26 weeks. The study showed that systemic complement inhibition with eculizumab was well-tolerated through 6 months but did not decrease the growth rate of GA significantly.

Zimura

Zimura is an aptamer that inhibits complement factor C5.[6] A phase IIa clinical trial (ClinicalTrials.gov identifier: NCT0070952) evaluating the safety and tolerability of Zimura administered in combination with ranibizumab was done for the treatment of wet AMD. Zimura was well-tolerated in combination with ranibizumab and there was a mean increase in visual acuity from baseline at all points of time. Based on results of this clinical trial, a phase II/III clinical trial investigating Zimura for treatment of geographic atrophy is planned by Ophthotech Corp, Princeton, NJ, USA.

Anti-oxidative Stress Therapies

Retinal pigment epithelium (RPE) layer is crucial for maintaining the homeostasis of the retina. Oxidative stress can lead to RPE cell degeneration. The critical role for oxidative stress in AMD is evident from cigarette smoking, which induces systemic oxidative stress, and is a proven risk factor for AMD. Metabolic wastes containing oxidative products and Amyloid-β have been shown to cause inflammatory response and lead to degeneration of photoreceptors and RPE cells.

Age-Related Eye Disease Study

Age-Related Eye Disease Study (AREDS) initially evaluated nutritional supplements, which contain vitamin C, vitamin E, β-carotene, zinc and copper, and showed reduced progression to advanced neovascular AMD by 25% over the 5-year study period. However, they had no effect on AMD GA. An increased of lung cancer was noted in smokers from β-carotene. Hence, an AREDS2 trial was designed to test whether adding lutein and zeaxanthin instead of β-carotene and/or omega-3 fatty acids could improve the AREDS formulation. The AREDS2 study showed that lutein and zeaxanthin together appeared to be safe and effective alternative to β-carotene in a median follow-up period of 5 years.[7] Furthermore, adding lutein and zeaxanthin provided about a 20% reduction in progression beyond the original AREDS formulation. The addition of omega-3 did not reduce the risk of progression. The development of cataract was not affected by any of the supplements.

OT-551

OT-551 is an antioxidant molecule. OT-551 is converted by intraocular esterases to its active metabolite, Tempol-H which is capable of reacting directly with free radicals and exerts potential antioxidant effects. A phase II study has been performed on a small group of 11 participants, aged 60 years and older, with GA present in both eyes. Topical OT-551 (at 0.45%) eye drops were given three times a day for up to 3 years. The primary and secondary outcomes included measuring BCVA and fundus autofluorescence (FAF), respectively. The study showed that topical administration of OT-551 was well-tolerated but did not exert a significant effect on lesion enlargement, retinal sensitivity or total drusen area.

Amyloid-β Targets

Amyloid-β targets[8] prevent accumulation and thereby modulate the levels. The investigational medications in this class include MRZ-99030, RN6G, and GSK933776.[9] MRZ-99030 is a dipeptide containing d-tryptophan and 2-amino-2-methylpropionic acid designed to modulate aggregation of amyloid-β and is formulated as eye drops. RN6G is a humanized antibody administered as an intravenous injection which prevents accumulation of amyloid β. Phase 1 studies have been completed on both medications. GSK933776 is a humanized monoclonal antibody intended to modulate levels of amyloid-β. A phase II trial to investigates the safety and efficacy of GSK933776 in patients with GA secondary to AMD is currently ongoing.

Visual Cycle Modifying Agents

Advanced glycation end products and byproducts of visual cycle such as A2E have been observed at the sites of RPE atrophy in GA eyes and associated with the GA pathogenesis. Furthermore, oxysterols are generated as byproducts of visual cycle by peroxidation of cholesterol, steroid and fatty acids, and metabolized in RPE cells. Excess accumulation of oxysterols in Bruch's membrane leads to RPE and photoreceptor cell death. It also causes migration of macrophages to induce inflammation.

Fenretinide (RT-101)

Fenretinide acts by inhibiting the formation of A2E and other lipofuscin fluorophores in vivo, with no deleterious effects on visual function or retinal morphology.[10] It thereby reduces the circulating levels of retinol and its carrier protein, the retinol binding protein. A phase II study to determine the efficacy of fenretinide did not show any benefit in reduction in progression of GA.

Emixustat

It is a nonretinoid compound that directly affects the biosynthesis of visual chromophores through inhibition of RPE-specific protein isomerase 65 (RPE65). RPE65 plays a key role in conversion of all-transretinal to 11-cis retinal so it can re-enter the visual cycle. Emixustat also acts as an antagonist of retinoid-binding proteins. Phase II/III clinical trial is underway to determine efficacy of orally delivered emixustat hydrochloride (ACU-4429) in GA progression.[11]

ALK-001

ALK-001 modulates vitamin A metabolism and there is sevenfold decrease in the formation of toxic vitamin A aggregates. A phase I study to assess the safety and pharmacokinetics of oral ALK-001 capsules in 40 healthy volunteers (21–70 years old) is ongoing.

Choroidal Blood Flow Enhancing Agents

Choroidal circulation is responsible for nutrition of outer retina and removal of metabolic wastes of the RPE. The reduced choroidal blood flow leads to accumulation of metabolic wastes in the outer retina, Bruch's membrane and RPE cells[12]. It can cause GA progression.

MC-1101

MC-1101 is an FDA-approved oral antihypertensive drug with hydralazine as its active ingredient. In animal studies, it has been shown to increase choroidal blood flow, prevent the rupture of the Bruch's membrane and also has anti-inflammatory and anti-oxidative effects.[12] Phase Ib clinical trial showed that topical instillation of 1% MC-1101 was safe and there were no serious ocular and systemic adverse events. Phase II/III trials are ongoing in patients with early to intermediate dry AMD who will receive topical 1% ophthalmic solution and be assessed for visual function over 24 months.

Stem Cell Therapy

Stem cell-based therapy has been a breakthrough in treating blindness due to degenerative retinal diseases. Stem cell-derived RPE cells can be transplanted in the subretinal space and can prevent photoreceptor death in GA. RPE cells can be derived from human embryonic stem cells (hESCs) or human induced pluripotent stem cells (iPSCs). In animal models these RPE cells have been shown to remain viable in subretinal space and improve retinal function.[13]

Based on these preclinical data, Phase I trial was designed to test the safety and tolerability of grafted hESC-derived RPE cells in patients with dry AMD and Stargardt's macular dystrophy. The data showed that transplanted RPE cells were viable at 4 months after transplantation with no signs of rejection or evidence of hyperproliferation or tumorigenesis. In addition, functional recovery was observed in patients receiving hESC-derived RPE. This initial success has led the way to phase I/II trials where patients were administered subretinal injections of 50,000–150,000 RPE cells and followed up for a median of 22 months (12–36 months). The results from this study showed improvement in BCVA compared with non-injected fellow eyes, and better vision-related quality-of-life in patients with atrophic AMD and Stargardt's disease. Thus, this study showed definitive evidence of the medium to long-term safety, survival and biological activity of the stem cell-derived cells in human disease. There are currently two other clinical trials using hESC-RPE cells in patients with dry AMD. Furthermore, the efficacy of clonogenic human central nervous system stem cells (HuCNS-SC) in the treatment of dry AMD is also being tested.

EMERGING THERAPEUTIC OPTIONS IN WET AMD

Intravitreal injection of anti-VEGF drugs is the standard of care in the management of wet AMD. The treatment regimen involves three initial monthly injections followed by maintenance injections. The treatment is extended as per protocol (Fig. 12.2). The 5 year results from the CATT study showed mean visual acuity decreased by 3 letters from baseline and 50% patients had 20/40 or better vision at 5 years. 20% patients were legally blind at 5 years. Thus prolonged anti-VEGF monotherapy is associated with vison loss from retinal thinning and progression of geographic atrophy. Furthermore, the patients and the caregiver have a significant treatment burden from multiple visits and repeated intravitreal injections. Hence there is a need to have newer treatment which can extend the duration of anti-VEGF medications and at the same time preserve retinal function. Other pharmacological agents and drug delivery options in clinical trials at this time include:

1. Steroids
2. Inhibitors of complement factors
3. Anti-platelet-derived growth factor agents (anti-PDGF)
4. New anti-VEGF drugs
5. Designed ankyrin repeat proteins
6. Sustained drug-delivery devices
7. Encapsulated cell technology
8. Adeno-associated virus vectors.

Steroids

Steroids have been used for treatment of various retinal disorders due to their anti-inflammatory, and anti-angiogenic properties.[14] There has been a huge evolution in delivery of steroid starting with retro-bulbar and posterior sub-tenon injections to intravitreal sustained delivery devices. Intravitreal triamcinolone was used as an adjunct to photodynamic therapy and it caused stabilization of the blood-retinal barrier, and decreased exudation. Since then combination of dexamethasone intravitreal implant (Ozurdex®, Allergan, Irvine, Calif, USA) and ranibizumab (Lucentis®, Genentech, Inc, South San Francisco, Calif, USA/ Novartis AG, Basel, Switzerland) has been used to treat patients with wet AMD. In this randomized clinical trial, use of dexamethasone implant reduced the total number of ranibizumab injections. Fluocinolone acetonide, is a longer acting steroid then dexamethasone. The Iluvien® implant (Alimera Sciences, Alpharetta, Ga, USA) is currently being evaluated in combination with ranibizumab in wet AMD. The major ocular adverse effects of steroids is progression of cataracts in phakic patients and intraocular pressure elevation needing anti-glaucoma eye drops or filtering surgery.

Inhibitors of Complement Factors

The role of Zimura® (Ophthotech Corp, Princeton, NJ, USA) in combination with ranibizumab has been already described earlier in the chapter. POT-4 is another potent inhibitor of complement factor C3 activation. Results from phase 1 trial of POT-4 in wet AMD patients suggest that it provides a good safety profile and drug tolerability. It is currently in Phase II clinical trials.

Anti-PDGF Agents

The 5-year results from CATT study and the SEVEN-UP study which analyzed the long-term results (7–8 years) of ANCHOR, MARINA and HORIZON studies show that there was plateau effect with anti-VEGF monotherapy in long term. There are also concerns of resistance to anti-VEGF and risks of progression of retinal atrophy. Hence use of anti-PDGF agents which acts on pericytes may serve as an adjuvant for CNVM regression.

Fovista (Ophthotech Corp, Princeton, NJ, USA) is an anti-PDGF agent.[15] A multicenter, randomized, double-masked, controlled phase IIb clinical trial has evaluated the efficacy and safety of Fovista in combination with ranibizumab. Patients receiving the combination therapy showed a significantly higher final visual acuity; a mean gain of 10.6 letters from baseline was achieved compared to a mean gain of 6.5 letters for patients in ranibizumab monotherapy. A phase III randomized, double-masked, controlled trial is currently underway to establish the safety and efficacy of intravitreal administration of Fovista in combination with ranibizumab compared to ranibizumab monotherapy in patients with wet AMD.

New Anti-VEGF Agents

Conbercept

KH902 (Chengdu Kanghong Biotech Co, Ltd, Sichuan, China) consists of the VEGF binding domains of the human VEGFR-1 and VEGFR-2 combined with the Fc portion of the human immunoglobulin G.[16] It binds VEGF-A, VEGF-B and placental growth factor. The AURORA study showed intravitreal conbercept was well tolerated and adverse systemic events were reported in the study. Conbercept seems to improve best-corrected visual acuity both with a PRN regimen and with monthly injections over a 12 month period.

Pazopanib
Pazopanib (GlaxoSmithKline, Brentford, UK) is a multi-tyrosine kinase inhibitor which has an effect on VEGFR-1, VEGFR-2, VEGFR-3, PDGFR-α, PDGFR-β and other receptors.[17] It was tested in a phase 1 trial in eye drop formulation on 70 patients with CNVM for 28 days. There was a significant decrease from baseline in central retinal thickness, however only a subset of patients showed an increase in best-corrected visual acuity.

Designed Ankyrin Repeat Protein Family
Designed ankyrin repeat proteins (DARPins) are small, single-domain molecules that can selectively bind to a target protein with high affinity and specificity. Abicipar pegol (Allergan), is a recombinant protein of the designed ankyrin repeat protein family.[18] Abicipar pegol has been evaluated in a phase I/II, open-label, multicenter, dose-escalation study and then in a phase II randomized double-blind clinical trial in patients with treatment naïve wet AMD. In phase 2 trial patients received abicipar pegol every month for 3 months while the control group received ranibizumab monthly for the entire duration of the study. The study was not powered enough to show statistically significant differences between the two drugs, however it showed good results in terms of efficacy and durability of abicipar pegol.

Sustained Drug-delivery Devices as an Alternative to Intravitreal Injections
Sustained delivery devices are able to release a drug in constant concentration and thereby reduce the burden of the repeated injections.[19] This not only reduces the overall costs but also lowers the incidence of risks of the injection procedure. The major hurdle in the use of anti-VEGF drugs in this platform is size of molecule and ability to remain viable in the reservoir. RTH258 (Alcon, Fort Worth, Tex, USA) is a single-chain antibody fragment which due to its small dimensions can permit use as a sustained drug-delivery devices. A phase I study was conducted to assess the safety, tolerability and the effects of treatment on ocular outcomes following a single intravitreal administration of RTH258 compared with ranibizumab in patients with wet AMD. A single injection of RTH258 or a single injection of ranibizumab 0.5 mg was administered to 194 patients in the prospective, randomized, multicentre study. Patients receiving RTH258 were divided into four cohorts, thus receiving four different doses. RTH258 demonstrated noninferiority compared with ranibizumab in mean change in CSFT from baseline to month 1 for the 4.5- and 6.0-mg dose groups. Changes in best-corrected visual acuity with RTH258 were comparable to those observed with ranibizumab.

Encapsulated Cell Technology
Encapsulated cell technology involves biocompatible implants that are able to produce continuously recombinant therapeutics.[19] NT-503 (Neurotech Pharmaceuticals, RI, USA), is an intraocular implant delivering anti-VEGF agent

and it is being tested in a prospective, multicenter two-stage study. Stage 1 (phase I) is open-label with all patients treated with the NT-503-3 encapsulated cell technology implant for 2 years. Stage 2 (phase II) is a separate, randomized, masked phase during which eligible patients will be randomized to the NT-503-3 group or the control group injected intravitreally with aflibercept (Eylea®; Regeneron, Tarrytown, NY, USA, and Bayer, Berlin, Germany) every 8 weeks.

Adeno-associated Virus Vectors

sFLT-1 (soluble fms-like tyrosine kinase-1) is a tyrosine kinase protein, which encodes for the VEGF receptor 1 and has anti-angiogenic properties. It also reduces vascular permeability. AAV2-sFLT01 (Genzyme, Cambridge, Mass, USA) is an adeno-associated virus vector that expresses a modified soluble Flt1 receptor.[19] A phase I clinical trial is currently ongoing to evaluate the safety and tolerability of this agent in patients with wet AMD. In this study a virus vector is used to transfer a gene into cells within the eye, which has anti-angiogenic effects. The duration of the gene effect is currently unknown, but can be long lasting. Similarly, AVA-101 (rAAV.sFLT-1 recombinant adeno-associated virus) contains a gene encoding sFLT-1 has been shown to have anti-VEGF activity. In a phase I study, AVA-101 was shown to be well-tolerated with no significant drug-related safety concerns. Furthermore, patients who received AVA-101 gained or maintained vision with minimal or no need for rescue treatment at 1 year.

CONCLUSION

Geographic atrophy is responsible for permanent vision loss in both dry and wet AMD patients. There is no definitive cure to halt the progression of GA. There is an immense effort being made through numerous clinica l trials to find a viable solution to prevent or minimize the progression of GA. These pharmacological agents target different aspects of GA, including inflammatory pathways, oxidative stress and RPE degeneration, byproducts of the visual cycle, restoration of choroidal perfusion, and replenishing RPE cells with stem cell-derived RPE cells. Until we have definitive evidence of benefit, the AREDS formulation remains the mainstay of treatment in patients with GA.

Anti-VEGF agents have revolutionized the treatment of wet AMD. However, anti-VEGF therapies are fraught with repeated treatments, drug resistance from chronic use and inducing atrophy. Combination treatment with steroids, anti-PDGF agents and DARPIN molecules will help overcome limitations of current anti-VEGF therapies. Moreover sustained drug delivery devices and encapsulated cell technologies may lower the treatment burden.

REFERENCES

1. Lambert NG, Singh MK, ElShelmani H, et al. Risk factors and biomarkers of age-related macular degeneration. Prog Retin Eye Res. 2016;54:64-102.
2. Rhoades W, Dickson D, Do DV. Potential role of lampalizumab for treatment of geographic atrophy. Clin Ophthalmol. 2015;9:1049-56.
3. Cao GF, Liu Y, Yang W, at al. Rapamycin sensitive mTOR activation mediates nerve growth factor (NGF) induced cell migration and pro-survival effects against hydrogen peroxide in retinal pigment epithelial cells. Biochem Biophys Res Commun. 2011;414(3):499-505.

4. Yehoshua Z, de Amorim Garcia Filho CA, Nunes RP, et al. Systemic complement inhibition with eculizumab for geographic atrophy in age-related macular degeneration: the COMPLETE study. Ophthalmology. 2014;21(3):693-701.
5. http://www.ophthotech.com/product-candidates/arc1905/.
6. Chew EY, Clemons TE, Sangiovanni JP, et al. Secondary analyses of the effects of lutein/zeaxanthin on age-related macular degeneration progression: AREDS2 report No. 3. JAMA Ophthalmol. 2014;132:142-9.
7. Wong WT, Kam W, Cunningham D, et al. Treatment of geographic atrophy by the topical administration of OT-551: results of a phase II clinical trial. Invest Ophthalmol Vis Sci. 2010;51(12):6131-9.
8. Parsons CG, Ruitenberg M, Freitag CE, et al. MRZ-99030—A novel modulator of Abeta aggregation: I—Mechanism of action (MoA) underlying the potential neuroprotective treatment of Alzheimer's disease, glaucoma and age-related macular degeneration (AMD). Neuropharmacology. 2015;92:158-69.
9. Mata N, Lichter JB, Vogel R, et al. Investigation of oral fenretinide for treatment of geographic atrophy in age-related macular degeneration. Retina. 2013;33:498-507.
10. Kubota R, Boman NL, David R, et al. Safety and effect on rod function of ACU-4429, a novel small-molecule visual cycle modulator. Retina. 2012;32:183-8.
11. Wei Jiang CG. Effects of hydralazine on ocular blood flow and laser-induced choroidal neovascularization. Int J Ophthalmol. 2009;2:324-7.
12. Kokkinaki M, Sahibzada N, Golestaneh N. Human induced pluripotent stem-derived retinal pigment epithelium (RPE) cells exhibit ion transport, membrane potential, polarized vascular endothelial growth factor secretion, and gene expression pattern similar to native RPE. Stem Cells. 2011;29:825-35.
13. Augustin AJ, Puls S, Oermann I. Triple therapy for choroidal neovascularization due to age-related macular degeneration: verteporfin PDT, bevacizumab, and dexamethasone. Retina. 2009;29:573-8.
14. http://www.ophthotech.com/product-candidates/fovista/.
15. Li X, Xu G, Wang Y, et al. AURORA Study Group: Safety and efficacy of conbercept in neovascular age-related macular degeneration: results from a 12-month randomized phase 2 study: AURORA study. Ophthalmology. 2014;121:1740-7.
16. Danis R, McLaughlin MM, Tolentino M, et al. Pazopanib eye drops: a randomized trial in neovascular age-related macular degeneration. Br J Ophthalmol. 2014;98:172-8.
17. Souied EH, Devin F, Mauget-Faÿsse M, MP0112 Study Group: Treatment of exudative age-related macular degeneration with a designed ankyrin repeat protein that binds vascular endothelial growth factor: a phase I/II study. Am J Ophthalmol. 2014;158:724-32.
18. Querques G, Capuano V, Frascio P, et al. Emerging therapeutic options in age-related macular degeneration. Ophthalmic Res. 2015;53(4):194-9.
19. Hanus J, Zhao F, Wang S. Current therapeutic developments in atrophic age-related macular degeneration. Br J Ophthalmol. 2016;100(1):122-7.

Chapter 13

Polypoidal Choroidal Vasculopathy

Lingam Gopal, Mayuri Bhargava, Su Xinyi

INTRODUCTION

Polypoidal choroidal vasculopathy (PCV) is a spectrum of disease involving the choroidal vasculature and usually affecting the adult population. Although described first in females of African American origin,[1] it is now known to be more common in the Asian population. The clinical presentations were initially described as 'posterior uveal bleeding syndrome'.[2] We now know that while hemorrhage is an important component of the manifestation, it is not a *sine qua non* of the disease entity. The incidence of PCV can be grossly underestimated if retinal surgeons do not routinely use indocyanine green angiography for evaluating sero-sanguinous maculopathy in adults.

DEMOGRAPHICS

The prevalence has been reported to be 22–25% among Japanese, Koreans and Chinese[3-5] while in countries like Italy, Belgium, Greece and US the prevalence has been reported to range from 4 to 9%.[6-8] In a report from Japan, up to 58.5% of the eyes presenting with neovascular age-related macular degeneration (AMD) was shown to have PCV.[9] Contrary to original description, PCV has been shown to occur in both genders and perhaps with equal frequency. The age at presentation is 1–2 decades earlier than the typical AMD. PCV tends to be bilateral although the presentation can be quite asymmetrical.

CLINICAL PRESENTATION

The PCV is primarily, a disease of the inner choroidal circulation. Two angiographic features—the polyps and branching vascular network (BVN) characterize PCV. Secondary features include the collection of fluid/blood/lipids in various spaces.

Symptomatology

The PCV and neovascular AMD can share common presenting symptoms such as reduced visual acuity especially for near and metamorphopsia. However, the incidence of sudden significant drop in vision is more common with PCV in view of its propensity to lead to large hemorrhagic detachments of the retina and retinal pigment epithelium. PCV can also remain asymptomatic if the lesions are extra-macular. The extent of vision disturbance obviously is related to the extent and location of the serous exudation and hemorrhage.

Ophthalmoscopic Features

- **Choroidal polyp:** Ophthalmoscopically, choroidal polyps can be seen as orange red nodules of variable size—most commonly located in the macular area (69.5%).[10] However, the lesions can also occur near arcades and in peripapillary area.
- **Serous exudation:** Hyperpermeability of the lesions leads to production of serous pigment epithelial detachments, retinal detachments as well as intra-retinal fluid. The extent of these serous detachments can vary from subtle lesions that are only detected on optical coherence tomography (OCT) to large retinal detachments involving several quadrants of the fundus. Large serous retinal detachments are usually associated with an episode of massive hemorrhage.
- **Hemorrhage:** The hallmark of PCV is the occurrence of hemorrhage in subretinal pigment epithelial space; subretinal space; and sometimes breakthrough vitreous hemorrhage. Massive hemorrhages are more often seen as a feature of PCV rather than AMD.
- **Fibrotic sequelae:** Contrary to AMD, PCV does not form large disciform scars, at least to start with.[11,12] Multiple hemorrhages lead to variable degree of fibrosis.
- **Role of antiplatelet agents and anticoagulants:** Patients who are on anti-coagulants are at increased risk of massive hemorrhages sometimes resulting in no perception of light. Patients on antiplatelet drugs (aspirin, clopidogrel) are also at increased risk of hemorrhage. These drugs may not cause the hemorrhage but perpetuate the same resulting in large bleeds.

Investigations

Currently, multi-modal imaging including fundus fluorescein angiography (FA), indocyanine green angiography (ICG) and optical coherence tomogoraphy (OCT) are becoming essential in differentiating PCV from choroidal neovascularization (CNV) secondary to age-related macular degeneration and lesions of retinal angiomatous proliferation (RAP).[13]

Fluorescein Angiography

On Fluorescein angiography (FA), PCV usually appears as leak similar to 'occult chroidal neovascular membrane' (CNVM), since the branching vascular networks are located in Bruch's membrane and are thus sub-RPE. Sometimes however, PCV can also present like a "classic" CNV with early well-defined hyper-fluorescence. This can be due to increased hyperfluorescence from atrophy of overlying RPE; subretinal fibrinous exudation or the occurrence of type 2 CNV secondary to PCV. The polyps can look like small PEDs on FA. Thus, macular PCV can be misdiagnosed as AMD if FA alone is performed.[14,15]

Indocyanine Green Angiography

Indocyanine green angiography (ICGA) is considered the gold standard for definitive diagnosis of PCV since it is primarily a pathology of the choroidal vasculature. ICG has high protein-binding capacity and fluoresces in the infrared range (790–805 nm). Considering this emission spectrum, lesions under RPE are better detected with ICG angiography.[16] The main characteristics of PCV on ICGA are the polyps and the branching vascular network (BVN). On ICGA, polyps (which are aneurysmal dilatations arising from inner choroidal vessels) are seen as hyperfluorescent spots with halo seen in the first 6 minutes. In the late phase the leak beyond the lesion remains, while the lesion itself can become hypofluorescent. Wash out phenomenon describes total disappearance of the dye from lesion in the very late phase. However, leaky lesions can retain the dye as hyperfluorescent rings.[17] Polyps may be single or multiple and when multiple can be seen as a cluster or at the terminals of a BVN.

Branching vascular network are seen as radiating vessels deep to RPE. Early-stage ICG video angiograms show filling of the network vessels and pulsatile polypoidal lesions are often observed in up to 10% of patients. Choroidal vascular hyperpermeability, (detected on ICGA as multifocal spots of hyperfluorescence in mid and late phases) is more often seen in eyes with PCV than with exudative AMD. ICG can also identify areas of pigment epithelial detachments (PEDs). A notch in PED can often represent the location of the polyp.

Tan et al.[18] described two varieties of abnormal vasculature in relation to PCV.
- A network of criscrossing vessels that have no specific identifiable origin.
- The typical BVN that have a point origin and subsequent sequential branching.

Types

Yuzawa et al.[19] classified PCV into two types based on ICG characteristics:
1. Polypoidal CNV, or type1 PCV, characterized by visible feeder and draining vessels and numerous network vessels or "interconnecting channels" on ICG video angiography. This type is considered to be the representative of CNV beneath the RPE.
2. In typical PCV, or type 2 PCV, neither feeder nor draining vessels is detectable and the number of network vessels is small similar to BVN. Mean subfoveal choroidal thickness is also noted to be thicker in typical PCV than in polypoidal CNV.
   Concept of late geographic hyperfluorescence (LGH): Kang et al.[20] have identified well-demarcated hyperfluorescent lesion in late-phase ICGA and believe that they are highly characteristic of PCV. These lesions typically are seen as clearly demarcated geographic areas of hyperfluorescence seen about 10 mts after injection of the dye. In contrast, in late onset hyperfluorescence due to AMD, the borders of the lesions are fuzzy. They believe that these areas of LGH may be predictive of future lesions and need close watch. On the flipside, disappearance of these lesions is believed to be a good prognostic indicator.

Optical Coherence Tomography

B-scan imaging with OCT shows the polypoidal lesions as steep dome-like elevations of highly reflective RPE layers with moderate reflectivity of the lesion. The elevations are sharper than what are noted in PEDs.[21] BVN is identifiable as two hyper-reflective lines (the double layer sign)—representing separation of RPE from Bruch's membrane by the BVN and generally corresponds to LGH on ICGA.[22] Treatment of BVN does not eliminate the double layer sign due to presence of fibrosis beneath RPE. A common feature noted is a notch in the PED where the polyps usually lie. PCV also tends to produce more serous retinal detachment and less intra retinal fluid compared to CNV-AMD.[23]

Choroidal hyperpermeability is very often associated with increased thickness of the choroid—termed 'pachy choroid'. Chung et al. have demonstrated thickened subfoveal choroid in eyes with PCV compared to those with AMD.[24,25] Pachy choroid has also been noted in conditions such as CSCR. The interpretation of thickened choroid can be difficult when the overall thickness is affected by relative thinning of one layer (choriocapillaris) along with thickening of another. Agarwal et al. have described the choroidal vascularity index (CVI) to define the ratio of luminal area to the total choroidal area.[26] This index is more robust. Vortex vein engorgement has also been noted to be more often seen in PCV eyes compared to controls.[27]

There is a suggestion that PCV could be a disease of choroidal congestion considering the observations of increased choroidal thickness and votex vein engorgement.

En-face OCT Imaging

High speed scanning with the present day machines permits en-face imaging. To visualize PCV complex, it is ideal to scan below the RPE and above Bruch membrane using slabs of 10 μm to 30 μm. Polyps are seen as round, ring-like structure and BVNs appear as mesh-like configuration.[28] PCV complexes may appear larger on en face imaging due to the ability of this technique to detect areas that may have no flow and due to the imaging of tissue that extends over and around the PCV vessels. Studies have demonstrated some correlation of en face OCT and ICGA in their ability to detect PCV complexes permitting en face imaging to be used in lieu of ICGA in follow up studies.

OCT Angiography

OCT angiography (OCT-A) is a noninvasive form of investigation that permits imaging of blood flow without a contrast dye being injected. In a study by Srour et al.[29] BVN was detected as a hyperflow lesion consistently, but the polyps were seen as hyperflow round lesions only in 25% and as hypoflow round structures in 75% indicating unusual blood flow through the polyps.

Fundus Autofluoresence

Fundus Autofluoresence (FAF) polyps show a central hypo-autofluorescence with a circumferential hyper-autofluoresent ring while the BVN shows granular hyperautofluorescence. Disappearance of the hyperautofluorescent ring tends to corresspond with closure of polyps on follow-up studies.[30] FAF is a useful addendum but does not replace the other investigations in the routine diagnosis and management of PCV.

Diagnosis

The Japanese study group of polyploidal choroidal vasculopathy[31] defined types of PCV as:

Definite PCV as presence of clinically evident orange red nodules or polyps identified with characteristic features on ICGA.

Probable PCV as abnormal vascular network or recurrent RPE detachments of hemorrhagic or serous nature.

An expert panel developed evidence based guidelines for clinical diagnosis of PCV. The summary of the guidelines are as follows:

- **Clinical suspicion:** Serous/sero-sanguinous or notched PED; massive sub-macular hemorrhage; presence of subretinal orange nodule; and non anti-VEGF responder.
- **Confirmatory (after ICGA):** Single or multiple focal nodular areas of hyperfluorescence from choroidal circulation within first 6 minutes after ICG injection. Nodular appearance on stereoscopic viewing; hypofluorescent halo; association with BVN; pulsatile filling of polyp on dynamic ICGA; focal hyperfluorescence corresponding to orange nodule seen on clinical examination; and association with massive submacular hemorrhage.

Age-related Macular Degeneration and Polypoidal Choroidal Vasculopathy

There is some confusion about AMD and PCV. Some questions remained unanswered:
- Whether AMD and PCV represent two different and distinct entities
- Are they variants of the same disease?
- What causes the polypoidal lesions to develop and how do we explain the observed racial differences?
- What is exactly the role of the pachychoroid?
- Is the treatment approach different for the two?
- Is the long-term prognosis different?

However, neovascular AMD and PCV present differences in epidemiology and and their clinical manifestations (Table 13.1).

TABLE 13.1: Showing differences between neovascular AMD and PCV

	CNV-AMD	PCV
Race	More in caucasians	More in Japanese, Chinese, Blacks
Age	Occurs 65 years and above usually	Occurs one decade earlier
Drusen	Important feature	Usually absent
Orange nodules	Absent	Pathognomonic
Large hemorrhagic PEDs	Less common	More common
Fluorescein angiography	Occult/Combined occult classic CNVM	Appearance similar to occult CNVM
ICG angiography	Plaque or ill-defined hyperfluorescence	Polyps and BVN
Fibrosis as sequelae	More common	Less common
Intra ocular VEGF levels	Higher	Lower than in AMD but higher than controls

MANAGEMENT

Considering the spectrum of manifestations; the confusion in clearly differentiating it from AMD; and the variable natural course, the approach to treatment is also fuzzy.

The treatment can be discussed under the following heads:
1. Management of PCV
2. Management of subretinal hemorrhage.

Management of PCV

The options available are thermal laser photocoagulation, photodynamic therapy (PDT) and intravitreal injection of anti-VEGF agents.

- **Thermal laser:**[32-33] Laser using green or yellow laser can be used to target the polyps directly. However, the collateral damage to the overlying and surrounding retina limits its use to extramacular lesions. Being an orange red lesion, diode laser is not ideally suited.
- **Photodynamic therapy (PDT):**[35] Photodynamic therapy involves intravenous infusion of the photosensitive dye 'Verteporfin' followed by treatment of the lesion of interest with 689 nm laser of low fluency. This results in damage to vascular endothelium by liberation of free oxygen radicals and not by heat generation. Hence collateral damage is avoided. This makes it possible to treat lesions within the macular area as well. The relative choroidal ischemia caused by the PDT is expected to reduce perfusion to the PCV lesion and encourage thrombosis and occlusion. While it is relatively straight forward to treat polyps, treating BVNs can pose a problem if the size of the BVN is large. Potential complications of PDT specific to PCV include tears in RPE, choroidal ischemia and perceived increased risk of sub retinal hemorrhage.[35,36] The larger the area treated, the more the risk of damage due to choroidal ischemia.
- **Anti-VEGF drugs:**[37] Currently experience is accumulating with use of both ranibizumab and aflibercept in PCV. There is in general agreement on the role of anti-VEGF drugs, although the levels of VEGF were found to be less than in AMD. The reduction in edema and subretinal fluid is prominently seen but polyp regression is less often noted.
- **Combination therapy:** It appeals to logic that a combination of PDT to the lesions combined with anti-VEGF drugs may perhaps give the best result in terms of recovery from this episode as well as reducing the risk of future recurrent hemorrhages. However, this is not a consistent observation clinically.

Figures 13.1A and B show a case of choroidal polyp identified on ICG but seen as occult CNVM on FFA. The effect of direct laser photocoagulation is evident in

Case 1 (Figs 13.1 and 13.2): A case of extramacular PCV.

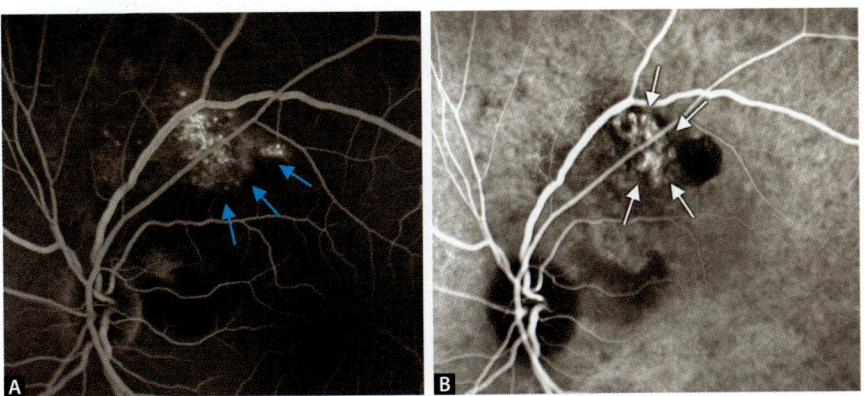

Figs 13.1A and B: (A) Shows fundus fluorescein angiogram that mimics occult CNVM (blue arrows). (B) ICG angiogram clearly depicting the polyps (white arrows)

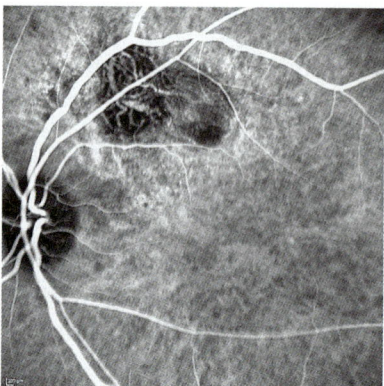

Fig. 13.2: Post focal laser ICG angiogram demonstrating successful closure of the polyps.

Case 2 (Figs 13.3 to 13.9): A case with multifocal polyps around macula.

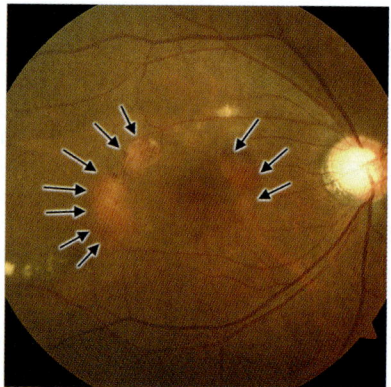

Fig. 13.3: Typical orange nodules are seen around the macula along with serous retinal detachment

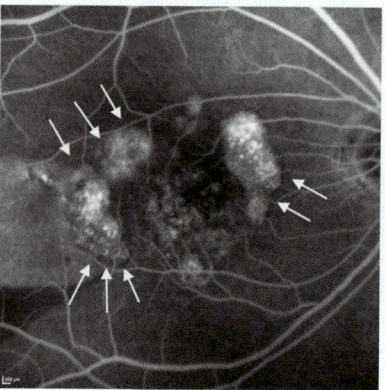

Fig. 13.4: Fundus fluorescein angiography reveals leaks corresponding to the nodules

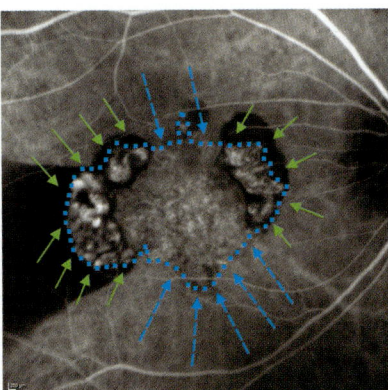

Fig. 13.5: The ICG angiogram clearly demarcates the polyps (green arrows) as well as the central branching vascular network (blue arrows). The whole PCV complex is outlined by the blue dotted line

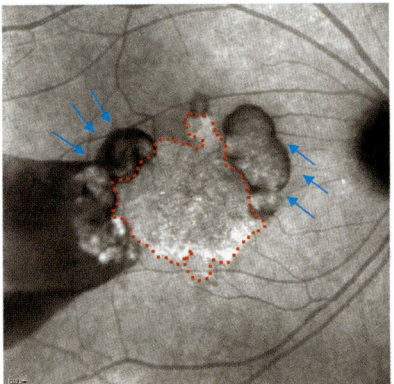

Fig. 13.6: In the late phase ICG angiogram showing the BVN more prominently and some of the polyps show fading of fluorescence while others retain the dye

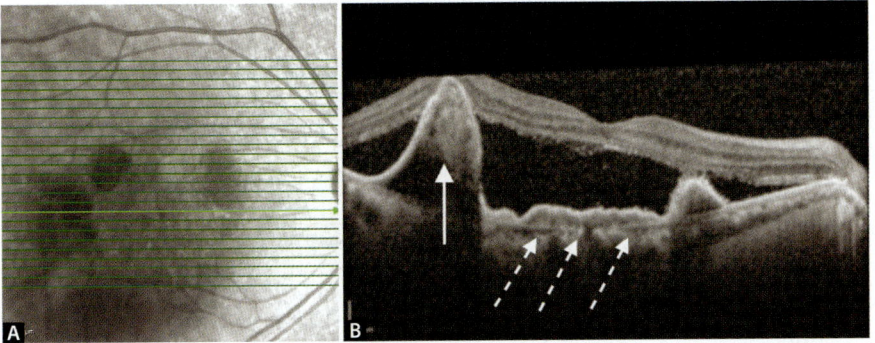

Figs 13.7A and B: The OCT features of the polyps (sharp dome shaped elevation of RPE with moderate intralesional reflectivity) and BVN (double layer sign). Note also the serous retinal detachment across the entire scan

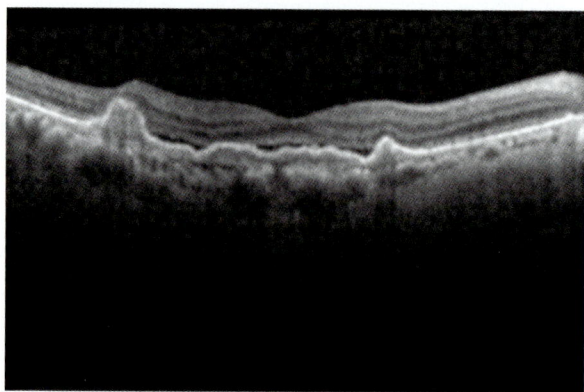

Fig. 13.8: The OCT after PDT depicting reduction in serous retinal detachment but persistence of the polyps and double layer sign of the BVN

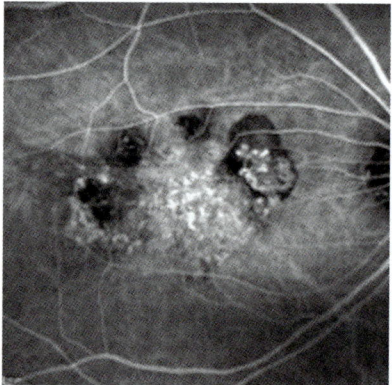

Fig. 13.9: Repeat ICG angiogram shows occlusion of temporal and superior polyps but persistence of nasal polyps and BVN

Figure 13.2. Figures 13.3 to 13.9 show the features of PCV on ICG and OCT in the form of multiple polyps and BVN. The partial closure of some of the polyps on PDT is also evident in the Figure 13.9.

Management of Subretinal Hemorrhage

Evaluation of the eye should include the extent of subretinal vs sub-RPE hemorrhage and their location in relation to center of macula. The principles of management are as follows:

1. If the hemorrhage is not extensive especially in terms of subfoveal thickness, it is best to ignore the hemorrhage and manage the PCV.
2. Sub-RPE hemorrhage is not amenable to be shifted away from posterior pole or removal surgically since the removal of these clots is associated with loss of RPE.
3. Subretinal hemorrhage can potentially be shifted away from posterior pole using a combination of gas tamponade and tissue plasminogen activator (TPA).

4. Large subretinal hemorrhages tend to breakthrough into vitreous cavity at some stage or other—more so after injection of gas.
5. Most often pars plana vitrectomy is performed to remove the vitreous component of the hemorrhage and sometimes to remove the subfoveal portion of the subretinal hemorrhage.
6. Small sub-RPE hemorrhage can sometimes resolve without affecting the overlying retinal function significantly.
7. Heroic surgeries with 360 degree retinotomy and removal of extensive hemorrhages are rarely associated with acceptable functional results, mostly due to extensive damage to the RPE as well risk of PVR.

End point of treatment: Ideally one would like to have no secondary effects in the form of retinal/subretinal/sub-RPE fluid or hemorrhage and closure of all polyps and BVN. Such a happy ending is unfortunately not the rule. In general:
- Continued treatment is definitely indicated if the lesions are active and symptomatic.
- Continued treatment is possibly indicated if the lesions are active although not symptomatic.
- No treatment is indicated if polyps are seen clinically and angiographically but have no activity (on OCT and clinically).

Results

The 'EVEREST' clinical trial has shown that polyp regression was greatest with combination of PDT and ranibizumab injection (77.8%) followed by PDT alone (71.4%) and least with Ranibizumab alone (28.6%).[38] Younger age, better presenting vision, smaller baseline hemorrhage and smaller lesion size were independent factors predictive of better visual outcomes after PDT monotherapy. PDT has not been as effective to cause regression of BVN or its exudative activity. Studies which compare visual outcomes between PDT and anti-VEGF therapy have generally reported better results with anti-VEGF therapy.[36] In the EVEREST study, despite higher rate of polypoidal lesion closure, the PDT arm achieved less visual gain.[38] Also, studies have shown that in PCV eyes treated with PDT, visual outcome was stable until 2 years, but worsened at 3 years, especially in eyes with recurrence.[39] Reduced fluence PDT has been proposed to reduce the risk of PDT-related complications.[40]

In LAPTOP study, patients with PCV were randomized to either ranibizumab monotherapy or PDT monotherapy. At month 12, a higher proportion of patients in the ranibizumab arm gained 0.2 log MAR units and visual improvement was maintained to month 24.[41]

Currently on-going randomized controlled trials for PCV (EVEREST 2 and PLANET) can provide further evidence regarding benefit of PDT in combination with ranibizumab or Aflibercept. 'EVEREST 2' is a 24-month, phase 4, randomized, double masked multicenter study of ranibizumab monotherapy or ranibizumab in combination with verteporfin photodynamic therapy on visual outcome in patients with symptomatic macular PCV. 'PLANET' is a randomized, double masked, sham-controlled phase 3b/4 study of the efficacy, safety, and tolerability of intravitreal Aflibercept monotherapy compared to Aflibercept with adjunctive photodynamic therapy as indicated in subjects with PCV.[42,43]

Cho HJ et al.[44] in a study compared Ranibizumab and Aflibercept in PCV. They reported a higher rate of polyp regression in eyes treated with Aflibercept (39.5%) than ranibizumab (21.6%), although the effect on central macular thickness and visual improvement was similar.

Recurrent Polypoidal Choroidal Vasculopathy

PCV is associated with frequent recurrences (64% at 2 years, 77% at 3 years and 78.6% at 5 years).[39] Hence, the long-term results are very often not satisfactory. Recurrences are characterized by hemorrhagic or exudative manifestation and are due to appearance of new polyps; polyps that did not close with treatment; or from BVN. Repeated PDT leads to cumulative damage to the normal choroidal vasculature and RPE. Thus, recurrent disease is treated with selective ablation of new or persistent polypoidal lesions with PDT or focal laser, while BVN activity can be managed using anti-VEGF monotherapy.

Treatment of Peripapillary PCV

Currently, there are no optimal guidelines for management of peripapillary PCV as these cases are generally excluded from randomised clinical trials. Ablative treatment with laser/PDT is associated with risk of damage to the optic nerve and papillomacular bundle, despite some studies suggesting that PDT even involving the disc is safe.[45] Hence, very often, these situations are managed with anti-VEGF monotherapy.

Prognosticating Factors

1. Presentation as serous detachments have better prognosis compared to presentation as hemorrhagic detachments of RPE and retina.
2. Multiple polyps have worse prognosis compared to isolated lesions.[46,47]
3. Type of abnormal vascular network; polyps supplied by interconnecting channels were found to have the best visual outcome following treatment, followed by PCV with non-leaking BVN while PCV with leaking BVN had the worst visual outcome.[18]
4. Pulsating PCV on ICG video angiography had a higher risk of extensive hemorrhagic events.
5. Choroidal vascular hyperpermeability on ICGA and thicker choroid on OCT may be a poor prognostic factor for response to anti-VEGF therapy in PCV.[48]

Genetics

In a recent meta-analysis of 66 published articles on the association of genetic variants with PCV identified 31 polymorphisms in 10 genes/loci.[49] These genes have been shown to be involved in the complement cascade (e.g. CFH), inflammatory pathway, extracellular matrix/basement membrane regulation pathway (ARMS2, HTRA1) and lipid metabolism (CETP). Several other studies have found CETP genetic variants to be associated with a high-risk of PCV[50-53] suggesting a possible role of the high-density lipoprotein pathway in the pathogenesis of PCV.

Interestingly, some studies have suggested genotypic-phenotypic correlation in PCV. The *ARMS2 LOC387715* rs10490924 variant has been shown to be associated with larger lesion size, higher risk of vitreous hemorrhage and worse visual outcome after PDT treatment.[54] In addition, the HTRA1-rs 11200638 is associated with poorer visual acuity 12 months after PDT treatment.[55] Certain risk genotypes (TT of rs10490924 and AA of rs11200638 at ARMS2/HTRA1) have been shown to have significantly poorer visual acuity outcome 1 year after combination therapy of PDT and intravitreal bevacizumab injection.[56] However, limitations of these pharmacogenomics studies include their small sample size and restrospective design, which have limited their clinical applicability. Of note, the *ARMS2 A69S* and *CFH 162V* polymorphisms are associated with increased choroidal thickness and choroidal vascular hyperpermeability, similar to central serous chorioretinopathy.[57]

Challenges and Future Direction

Substantial uncertainty still remains whether PCV is part of the AMD spectrum, or a completely separate clinical entity. More importantly, the pathogenesis of PCV remains unclear. The exact role of VEGF in PCV is unclear, though it is widely believed that VEGF is less crucial in PCV than in CNV-AMD. This may partially explain the limited efficacy of anti-VEGF monotherapy in PCV. Also, although multiple pathways have been eluded to play a role in PCV pathogenesis, such as complement activation, extracellular regulation, lipid metabolism and angiogenesis, how they contribute exactly to PCV formation remains unclear. Moreover, we still do not know what causes the branching vascular network, and why they do not respond well to either PDT or anti-VEGF agents.

As can be seen, this lack of understanding of the underlying pathogenesis has resulted in unclear treatment strategies for the various components of PCV. Addressing these gaps in our knowledge will allow us to develop targeted and effective treatment for PCV.

REFERENCES

1. Stern RM, Zakov ZN, Zegarra H et al. Multiple recurrent serosanguineous retinal pigment epithelial detachments in black women. Am J Ophthalmol. 1985;100:560-9.
2. Kleiner RC, Brucker AJ, Johnston RL. The posterior uveal bleeding syndrome. Retina. 1990;10:9-17.
3. SHo K, Takahashi K, Yamada H, et al. Ploypoidal choroidal vasculopathy: incidence, demographic features and clinical characteristics. Arch Ophthalmol. 2003;121:1392-6.
4. Wen F, Chen C, Wu D, et al. Polypoidal choroidal vasculopathy in elderly Chinese patients. Graefes Arch Clin Exp Ophthalmol. 2004;242:625-9.
5. Byeon SH, Lee SC, Oh HS, et al. Incidence and clinical patterns of polypoidal choroidal vasculopathy in Korean patients. Japan Journal of Ophthalmol. 2008;52:57-62.
6. Scasellat-Sforzolini B, Mariotti C, Bryan R, et al. Polypoidal choroidal vasculopathy in Italy. Retina. 2001;21:121-5.
7. Ladas ID, Rouvas AA, Moschos MM, et al. Polypoidal choroidal vasculopathy and exudative age related macular degeneration in Greek population. Eye (London). 2004;18:455-9.
8. Lafaut BA, Leys AM, Snyers B, et al. Polypoidal choroidal vasculopathy in Caucasians. Greaefes Arch Clin Exp Ophthalmol. 2000;238:752-9.
9. Imaizumi H, Takeday M. Knobby-like choroidal neovascularization accompanied with retinal pigment epithelial detachment. Nippon Ganka Gakkai Zasshi. 1999;103:527-37.
10. Hou J, Tao Y, Li XX, et al. Clinical characteristics of polypoidal choroidal vasculopathy in Chinese patients. Graefes Arch Clin Exp Ophthalmol. 2011;249:975-9.
11. Spaide RF, Yannuzzi LA, Slakter JS. Indocyanine green videoangiography of idiopathic polypoidal choroidal vasculopathy. Retina. 1995;15:100-10.
12. Yannuzzi LA, Sorenson J, Spaide RF, Lipson B. Idiopathic polypoidal choroidal vasculopathy. Retina. 1990;10:1-8.
13. Coscas G, Yamashiro K, Coscas F, DeBenedetto U, Tsujikawa A, Miyake M, et al. Comparison of exudative age-related macular degeneration subtypes in Japanese

and French patients: multicenter diagnosis with multimodal imaging. Am J Ophthalmol. 2014;15:309-18.
14. Otsuji T, Tsumura A, Takahashi K, Sho K, Nagai Y, Fukuchi T, et al. Evaluation of cases of polypoidal choroidal vasculopathy showing classic choroidal neovascularization in their natural course. Nippon. Ganka Gakkai Zasshi. 2006;110:454-61.
15. Maruko I, Iida T, Saito M, Nagayama D. Combined cases of polypoidal choroidal vasculopathy and typical age-related macular degeneration. Graefe's Arch Clin Exp Ophthalmol. 2010;248:361-8.
16. Desmettre T, Devoisselle JM, Mordon S. Fluorescence properties and metabolic features of indocyanine green (ICG) as related to angiography. Surv Ophthalmol. 2000;45:15-27.
17. Koh AK. On behalf of The expert PCV panel. Polypoidal choroidal vasculopathy-Evidence based guidelines for clinical diagnosis and treatment. Retina. 2013;33: 686-716.
18. Tan CSH, Ngo WK, Lim LW, Lim TH. A novel classification of the vascular patterns of polypoidal choroidal vasculopathy and its relation to clinical outcomes. Br J Ophthalmol. 2014;98:1528-33.
19. Yuzawa M, Mori R, Kawamura A. The origins of polypoidal choroidal vasculopathy. Br J Ophthalmol. 2005;89:602-7.
20. Kang SW, Chung SE, Shin WJ, Lee JH. Polypoidal choroidal vasculopathy and late geographic hyperfluorescence on indocyanine green angiography. Br J Ophthalmol. 2009;93:759-64.
21. Lijima H, Iida T, Imai M, Gohdo T, Tsukahara S. Optical coherence tomography of orange-red subretinal lesions in eyes with idiopathic polypoidal choroidal vasculopathy. Am J ophthalmol. 2000;129:21-6.
22. Sato T, Kishi S, Watanabe G, et al. Tomographic features of branching vascular networks in polypoidal choroidal vasculopathy. Retina. 2007;27: 589-94.
23. Ozawa S, Ishikawa K, Ito Y, Nishihara H, Yamakoshi T, Hatta Y, et al. Differences in macular morphology between polypoidal choroidal vasculopathy and exudative macular degeneration detected by optical coherence tomography. Retina. 2009;29: 793-802.
24. Chung SE, Kang SW, Lee JH, Kim YT. Choroidal thickness in polypoidal choroidal vasculopathy and exudative age related macular degeneration. Ophthalmology. 2011;118:840-5.
25. Jirarattanasopa P, Ooto S, Nakata I, Tsujikawa A, Yamashiro K, Oishi A, et al. Choroidal thickness, vascular hyperpermeability, and complement factor H in age related macular degeneration and polypoidal choroidal vasculopathy. Invest ophthalmol. 2012;53:3663-72.
26. Agarwal R, Gupta P, Tan KA, Cheung CM, Wong TY, Cheng CY. Choroidal vascularity index as a measure of vascular status of the choroid: Measurements in healthy eyes from a population-based study. Sci Rep. 2016;12:6.
27. Chung SE, Kang SW, Kim JH, Kim YT, Park Do Y. Engorgement of vortex vein and polypoidal choroidal vasculopathy. Retina. 2013;33:834-40.
28. Saito M, Iida T, Nagayama D. Cross sectional and enface optical coherence tomographic features of polypoidal choroidal vasculopathy. Retina. 2008;28:459-64.
29. Srour M, Querques G, Semoun O, El Ameen A, Miere A, Sikorav A, et al. Optical coherence tomography angiography characteristics of polypoidal choroidal vasculopathy. Br J Ophthalmol. 2016; Epub: bjophthalmol-2015-307892.
30. Yamagishi T, Koizumi H, Yamazaki T, Kinoshita S. Changes in fundus autofluorescence after treatments for polypoidal choroidal vasculopathy. Br J Ophthalmol. 2014;98: 780-4.

31. Japanese Study Group of Polypoidal Choroidal Vasculopathy. Criteria for diagnosis of polypoidal choroidal vasculopathy. Nippon Gangka Gakkai Zasshi. 2005;109:417-27.
32. Lee MW, Yeo I, Wong D, Ang CL. Argon laser photocoagulation for the treatment of polypoidal choroidal vasculopathy. Eye (Lond). 2009;23(1):145-8.
33. Yuzawa M, Mori R, Haruyama M. A study of laser photocoagulation for polypoidal choroidal vasculopathy. Jpn J Ophthalmol. 2003;47:379-84.
34. Wong RL, Lai TY. Polypoidal choroidal vasculopathy: an update on therapeutic approaches. J Ophthalmic Vis Res. 2013;8:359-71.
35. Hirami Y, Tsujikawa A, Otani A, Yodoi Y, Aikawa H, Mandai M, et al. Hemorrhagic complications after photodynamic therapy for polypoidal choroidal vasculopathy. Retina. 2007;27:335-41.
36. Fan NW, Lau LI, Chen SJ, Yang CS, Lee FL. Comparison of the effect of reduced-fluence photodynamic therapy with intravitreal bevacizumab and standard-fluence alone for polypoidal choroidal vasculopathy. J Chin Med Assoc. JCMA. 2014;77:101-7.
37. Inoue M, Arakawa A, Yamane S, Kadonosono K. Long-term outcome of intravitreal Ranibizumab treatment compared to photodynamic therapy in eyes with polypoidal choroidal vasculopathy. Eye (Lond). 2013;27:1013-20.
38. Koh A, Lee WK, Chen LJ, et al. EVEREST study: efficacy and safety of verteporfin photodynamic therapy in combination with ranibizumab or alone versus ranibizumab monotherapy in patients with symptomatic macular polypoidal choroidal vasculopathy. Retina. 2012;32:1453-64.
39. Wong CW, Cheung CM, Mathur R, Li X, Chan CM, Yeo I, et al. Three-year results of polypoidal choroidal vasculopathy treated with photodynamic therapy: retrospective study and systematic review. Retina. 2015;35:1577-93.
40. Yoshida Y, Kohno T, Yamamoto M, Yoneda T, Iwami H, Shiraki K. Two-year results of reduced-fluence photodynamic therapy combined with intravitreal ranibizumab for typical age-related macular degeneration and polypoidal choroidal vasculopathy. Jpn J Ophthalmol. 2013;57:283-93.
41. Oishi A, Tsujikawa A, Yamashiro K, Ooto S, Tamura H, Nakanishi H, et al. Comparison of the effect of ranibizumab and verteporfin for polypoidal choroidal vasculopathy: 12-month LAPTOP study results. Am J Ophthalmol. 2013;156: 644-51.
42. Visual Outcome in Patients with Symptomatic Macular PCV Treated with Either Ranibizumab as Monotherapy or Combined with Verteporfin Photodynamic Therapy. (EVEREST II). Retrieved August 22, 2014, from https:// clinicaltrials.gov/ct2/show/NCT01846273.
43. Aflibercept in Polypoidal Choroidal Vasculopathy (PLANET). Retrieved August 22, 2014, from https://clinicaltrials.gov/ct2/show/NCT02120950.
44. Cho HJ, Kim KM, Kim HS, Han JI, Kim CG, Lee TG, et al. Intravitreal aflibercept and ranibizumab injections for polypoidal choroidal vasculopathy. Am J Ophthalmol. 2016;165:1-6.
45. Bernstein PS, Horn RS. Verteporfin photodynamic therapy involving the optic nerve for peripapillary choroidal neovascularization. Retina. 2008;28:81-4.
46. Suzuki M, Nagai N, Shinoda H, Uchida A, Kurihara T, Tomita Y, et al. Distinc responsiveness to intravitreal Ranibizumab therapy in Polypoidal choroidal vasculopathy with single or mutliple polyps. Am J Ophthalmol. 2016;166:52-9.
47. Uyama M, Wada M, Nagai Y, et al. Polypoidal choroidal vasculopathy: natural history. Am J Ophthalmol. 2002;133:639-48.
48. Kim H, Lee SC, Kwon KY, Lee JH, Koh HJ, Byeon SH, et al. Subfoveal choroidal thickness as a predictor of treatment response to anti-vascular endothelial growth factor therapy for polypoidal choroidal vasculopathy. Graefes Arch Clin Exp Ophthalmol. 2015;254(8):1497-503.

49. Ma L, Li Z, Liu K, Rong SS, Brelen ME, Young AL, et al. Association of Genetic Variants with Polypoidal Choroidal Vasculopathy: A Systemic Review and Updated Meta-analysis. Ophthalmology. 2015;122(9):1854-65.
50. Liu K, Chen LJ, Lai TY, Tam PO, Ho M, Chiang SW, et al. Genes in the high-density lipoprotein metabolic pathway in age-related macular degeneration and polypoidal choroidal vasculopathy. Ophthalmology. 2014;121:911-6.
51. Nakata I, Yamashiro K, Yamada R, Gotoh N, Nakanishi H, Hayashi H, et al. Genetic variants in pigment epithelium-derived factor influence response of polypoidal choroidal vasculopathy to photodynamic therapy. Ophthalmology. 2011;118:1408-15.
52. Nakata I, Yamashiro K, Kawaguchi T, Gotoh N, Nakanishi H, Akagi-Kurashige Y, et al. Association between the cholesteryl ester transfer protein gene and polypoidal choroidal vasculopathy. Invest Ophthalmol Vis Sci. 2013;54:6068e6073.
53. Zhang X, Li M, Wen F, Zuo C, et al. Different impact of high-density lipoprotein-related genetic variants on polypoidal choroidal vasculopathy and neovascular age-related macular degeneration in a Chinese Han population. Exp Eye Res. 2013;108:16-22.
54. Chen H, Liu K, Chen LJ, Hou P, Chen P, Pang CP. Genetic associations in polypoidal choroidal vasculopathy: a systematic review and metaanalysis. Mol Vis. 2012; 18:816-29.
55. Tsuchihashi T, Mori K, Horie-Inoue K, Okazaki Y, Awata T, Inoue S, et al. Prognostic phenotypic and genotypic factors associated with photodynamic therapy response in patients with age-related macular degeneration. Clin Ophthalmol. 2014;8: 2471-78.
56. Park DH, Kim IT. LOC387715/HTRA1 variants and the response to combined photodynamic therapy with intravitreal bevacizumab for polypoidal choroidal vasculopathy. Retina 2012;32(2):299-307.
57. Yoneyama S, Sakurada Y, Kikushima W, Sugiyama A, Tanabe N, Mabuchi F, et al. Genetic factors associated with choroidal vascular hyperpermeability and subfoveal choroidal thickness in polypoidal choroidal vasculopathy. Retina. 2016;38(8): 1535-41.

Chapter 14

Macular Phototoxicity

Dhananjay Shukla

INTRODUCTION

While the primary function of eyes is to perceive the light produced or reflected from the material world we "see;" more the light is certainly not the merrier for the vision. In fact, suboptimal light is way better than supraoptimal light in terms of comfortable visibility and safety. Too bright a light, when seen for too long, can permanently damage the ocular media and retina. The "too bright" is defined by two parameters: intensity of the light and duration of the ocular exposure.[1] An extremely bright flash of light can vaporize the target ocular tissue in the fraction of a second, such damage is called *photomechanical injury*, e.g. accidental exposure to industrial or military Q-switched lasers (this effect is also used therapeutically in posterior capsulotomy by Nd:YAG laser).[1-2] These acute and severe injuries usually have a clear cut cause, and are fortunately rare. Subacute light injuries occur over a longer exposure, usually in seconds, and cause retinal burn by raising the tissue temperature to about 10–20°C.[1-2] The classic examples of *photothermal injuries* are retinal photocoagulation (intentional or accidental, depending on the target area) or laser pointer injuries by staring into the pointer. Though more common than photomechanical accidents, they are also relatively rare.[1,3] The most common, and insidious light injuries are those caused by long-term exposure to light at intensity considered safe for a brief duration. These are *photochemical injuries* (also called *phototoxic* or simply, *photic* injuries), and cause subtle but cumulative damage, which therefore goes undetected, unreported and underdiagnosed to a large extent.[1-3] Further, while the photic damage to the transmission media is reversible or manageable to a large extent, retinal phototoxicity tends to be permanent and irreversible. This review therefore focuses on the retinal photic injuries, and elaborates on the key offenders in the visible spectrum, the hazardous environmental settings, the risk factors, the early diagnostic signs and the preventive measures.

Photochemical Injuries: Pathogenetic Mechanism

Photochemical toxic reactions occur at temperatures too low to cause thermal burns (so it is technically wrong to call the resultant skin or retinal lesions as *sunburns* or eclipse *burns*), at light brightness above the normal physiological levels, and exposure times in seconds to minutes.[1,3] The injury occurs only when the above parameters of light exposure are so excessive that they overwhelm the retinal repair mechanisms. The extent of damage is influenced by coexistent ocular disease, clarity of crystalline lens, the subject's age, diet and body temperature (fever *primes* retina for the low-intensity burns) as well as systemic intake of certain photosensitizing drugs (see below).[1-3]

Phototoxicity is mediated through free radical release when the energy in the photons of the incident light excites the atoms of the substrate tissue, damaging the cell membranes, proteins, and nucleic acids. The higher the energy in photons, the more is the photochemical damage.[2] As the lower wavelengths of light have greater energy, they are more phototoxic. Very low to low wavelengths (UV-A and UV-B, violet) are absorbed to a large extent by the cornea and crystalline lens.[1,4,5] The prominent type of photochemical injury is therefore also referred to as *blue-light hazard*. The substrate for blue light absorption is retinal pigment epithelium (RPE), specifically, the lipofuscin pigment. The toxicity develops over 1–2 days.[1,2,4] To a lesser extent, slightly higher wavelength (500 nm, blue-green) can also directly damage the photoreceptors, mainly rods. This type of damage requires repetitive exposure over several days.[2-5]

Agents of Phototoxicity

Sunlight and Welding Arc

Looking up at the sun momentarily, even on a sunny day, is unlikely to cause retinal damage due to instinctive aversion of gaze and pupillary constriction, which limit both the retinal exposure and heating.[1] However, sun worshippers (a centuries old practice indeed, cutting across religions) who erroneously believed that *sun-gazing* was good for their eyes, and practiced it every day for several years. All these subjects had significant RPE mottling with corresponding visual decline (which they refused to admit). A similar picture has been reported in psychiatric patients and addicts with altered consciousness due to hallucinogenic drugs.[6,7] A more common presentation in saner, general population is observed after watching a solar eclipse, where the damage is enhanced by a greater pupillary dilatation and ability to watch the darkened sun for a longer period. The typical acute lesion is a subtle yellow white foveolar spot (Figs 14.1A and B), which could be missed unless looked for.[8] The lesion may fades away over a few months, generally leaving no clinical traces or subtle RPE mottling. The children are more vulnerable to damage due to their clear lenses (which allow more short wavelengths) and lack of awareness.[8,9] An important aspect in diagnosis is proactive history taking about solar exposure, which the patient may dismiss as insignificant, especially in chronic solar retinopathy with mild-moderate visual symptoms (blurred vision, central scotoma).[10] Reflection of bright sunlight from large surfaces like lakes and snow-covered landscapes can also predispose mountain trekkers and skiers to chronic indirect solar retinopathy.[4,11]

Welders experience both acute painful corneal erosions (photophthalmia) and chronic photic injuries from the occupational exposure to near UV wavelengths in welding arc light (CJO). The chronic injuries are probably very common, and largely underreported globally,[12] most pertinently in India, where it is common to see welders not wearing protective glasses (Figs 14.2A and B). The younger (<30 years) welding apprentices are more vulnerable due to the clear lens permitting more UV-A light.[4,12] The fundus picture is similar to solar retinopathy in both acute and chronic stages.[1,4,12]

Phototoxicity from Microscope, Endoilluminators and Ambient Light

Improved brighter lighting during intraocular surgery has improved surgical outcomes; but ironically has also increased the scope of retinal phototoxicity.[1]

Macular Phototoxicity

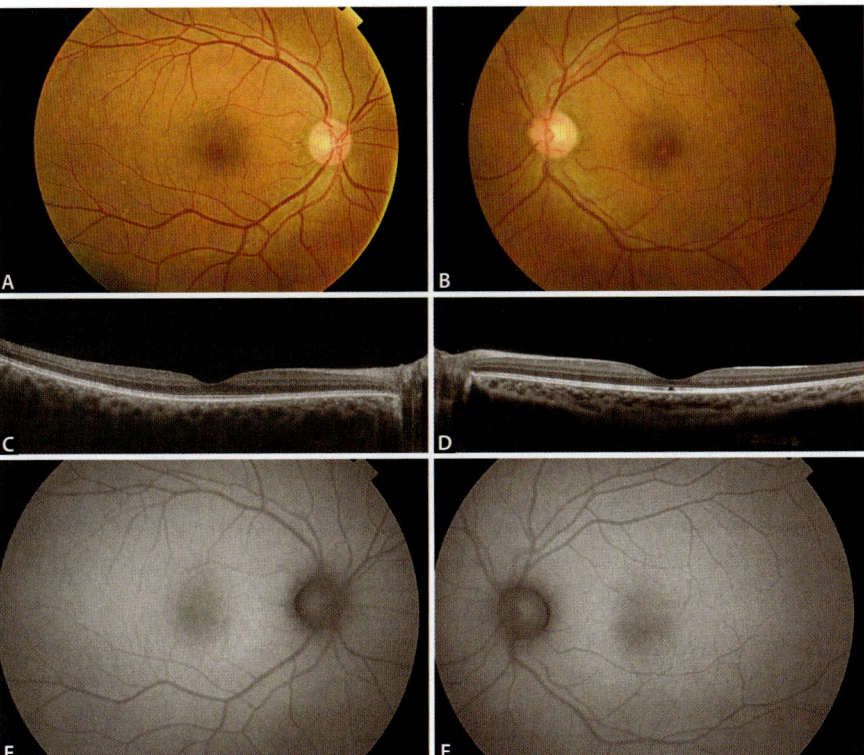

Figs 14.1A to F: This 62-year-old physician accidentally noted distorted and subnormal vision in his left eye a week back. Best-corrected visual acuity was 6/6 in the right eye and 6/18 in the left. On asking a leading question, he confessed to having seen an eclipse several years back, squinting with his right eye. (A) Right fundus showed only a few drusen; (B) while the left fovea had a central depigmented spot; (C) Spectral domain optical coherence tomography (SD-OCT, grid view) showed a normal foveal contour in the right eye; (D) SD-OCT of the left eye (cross line) revealed a disruption of the outer retinal lines corresponding to the ellipsoid zone and the interdigitation zones (see text for details); the external limiting membrane was intact. Central foveal thickness was reduced to 143 microns (normal range: 220-260 microns approximately); (E) Fundus autofluorescence imaging was normal in the right eye; (F) Left showed a central speck of increased hypoautofluorescence, with hyperautofluorescent parafoveal area

The spectral components of white light (blue, green and yellow) which are most helpful for tissue identification by the surgeon are also unfortunately most damaging to the retina of the eye under scalpel.[13] Light injuries have been reported after cataract, glaucoma, corneal and retinal surgeries. The latter two are more vulnerable due to longer duration (>30 minutes).[1] Cataract surgery, however is the one most commonly performed, and when accidentally or inherently complicated and therefore longer (e.g. trans-scleral fixation of PCIOL), can result in phototoxicity in close to 10% of cases, with adverse visual outcomes in half the subjects.[14] Retinal surgeries are however, inherently vulnerable due to use of endoscopic lights. This concern is more relevant now with use of small-gauge endoilluminators, which require double the power in light source as compared to 20G endo-lights.[13] The risk is further increased in macular surgeries, use of dyes (especially Indocyanine green), immobile chandeliers (which do not allow

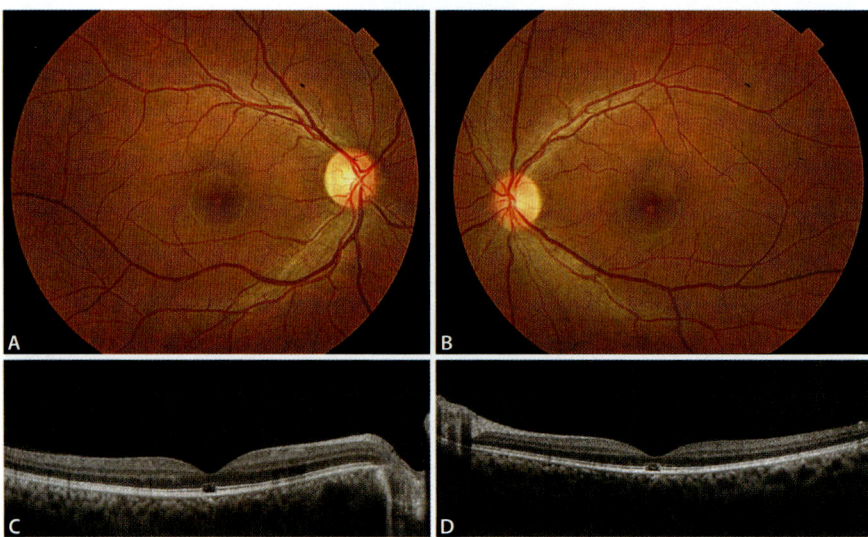

Figs 14.2A to D: This 30-year-old man has been a welder for more than 10 years, and has been stoically living with a best-corrected Snellen visual acuity of 6/18 in both eyes. (A and B) Fundi revealed a central identical pale spot at fovea in both eyes; (C and D) SD-OCT revealed disruption of the outer retinal lines corresponding to the ellipsoid and interdigitation zones; the external limiting membrane was intact in both eyes. Central foveal thickness was subnormal in both right (171 microns) and left eyes (163 microns).

retinal recovery from constant exposure), surgical video making (which multiply the light requirement) and trainee surgeons taking more time in surgery.[13,15]

Though less common, such damage can also follow prolonged exposure to fundus camera, indirect ophthalmoscope, and imaging devices. This should be remembered especially during examination of vulnerable eyes.[1] The light-emitting diodes (LED), which are fast becoming the preferred source of domestic lighting, emit much more blue light than the conventional lamps. An experimental study reported photochemical damage from the "white light" LED designs in albino rats and recommended further investigation on pigmented human retina.[16] Cases of macular phototoxicity of macula due to excessive, continued exposure to a video gaming device or computer screen, which are known to emit blue light from LED screens have been documented (unpublished data).

Factors Affecting Vulnerability to Phototoxicity

Aging
Ocular media, mainly the cornea and the lens, are the most important protectors against photic injuries. The protection by cornea against UV light remains uniform throughout life, while the crystalline lens becomes more protective as the age advances. We have already seen how welders above the age of 30 years are more protected from the UV light of welding arc. With further yellowing of the aging lens, it starts blocking the visible blue light too, which remains a threat through life. This protection is partly offset by the accumulation of lipofuscin pigment in RPE which increases phototoxic vulnerability.[1,3] Cataract surgery therefore has the potential to increase the retinal exposure to blue light, besides the potential

for intraoperative phototoxicity. There has been a prolonged debate on the use of UV- or blue-blocking intraocular lenses (IOLs) to mimic the protection of the aging lens.[1,17] On the other hand, blue-blocking IOLs have been accused of disturbing the circadian rhythm and quality of sleep of the elderly.[18] These fears have been put to rest by recent trials;[19] there are however insufficient data to show tangible benefits of these IOLs either, particularly in terms of phototoxic damage resulting in age related macular degeneration (AMD).[20]

Retinal Disease
Like aging, the diseases that result in lipofuscin accumulation in the RPE, such as best disease and Stargardt's disease, make the retina more susceptible to light damage. Other diseases that affect the photo-pigment regeneration, like retinitis pigmentosa, have also shown the potential for photic damage in animals though this potential is so far unproven in human subjects.[3] On the other hand, the role of cumulative phototoxic damage by short wavelengths, in the causation of AMD has been discussed and debated for close to a century.[1] Though a large body of experimental evidence is available in favor of this causative link, it remains unproven till date.[1]

Diet, Supplements and Drugs
Retina being the most metabolically active tissue in the body, is highly vulnerable to oxidative injury.[21] An antioxidant rich diet has been proposed to make the retina resistant to light damage;[22] however the modern diet is woefully deficient in macular carotenoids lutein and zeaxanthin, which could easily be provided by a diet rich in fruits and vegetables.[21]

Photosensitizing drugs are typically composed of tricyclic, heterocyclic or porphyrin rings, which allow them to bind to melanin in the RPE, and make ordinarily harmless visible light (400–600 nm) phototoxic.[23] In view of the vast range of pharmacotherapeutic drugs, including antibiotics (e.g. tetracycline), antimalarials (e.g. hydroxychloroquine) psychoactive drugs (benzodiazepines), antiarrhythmic drugs (amiodarone), diuretics (furosemide, hydrochlorothiazide), NSAIDs (indomethacin) and even herbal supplements (St John's wort), the incidence of drug-induced phototoxicity appears to be grossly under-reported.[1,3,23]

Diagnosis of Acute and Chronic Macular Phototoxicity
Irrespective of the cause, the most common retinal lesion is a faint yellow dot at central macula in most cases of acute phototoxicity (Figs 14.1B, 14.2A and B); a more dramatic blanching of retina has been described, but rare.[1] The most important diagnostic clue is an exposure to a source of bright light immediately preceding the drop in vision. If the intensity of the exposure does not appear to match the severity of the macular lesion, it is instructive to look at the systemic status (febrile illness, diabetes, and hypertension), use of photosensitizing drugs, and associated intraocular disease (heredomacular degenerations).[1,3,23] Associated photokeratitis (as in welding arc exposure) is a simple giveaway.[1,12] The lesion fades quickly, leaving no footprints or a faint RPE stippling, and partial or complete visual recovery. Subacute and chronic cases are therefore much more difficult to diagnose: the fundus may look normal, the visual complaint vague and non-specific, and the patient may not remember the exposure (e.g., looking at an eclipse).[10,11] In this scenario, leading questions must be asked about the

occupation (welder, mountaineer, sun-worshipper) and residence (mountains, cold regions), besides the usual suspects.

The key investigation, especially in the more obscure chronic cases, is spectral domain optical coherence tomography (SD-OCT). Previous versions of OCT are unable to demonstrate the finer details in the outer retina that characterize photic retinopathy.[11] In the acute phase, OCT shows a central triangular or vertical zone of hyperreflectivity in the outer nuclear layer,[24,25] with or without the interruption of the bright lines corresponding to the inner segment-outer segment junction (IS-OS junction, now called *ellipsoid zone*) of photoreceptors (cones), and their apices (COST line or Verhoeff's line, now called *Interdigitation zone*).[24,26] The chronic picture however characteristically shows an interruption of the outer retinal lines (the interdigitation and the ellipsoid zones) with intact external limiting membrane, with or without the central foveal thinning/atrophy (Figs 14.1C and D, 14.2C and D).[24]

The OCT findings are well supplemented by the fundus autofluorescence (FAF) imaging, which reveals the loss of the characteristic hypo-autofluoroscent signal at central fovea in the acute phase.[10,24,25] After a few months, FAF shows recovery of the normal central hypo- signal. In some cases with recurrent photic insults (e.g., welders), the spot corresponding to outer retinal interruption develops accentuated punctate hypo-autofluorescence (typically, but not universally at the central fovea), while the surrounding region shows hyperautofluorescence (Figs 14.1E and F).[10,11,24] Multiple hypo- signals can be found scattered around fovea in some chronic cases.[11] Fluorescein angiography is a less informative investigation, which reveals nothing in subtle cases; window defects occur only at the stage where clinical RPE stippling is anyway clinically evident.[27]

In conclusion, SD-OCT is the key investigation in acute and chronic, proven or suspected photic retinopathy, particularly that secondary to chronic recurrent exposure, like solar and welding arc retinopathy. The outer retinal findings, while characteristic, are not pathognomonic of photochemical damage, and could be mimicked by type 2 macular telangiectasia, maculopathy due to tamoxifen (early changes in vitreomacular traction and postoperative images of a closing macular hole.[28] Some of the mimics can be ruled out by history alone (tamoxifen use, macular hole surgery), others by additional OCT findings in the affected and fellow eye (macular telangiectasia and vitreomacular traction), or by additional investigations like fluorescein angiography and FAF imaging (macular hole and telangiectasia).[28]

The General Assembly of the United Nations proclaimed 2015 as the *International Year of Light and Light-based Technologies*.[29] It's therefore high time for us to review the effect of light on the eyes. In the modern times, young women are rightly conscious of the sun-tan and sunburn, and often take protective measures. We however remain woefully ignorant of the several ways light can damage the eyes, where the most insidious and permanent damage is often at the retinal level. The threat of chronic phototoxicity has ironically become more real and relevant today in spite of reduced outdoor activities, due to increasing exposure of children and young adults (with clear lenses, and therefore more vulnerable retina) to LED light of electronic media, as well as domestic bulbs, the duration of exposure further increased by our greater life expectancy.[16,29] Marshall has poetically labeled the global light levels as approaching what could be described as *Light Pollution*.[29] While waiting for technological improvements in these devices to make them safer, it is wise to recognize and limit exposure to the blue-light sources; even though a recent review absolves the current electronic media (TV, computers, tablets and smartphones) and LED lights of the blame for phototoxicity.[30] On the other hand, outdoor workers in general, and mountain trekkers and welders in particular, need to be educated about the hazards of chronic and repetitive exposure to reflected sunlight and the welding arc, and the imperative need for protective eye gear in hazardous occupations.[1-4,11,12,16] Acceptable levels of light exposures need to be defined by regulatory authorities, esp. in India, where laborers toil away in largely unprotected environment, both physically and legally.[3,11] UV protecting sunglasses esp. for individuals with fever, on photosensitizing drugs, diabetes and hypertension, and after cataract surgery offer a reasonable protection.[1] As eye surgeons, we ourselves should exercise precautions like minimal lighting compatible with comfortable intraocular surgery, avoiding routine oxygen intubation, and checking out sensitizing drugs, etc. preoperatively.[1,13,20,23] While we march towards a digital age in a technology-savvy India, prudent use of safety measures and precautions inside and outside our homes shall allow us to enjoy the comforts of modern life without getting burnt by the very light that illuminates and nurtures our lives.

REFERENCES

1. Mainster MA, Turner PL. Photic retinal injuries: *Mechanisms, Hazards, and Prevention*, 5th (Edn). In: Ryan SJ (Ed.). *Retina*. Elsevier: St. Louis. 2013;2:1551-63.
2. Wu J, Seregard S, Algvere PV. Photochemical damage of the retina. Surv Ophthalmol. 2006;51:461-81.
3. Hunter JJ, Morgan JI, Merigan WH, Sliney DH, Sparrow JR, Williams DR. The susceptibility of the retina to photochemical damage from visible light. Prog Retin Eye Res. 2012;31:28-42.
4. Söderberg PG. Optical radiation and the eyes with special emphasis on children. Prog Biophys Mol Biol. 2011;107:389-9.
5. Youssef PN, Sheibani N, Albert DM. Retinal light toxicity. Eye. 2011;25:1-14.
6. Kamp PS, Dietrich AM, Rosse RB. Sun gazing by psychiatric patients. Am J Psychiatry. 1990;147:810-1.
7. Schatz H, Mendelblatt F. Solar retinopathy from sun-gazing under the influence of LSD. Br J Ophthalmol. 1973;57:270-3.
8. Khatib N, Knyazer B, Lifshitz T, Levy J. Acute eclipse retinopathy: a small case series. J Optom. 2014;7:225-8.
9. Gregory-Roberts E, Chen Y, Harper CA, Ong T, Maclean MA, Fagan XJ, et al. Solar retinopathy in children. J AAPOS. 2015;19:349-51.
10. dell'Omo R, Konstantopoulou K, Wong R, Pavesio C. Presumed idiopathic outer lamellar defects of the fovea and chronic solar retinopathy: an OCT and fundus autofluorescence study. Br J Ophthalmol. 2009;93:1483-7.
11. Shukla D. Optical coherence tomography and autofluorescence findings in chronic phototoxic maculopathy secondary to snow-reflected solar radiation. Indian J Ophthalmol. 2015;63:455-7.
12. Yang X, Shao D, Ding X, Liang X, Yang J, Li J. Chronic phototoxic maculopathy caused by welding arc in occupational welders. Can J Ophthalmol. 2012;47:45-50.
13. Charles S. Illumination and phototoxicity issues in vitreoretinal surgery. Retina 2008;28:1-4.
14. Kweon EY, Ahn M, Lee DW, You IC, Kim MJ, Cho NC. Operating microscope light-induced phototoxic maculopathy after transscleral sutured posterior chamber intraocular lens implantation. Retina. 2009;29:1491-5.

15. Siu TL, Morley JW, Coroneo MT. Toxicology of the retina: advances in understanding the defence mechanisms and pathogenesis of drug- and light-induced retinopathy. Clin Experiment Ophthalmol. 2008;36:176-85.
16. Shang YM, Wang GS, Sliney D, Yang CH, Lee LL. White light–emitting diodes (LEDs) at domestic lighting levels and retinal injury in a rat model. Environ Health Perspect. 2014;122:269-76.
17. Mainster MA. Violet and blue light blocking intraocular lenses: photoprotection versus photoreception. Br J Ophthalmol. 2006;90:784-92.
18. Henderson BA, Grimes KJ. Blue-blocking IOLs: a complete review of the literature. Surv Ophthalmol. 2010;55:284-9.
19. Brøndsted AE, Sander B, Haargaard B, Lund-Andersen H, Jennum P, Gammeltoft S, et al. The Effect of Cataract Surgery on Circadian Photoentrainment: A Randomized Trial of Blue-Blocking versus Neutral Intraocular Lenses. Ophthalmology. 2015;122:2115-24.
20. Yang H, Afshari NA. The yellow intraocular lens and the natural ageing lens. Curr Opin Ophthalmol. 2014;25:40-3.
21. Hammond BR, Johnson BA, George ER. Oxidative photodegradation of ocular tissues: beneficial effects of filtering and exogenous antioxidants. Exp Eye Res. 2014;129:135-50.
22. Vaughan DK, Nemke JL, Fliesler SJ, Darrow RM, Organisciak DT. Evidence for a circadian rhythm of susceptibility to retinal light damage. Photochem Photobiol. 2002;75:547-53.
23. Siu TL, Morley JW, Coroneo MT. Toxicology of the retina: advances in understanding the defence mechanisms and pathogenesis of drug- and light-induced retinopathy. Clin Experiment Ophthalmol. 2008;36:176-85.
24. Shukla D, Sharan A, Venkatesh R. Optical coherence tomography and autofluorescence findings in photic maculopathy secondary to distant lightning strike. Arch Ophthalmol. 2012;130:656-8.
25. Bruè C, Mariotti C, De Franco E, Fisher Y, Guidotti JM, Giovannini A. Solar retinopathy: a multimodal analysis. Case Rep Ophthalmol Med. 2013;2013:906-20.
26. Staurenghi G, Sadda S, Chakravarthy U, Spaide RF. International Nomenclature for Optical Coherence Tomography (IN•OCT) Panel. Proposed lexicon for anatomic landmarks in normal posterior segment spectral-domain optical coherence tomography: the IN•OCT consensus. Ophthalmology. 2014;121:1572-8.
27. Jain A, Desai RU, Charalel RA, Quiram P, Yannuzzi L, Sarraf D. Solarretinopathy: comparison of optical coherence tomography (OCT) and fluorescein angiography (FA). Retina. 2009;29:1340-5.
28. Comander J, Gardiner M, Loewenstein J. High-resolution optical coherence tomography findings in solar maculopathy and the differential diagnosis of outer retinal holes. Am J Ophthalmol. 2011;152:413-9.
29. Marshall J. Light in man's environment. Eye. 2016;30:211-4.
30. O'Hagan JB, Khazova M, Price LL. Low-energy light bulbs, computers, tablets and the blue light hazard. Eye. 2016;30:230-3.

Chapter 15

Retinoblastoma

Fairooz P Manjandavida, Santosh G Honavar

INTRODUCTION

Retinoblastoma is the most common intraocular childhood malignancy that is completely curable if detected and treated early. Usually presenting in children at 18 to 36 months of age. Adult onset retinoblastoma is reported but rare. Retinoma or retinocytoma is considered the benign counterpart of retinoblastoma.[1]

The pathogenesis of retinoblastoma has been recently explained in terms of molecular genetics and stem cell biology. It is known to originate from the cells of neuroectodermal origin from the inner layer of the optic cup. The cell of origin of retinoblastoma is still debated. Earlier it was thought that retinoblastoma arises from the photoreceptors. They may have different cellular origin including retinal progenitor cells, cone precursor cells and rod precursor cells. It is also hypothesized that retinoblastoma arising from retinal progenitor cells possess higher grades of anaplasia than those arising from cone rod cell origin.[2]

Incidence of retinoblastoma has wide geographical variation, so is the survival and prognosis. It occurs in 1 in every 15,000 to 20,000 live births. The estimated number of new cases of retinoblastoma diagnosed globally is 7000–8000 each year.[3] Outcome of retinoblastoma is favorable in countries like USA, Europe, Australia, New Zealand and Japan, where mortality is <5%. In these countries, tremendous efforts are being made towards preserving vision with innovative treatments and also reducing treatment-related complications. In contrast, countries in Asia, Africa and South America where the reported mortality rate is as high as 20–60%, it is primarily a fight to save life.[4,5] It is estimated that 3000–3400 children die annually due to this eye cancer.[3,4]

GENETICS

Retinoblastoma gene (RB1 gene) is the first tumor suppressor gene to be identified. The genetics of retinoblastoma has been accepted as the prototype of numerous cancers in the human race. Two step biallelic inactivation of human retinoblastoma susceptibility gene, RB1 on chromosome 13q14 that codes for retinoblastoma protein represents the key event in the pathogenesis of retinoblastoma.[6,7] According to Knudson's two hit hypothesis, development of retinoblastoma requires mutation of both copies of RB1 gene. It is also found that retinoblastoma can arise from MYC mutation in the absence of RB1 mutation.[6] It was recently found that loss of both copies of RB1 may lead to retinoma, but further genomic instability leads to development of retinoma to retinoblastoma. It manifests as two forms, sporadic non-hereditary and familial hereditary due to somatic and germline mutations respectively.[8,9] In the non-hereditary form (60%), the mutation occurs at the cellular level during the development of retina leading to unilateral sporadic form often presenting late after the first year of life. In hereditary retinoblastoma (40%), one allele is mutated in the germline and the other at the cellular level. The heritable form of retinoblastoma often has an early onset presenting as bilateral, multiple tumors and is transmitted to successive generations in an autosomal dominant fashion.[6,10-12] Approximately 5-10% of patients have one or more affected member in the family. It also increases the risk of development of second non-ocular cancers namely osteosarcoma in the long bones of arms and legs and soft tissue sarcomas of head and neck. Furthermore, patients undergoing radiotherapy before 1 year of age are at higher risk of developing the tumor of the irradiated field. More profound and lethal is the occurrence of primitive neuroectodermal tumors (PNET) in the pineal gland—so called trilateral retinoblastoma.[13-14] The prognosis of pineoblastoma is invariably poor and children succumb to the disease. It is essential to identify the genetic mutation in retinoblastoma for modification of management and identifying the generation at risk at an early stage. Genetic counseling is as important as treating the disease in a broader perspective. Molecular testing of the family members at risk allows for prompt management and screening of the disease. In the recent past, many centers in the developed world has successfully introduced genetic testing as a part of retinoblastoma management.[11,13] The breakthrough research in the genetics of retinoblastoma was the recent availability of pre-implantation genetic diagnosis in combination with in-vitro fertilization.[15,16] Apart form the established genetic mechanism, epigenetics also plays a role in the development of retinoblastoma, and is being explored. Yet another mechanism, named parental gonadal mosaicism has been identified in children developing sporadic heritable retinoblastoma, and should be considered in suspected genetic disease with negative serum genetic analysis.[11,17,18]

CLASSIFICATION AND STAGING

The initial step in the management of retinoblastoma is categorizing the eyes depending on the clinical features to predict treatment success in terms of visual potential and eye salvage. The most popular classification proposed by Reese and Ellsworth in 1963, five decades ago was an initiative to predict globe salvage during the era of external beam radiotherapy, which is no more accurate in the contemporary era of chemoreduction and other advanced techniques.[19] The Essen classification in 1983 by Hopping tried to address the emerging newer treatment, but failed to be widely accepted.[20] Shields et al. evaluated the eyes undergoing chemoreduction using Reese-Ellsworth classification and showed erratic correlation with treatment success. Subsequently it paved the way for the newer classification of intraocular retinoblastoma.[21-23] The International Society of Retinoblastoma and Genetic Eye Disease in Paris (2003) formulated the current classification system—International Classification of Retinoblastoma (ICRB) that includes clinical grouping depending on the natural course and severity, emerging from the previous Philadelphia classification by Shields et al. and the Children's Hospital Los Angeles (CHLA) by Murphree et al.[23,24] (Table 15.1) Recently the vitreous seeds were morphologically classified as spherules, clouds and dusting.[25]

TABLE 15.1: International Grouping of Intraocular Retinoblastoma [22,24]

Group	Clinical features
Group A	Any tumor <3 mm in size
Group B	Any tumor >3 mm Any tumor with subretinal fluid Any tumor in macular location
Group C	Any tumor >3 mm in size, occupying <50% of the globe with focal subretinal and vitreous seeds
Group D	Any tumor >3 mm in size, occupying <50% of the globe with diffuse subretinal and vitreous seeds
Group E	Any tumor >50% of globe, diffuse infiltrating, secondary glaucoma, hyphema, anterior segment seeds, vitreous hemorrhage, aseptic orbital cellulitis, phthisis bulbi

The recent International Retinoblastoma Staging System by Chantada et al. is widely accepted and incorporates intraocular and extraocular disease under five distinct stages based on collective information on clinical evaluation, ocular imaging, histopathology and systemic survey (Table 15.2).[26] The staging system predicts life salvage and long-term survival. As in any other cancers, the TNM classification was applied to retinoblastoma by the International Union Against Cancer and modified in 2010. The TNM is further subclassified as clinical TNM and pathological TNM classification.[27]

CLINICAL FEATURES

The most common symptom of retinoblastoma is white reflex (Fig. 15.1). Others include squint (exotropia or esotropia), redness, pain and buphthalmos. In advanced stages with extraocular extension, children may present with proptosis or a protruding fungating mass. Ocular signs include white mass behind the

TABLE 15.2: International Staging System for Retinoblastoma [26]

Stage	Feature
Stage 0	No enucleation
Stage 1	Enucleation, tumor completely resected
Stage 2	Enucleation with microscopic residual tumor
Stage 3	Regional extension • Overt orbital disease • Pre auricular or cervical lymph node extension
Stage 4	Metastatic disease

	• Hematogenous metastasis
	  – Single lesion
	  – Multiple lesion
	• CNS Extension
	  – Pre-chiasmatic lesion
	  – CNS mass
	  – Leptomeningeal disease

lens. Clumps of tumors cells in the anterior chamber and hypopyon are seen with anterior segment extension. Diffuse anterior segment retinoblastoma is a rare entity without involvement of retina but only the anterior chamber. In the presence of secondary glaucoma, they may present with cloudy cornea, iris neovascularization, ectropion uveae and buphthalmos. Warning signs in RB include redness, buphthalmos, hyphema, hypopyon, iris neovascularization, vitreous hemorrhage, eyelid edema, proptosis and unexplained phthisis bulbi.

On detailed fundus evaluation, retinoblastoma appears as a yellowish white vascular retinal mass with associated calcification and subretinal fluid with dilated feeder vessels. It can be solitary or multiple. Sporadic retinoblastoma presents as solitary mass, whereas familial (germline) retinoblastoma is multifocal and bilateral. Tumor growth pattern incudes exophytic (tumor growing under the retina towards choroid associated with exudative retinal detachment), endophytic (tumor growing towards the vitreous), mixed (both exophytic and endophytic), diffuse infiltrating (grayish thickening of the retina) and anterior segment retinoblastoma (tumor involving the anterior segment structures with or without involvement of the peripheral retina). Subretinal seeds and vitreous seeds are frequent and these may be focal or diffuse.[1,2] Vitreous seeds are further morphologically classified as spherule, dust and cloud. The benign counterpart of retinoblastoma, retinoma/retinocytoma appears as regressed retinoblastoma, calcified or fleshy with surrounding choroidal atrophy and sheathing of vessels. The clinical differential diagnoses are Coats' disease, persistent fetal vasculature (PFV), vitreous hemorrhage, ocular toxocariasis, familial exudative vitreoretinopathy, coloboma, astrocytic hamartoma and endogenous endophthalmitis.[1,2]

DIAGNOSIS

Apart from clinical diagnosis, the most common diagnostic tool in confirming the diagnosis is B-scan ultrasonography showing a characteristic intraocular mass with calcification as indicated by high internal reflectivity.[28] Other modalities that give supporting information are fluorescein angiography, autofluorescence and optical coherence tomography.[29,30] Radiological imaging is indicated in identifying the extension of tumor outside the confines of the eyeball. Magnetic resonance imaging (MRI) is preferred over computerized tomography scan (CT scan) especially in patients of retinoblastoma with germline mutation.[31]

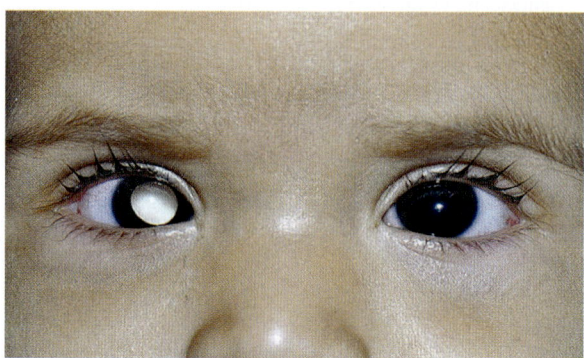

Fig. 15.1: The most common clinical feature is white reflex in retinoblastoma

MRI provides superior soft tissue details. The tumor characteristically appears hyperintense in T1 and hypointense in T2 whereas calcification remains markedly hypointense.[32] MRI is considered more valuable as compared to CT scan in detecting optic nerve invasion and intracranial extension. In addition, it also helps in screening and detecting midline lesions associated with trilateral retinoblastoma-pineoblastoma. It is wise to recommend yearly MRI in children harboring bilateral and or hereditary retinoblastoma at least up to 5 years of age. CT-scan of the orbit can confirm intraocular calcification and delineate extraocular extension.

MANAGEMENT

Untreated retinoblastoma is uniformly fatal. The primary goal remains life salvage. The secondary and tertiary goals are eye salvage and vision salvage respectively. Enucleation was considered the treatment of choice of retinoblastoma a century ago, and was replaced by more conservative external beam radiation with its well-recognized complications. Since the mid-1990s, the management of retinoblastoma has undergone a paradigm shift owing to better alternatives to save life, eye and vision.[33] The introduction of systemic intravenous chemotherapy was a breakthrough and to a larger extent has helped avoid enucleation in bilateral as well as unilateral retinoblastoma.[33,34] Chemotherapy alone is not curable, without additional focal treatment such as cryotherapy and transpupillary thermotherapy. The more localized and targeted treatment involves plaque brachytherapy. The most recent additions to the armamentarium are intraarterial and intravitreal chemotherapy.[35-38] In short, the management of retinoblastoma is highly individualized and requires a multidisciplinary team comprising trained ocular oncologist, oncopathologist, pediatric oncologist, radiation oncologist, interventional radiologist, neurosurgeon and a geneticist. The available management modalities are briefly outlined below.

- Chemotherapy
    - Systemic intravenous chemotherapy
    - Local
        - Intraarterial chemotherapy
        - Intravitreal chemotherapy
        - Periocular subtenon's chemotherapy
- Radiotherapy
    - Plaque brachytherapy
    - External beam radiotherapy
    - Proton beam radiotherapy
- Focal therapy
    - Cryotherapy
    - Laser transpupillary thermotherapy
- Enucleation (with orbital implant).

Chemotherapy

Systemic Intravenous Chemotherapy

The introduction of intravenous chemotherapy (IVC)–'chemoreduction' changed the outlook towards the dreadful childhood cancer, essentially increasing the survival rate and preserving the eye and vision. Chemoreduction reduces the size of the tumor and makes it amenable for focal treatment. IVC alone is not curative, but is used synergistically with intensive focal therapy with cryotherapy and laser treatment.[34,39,40]

Though there exist many protocols, the most widely accepted is the triple drug regimen consisting of vincristine (1.5 mg/m^2), etoposide (150 mg/m^2) and carboplatin (560 mg/m^2) for 6 cycles, given 3–4 weeks apart. With this current protocol of chemoreduction and sequential consolidation with focal therapy, most eyes are salvageable with functional vision with excellent life salvage. It was observed that there was 100%, 93% and 90% tumor control in group A, B and C eyes respectively.[34] The eye salvage was <50% in advanced group D and E eyes; however, use of high-dose IVC regimen with local delivery of subtenon's chemotherapy and low dose radiotherapy could still salvage about 83% of eyes (Figs 15.2A and B).[41]

IVC is safe if administered under the supervision and care of pediatric oncologist. Most commonly identified complications are reversible myelo-suppression, neurotoxicity, ototoxicity, and non-specific gastrointestinal toxicity. Apart from gaining control over the tumor, the major advantages of IVC lies in preventing the more devastating systemic micrometastasis, pineoblastoma and second malignant neoplasm.

Periocular Subtenon's Chemotherapy

The major disadvantage of IVC is the poor penetration of the chemotherapeutic agents into the vitreous and achieving higher drug concentration. Periocular chemotherapy was initially explored to achieve high drug concentration locally.[41] It is indicated in eyes with vitreous seeds. The drugs used are carboplatin (10 to 15 mg) and topotecan (1 to 2 mg). Most common complication is periocular edema and conjunctival scarring, and less common are extraocular muscle fibrosis and optic atrophy. Associated complications with topotecan are known to be less severe when compared to carboplatin and is therefore preferred.[41-45]

Intra-arterial Chemotherapy

Intra-arterial chemotherapy (IAC) is a targeted therapy of administering chemotherapeutic agent directly into the main blood vessel supplying the tumor.[36] IAC is currently used in many centers as the primary modality of treatment in advanced unilateral retinoblastoma. It is technologically challenging, requiring a highly skilled interventional radiologist or a neurosurgeon. The introduction of this

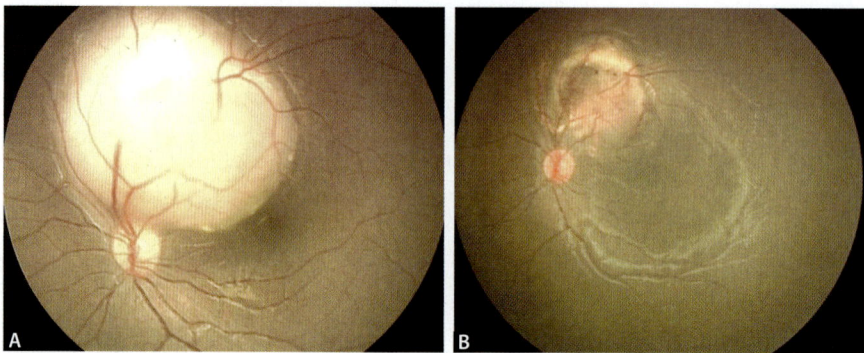

Figs 15.2A and B: Systemic intravenous chemotherapy in group B retinoblastoma. (A) Showing a macular tumor overlying the fovea; (B) Chemoreduction and consolidation with laser therapy spared the fovea with 20/20 vision post-treatment

technique dates back to 1955, when Reese and co-workers treated retinoblastoma with direct catheterization and infusion of triethylenemelamine into the internal carotid artery. Kaneko and Yamane developed a targeted approach of selective ophthalmic artery infusion (SOAI)—balloon occlusion technique using melphalan, in an effort to reduce complications.[46] But the authors failed to provide adequate data on tumor control and ocular complications. Abramson and Gobin further modified the technique into superselective ophthalmic artery infusion by directly entering the ophthalmic artery.[47] The drugs infused were topotecan, carboplatin and melphalan. It is emerging as the treatment of choice in unilateral advanced retinoblastoma (Figs 15.3A to D). The most common complications of IAC include periocular edema, mechanical ptosis and forehead hyperemia. Major complications of IAC are related to vascular toxicity and or occlusion of ophthalmic artery and retinal and choroidal vessels, leading to central retinal artery occlusion, choroid atrophy and vitreous hemorrhage.[36,48,49]

Intravitreal Chemotherapy

The outcome of advanced group D eyes with diffuse vitreous seeds remains a challenge, with high rate of recurrence and systemic chemotherapy failure, often requiring external beam radiotherapy. The globe salvage with EBRT is not more than 20–30%, offering suboptimal control of the disease with associated complications especially in children with the only seeing eye in heritable bilateral retinoblastoma. The direct delivery of chemotherapeutic agents into the vitreous cavity was assumed to provide adequate tumor control.[38,50,51] Inomata and

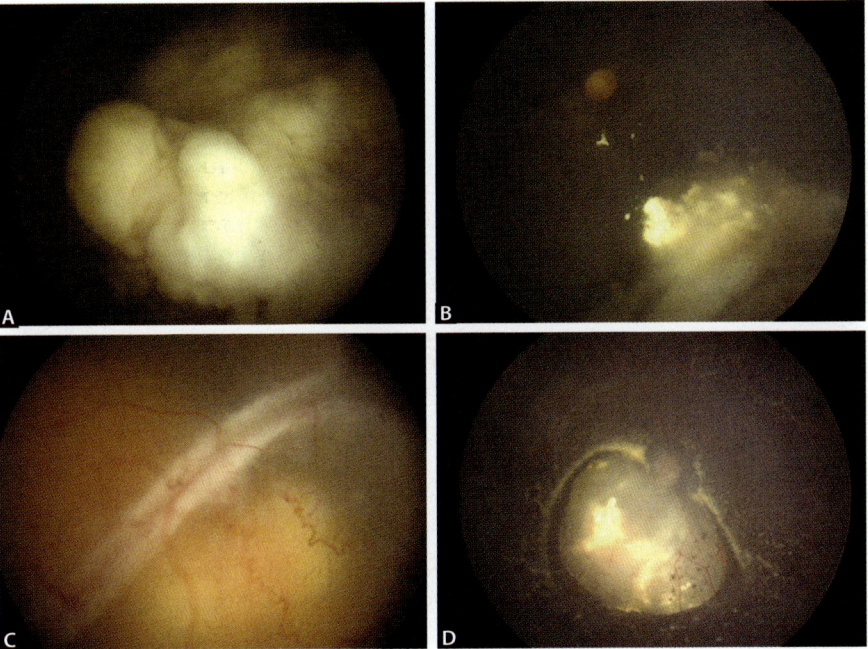

Figs 15.3A to D: Intra-arterial chemotherapy in advanced retinoblastoma. (A) A group D eye with diffuse vitreous seeds; (B) After 3 cycles of intra-arterial chemotherapy; (C) A group E eye with a very large tumor and diffuse subretinal fluid; (D) After 3 cycles of intra-arterial chemotherapy

Kaneko found melphalan to be the most effective and relatively less toxic agent intravitreally as supported by the in-vitro experiment in the rabbit model.[52] The most common chemotherapeutic drug used is melphalan, although topotecan is also found to provide equally encouraging results.[38,50,51] The only complication observed was salt and pepper retinopathy noticed in 43% of eyes due to localized toxicity at the site of injection.[52] The initial results are encouraging; however, the results of a prospective phase II trial are still awaited and the long-term local and systemic complications are unknown. It was also observed that eyes receiving 8–10 µg showed suboptimal response and higher doses of >50 µg led to phthisis bulbi.[53]

Radiotherapy

Plaque Brachytherapy

Focal application of radioactive device enables targeted treatment—delivery of radiation locally, and reducing ocular side effects. Plaque brachytherapy is the method of placing a radioactive plaque on the sclera corresponding to the base of the tumor and rendering trans-scleral irradiation to the tumor. Mostly commonly used radioactive materials are Iodine 125 and ruthenium 106. The main indication is recurrent or residual tumor following chemoreduction and focal treatment. Shields et al analyzed the outcome of plaque brachytherapy as a primary treatment (29%) and secondary treatment (79%). The average tumor size was 8 mm in basal diameter and 4 mm in thickness. The dosage delivered to the tumor apex ranges from 3500–4000 cGy, and mandates precise tumor localization and measurement of tumor dimensions for optimal treatment. The tumor control with Iodine 125 plaque brachytherapy has been reported as 95% at 5 years[37, 54]

External Beam Radiotherapy

The once popular modality is now less preferred owing to the short-term and long-term adverse effects. The most common complications include dry eye, radiation cataract, neovascular glaucoma, radiation retinopathy, and orbital and midfacial growth retardation. The most dreaded complication is the risk of development of second malignant neoplasm, especially in patients with hereditary forms of retinoblastoma and mostly radiation dose dependant.[55] The risk is as high as 50% in this group when compared to 6% in patients with non-heritable tumor. It is estimated that patients undergoing EBRT at <12 months of age are at greater risk when compared to those >12 months.[56]

Focal Therapy

These are focal techniques such as cryotherapy and laser treatment applied directly to the tumor either as a primary modality, but most often as adjunctive to chemoreduction for consolidation.[1,33]

Cryotherapy is effective in small equatorial and peripheral retinal tumors measuring up to 2 mm in thickness and 4 mm basal diameter. The cryoprobe is applied transclerally and classically triple freeze thaw protocol is used. Cryotherapy applied prior to chemotherapy has synergistic effect by increasing the delivery of chemotherapeutic agents across the blood retina barrier.[1,33,571]

Laser treatment plays a major role in tumor control. The use of diode laser transpupillary thermotherapy (TTT) is the most common and widely used technique with minimal complications. The focused heat generated by the infrared radiation is applied over the tumor at a sub-photocoagulation level to induce tumor cell apoptosis sparing damage to the retinal vessels. The laser is applied with a 1300-micron spot until the tumor turns subtle grey in color. This technique provides satisfactory control for small tumors with <2 mm in thickness. Multiple sessions are administered, until the tumor is reduced to a flat chorioretinal scar. Major advantage is its adjunctive role during chemoreduction, where the heat amplifies the cytotoxic effect of systemic carbopaltin—the term known as chemothermotherapy. The known complications are focal iris atrophy, peripheral lens opacification, retinal traction, retinal vascular obstruction and transient localized serous detachment.[58]

Enucleation

Despite the several advancements in the management of retinoblastoma as mentioned and discussed, enucleation is still considered the primary treatment of advanced retinoblastoma and is life-saving. In the last few decades, the frequency of enucleation has steadily decreased in favor of conservative modalities, and because of relatively early detection of tumors. It is not uncommon in the developing countries where >50% of children present with advanced retinoblastoma requiring primary enucleation.[59] The indication of enucleation are eyes belonging to group E, anterior chamber tumor seeding, neovascular glaucoma and hyphema, necrotic tumor with secondary orbital inflammation, and vitreous hemorrhage precluding visualization of the tumor. The technique requires modification to avoid the risk of accidental perforation and orbital tumor seeding. The preferred method is minimal manipulation enucleation with long optic nerve stump, ideally >15 mm. Placement of an orbital implant is advised in all children undergoing enucleation, primarily to stimulate orbital growth and thereby improving cosmesis and enable fitting a custom made prosthesis.[1,2]

Enucleation is not the end of retinoblastoma management and does not imply that the life is saved. The eyes undergoing enucleation may carry histopathological high-risk factors for systemic metastasis (Table 15.3). Histopathological high-risk factors in enucleated eyes are retrolaminar optic nerve invasion, choroidal invasion of 3 mm or greater, anterior segment invasion, any degree of optic nerve plus choroidal invasion, scleral invasion and extrascleral extension.[60,61] (Table 15.3) In the presence of high-risk features, patients undergo adjuvant chemotherapy to reduce the risk of systemic metastasis.

Multimodal treatment protocol is followed in advanced cases with orbital extension of intraocular tumor. It includes initial neoadjuvant chemotherapy, enucleation, followed by radiation and adjuvant chemotherapy. This has improved the survival in locally advanced disease (Figs 15.4A and B). Metastatic retinoblastoma has poor prognosis especially central nervous system metastasis and is the major cause of death in retinoblastoma.[62]

TABLE 15.3: Post-enucleation histopathological high-risk features in retinoblastoma[1,2,61]

Histopathological high-risk features
1. Postlaminar optic nerve invasion
2. Choroidal invasion ≥3mm in diameter or thickness
3. Anterior segment invasion
4. Any degree of optic nerve + choroidal invasion
5. Optic nerve transection involvement
6. Extrascleral extension

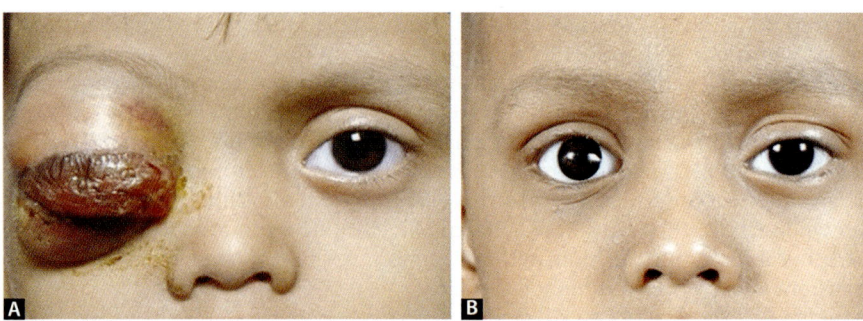

Figs 15.4A and B: Intensive multimodal treatment protocol in orbital retinoblastoma. (A) Right eye showing secondary orbital recurrence of retinoblastoma after enucleation; (B) After completion of high-dose neoadjuvant chemotherapy, followed by radiation and adjuvant chemotherapy, the tumor is seen to have completely regressed thereby preventing exenteration with optimal cosmesis and improved survival

CONCLUSION

To summarize, retinoblastoma is curable if recognized early and managed appropriately. The choice of chemotherapeutic agents and route of administration continue to evolve. However, the management varies from patient-to-patient, depending on the stage of the disease, availability of technical skills and optimal cost-effective therapeutic modalities. The art of management lies in early detection, selection of appropriate management strategy and long-term follow up to assess recurrence and treatment-related complications. Above all, it is the family whom we treat, not the patient alone.

REFERENCES

1. Ramasubramanian A, Shields CL. Epidemiology and magnitude of the problem. In: Ramasubramanian A, Shields CL (eds). Retinoblastoma. Jaypee Brothers Medical Publishers: New Delhi, India, 2012, pp. 10-15.
2. Grossniklaus HE. Retinoblastoma. Fifty years of progress. The LXXI Edward Jackson Memorial Lecture. Am J Ophthalmol. 2014;158(5):875-91.
3. Kivela T. The epidemiological challenge of the most frequent eye cancer: retinoblastoma, an issue of birth and death. Br J Ophthalmol. 2009;93:1129-31.
4. Dimaras H, Dimba EAO, Gallie BL. Challenging global retinoblastoma survival. Br J Ophthalmol. 2010;95:1451-2.
5. Chantada GL, Qaddoumi I, Cantruk S, et al. Strategies to manage retinoblastoma in developing countries. Pediatr Blood Cancer. 2011; 56:341-8.
6. Knudson AG. Mutation and cancer: statistical study of retinoblastoma. Proc Natl Acad Sci USA. 1971;68:820-3.
7. Friend SH, Bernards R, Rogelj S, et al. A human DNA segment with properties of the gene that predisposes to retinoblastoma and osteosarcoma. Nature.1986;323: 643-6.
8. Gianciati C, Giordiano A. RB and cell cycle progression. Oncogene. 2006;25:5220-7.
9. Dimaras H, Khetan V, Halliday W, et al. Loss of RB1 induces non-proliferative retinoma: increasing genomic instability correlates with progression to retinoblastoma. Hum Mol Genet. 2008;17(10):1363-72.

10. Ganguly A, Shileds CL. Differential gene expression profile of retinoblastoma compared to normal retina. Mol Vis. 2010;16:1292-303.
11. Chakraborthy S, Khare S, Dorairaj SK, et al. Identification of genes associated with tumorogenesis of retinoblastoma by microarray analysis. Genomics. 2007;90:344-53.
12. Reis AH, Vargas FR, Lemos B. More epigenetic hits than meets the eye: micro RNAs and genes associated with tumorigenesis of retinoblastoma. Front Genet 2012;3:284. 2102.00284. Epub 2012.
13. Lohman DR, Gallie BL. Retinoblastoma: revisiting the model prototype of inherited cancer. Am J Med Genet C Semin Med Genet. 2004;129:23-8.
14. Meadows AT, Leahey AM. More about second cancers after retinoblastoma. J Natl Cancer Inst. 2008;100:1743-5.
15. Gallie BL, Hei YJ, Dunn JM. Retinoblastoma treatment in premature infants diagnosed prenataly by the ultrasound and molecular diagnosis. Am J Hum Genet. suppl 65, A62.
16. Xu K, Rosenwaks Z, Beaverson K, et al. Preimplantation genetic diagnosis for retinoblastoma: the first reported live born. Am J Ophthalmol. 2004;137:18-23.
17. Murphree AL, Triche TJ. An epigenomic mechanism in retinoblastoma: the end of the story? Genome Med. 2012;4:15.
18. Livide G, Epistolato MC, Amenduni M, et al. Epigenetic and copy number variation analysis in retinoblastoma by MS- MLPA. Pathol Oncol Res. 2012;18:703-12.
19. Reese AB, Ellsworth RM. The evaluation and current concept of retinoblastoma therapy. Trans Am Acad Ophthalmol Otolaryngol. 1963;67:164-72.
20. Hopping W. The new Essen prognosis classification for conservative sight-saving treatment of retinoblastoma. In: Lommatzsch PK, Blodi FC (eds). Intraocular Tumors: International Symposium Under the Auspices of the European Ophthalmoloigcal Society. Berlin, Germany: Springer-Verlag; 1983. Pp. 497-505.
21. Shields CL, Mashayakhi A, Demirci H, et al. Practical approach to management of retinoblastoma. Arch Ophthalmol. 2004;122(5): 729-35.
22. Shields CL, Shields JA. Basic understanding of current classification and management of retinoblastoma. Curr Opin Ophthalmol. 2006;17:228-34.
23. Shields CL, Mashayakhi A, Au AK, et al. The International Classification of Retinoblastoma predicts chemoreduction success. Ophthalmology. 2006;113:276-80.
24. Murphree AL. Intraocular retinoblastoma: the case for a new group classification. Ophthalmol Clin North Am. 2005;18:41-53.
25. Munier FL. Classification and management of seeds in retinoblastoma. Ellsworth Lecture Ghent August 24th 2013. Ophthalmic Genet. 2014;35(4):193-207.
26. Chantada G, Doz F, Antoneli CB, et al. A proposal for an international retinoblastoma staging system. Pediatr Blood Cancer. 2006;47:801-5.
27. Edge SB, Byrd DR, Compton CC, Fritz AG, Greene FL, Trotti A. AJCC Cancer Staging Manual and Handbook, 7th (Edn). New York, NY: Springer. 2010:623-9.
28. Shields JA, Shields CL. Diagnostic approaches to Retinoblastoma. In: Intraocular Tumors. A Text and Atlas, Shields JA, Shields CL (Eds). WB Saunders: Philadelphia; 1992: 363-76; author reply-5.
29. Sony P, Garg SP. Optical coherence tomography in children with retinoblastoma. J Pediatr Ophthalmol Strabismus. 2005;42:134.
30. Bianciotto C, Shields CL, Iturralde JC, et al. Fluorescein angiographic findings after intra-arterial chemotherapy for retinoblastoma. Ophthalmology. 2012;119(4):843-9.
31. Pearce MS, Salotti JA, Little MP, et al. Radiation exposure from CT scans in childhood and subsequent risk of leukemia and brain tumours: a retrospective cohort study. Lancet. 2012;380:499-505.
32. De Potter, Shields CL, Shields JA, Flanders AE. The role of MR imaging in children with intraocular tumors and simulating lesions. Ophthalmology. 1996;103:1774-83.

33. Shields CL, Fulco EM, Arias JD, et al. Retinoblastoma frontiers with intravenous, intra-arterial, periocular, and intravitreal chemotherapy. Eye. 2012;27:253-64.
34. Shields JA, Shields CL, Meadows AT. Chemoreduction in the management of retinoblastoma. Am J Ophthalmol. 2005;140:505-6.
35. Abramson DH, Dunkel IJ, Brodie SE, et al. A phase I/II study of direct intra-arterial (ophthalmic artery) chemotherapy with melphalan for intraocular retinoblastoma initial results. Ophthalmology. 2008;115:1398-404.
36. Shields CL, Manjandavida FP, Lally SE, Pieretti G, Arepalli SA, Caywood EH, et al. Intra-arterial chemotherapy for retinoblastoma in 70 eyes: outcomes based on the international classification of retinoblastoma. Ophthalmology. 2014;121(7):1453-60.
37. Shields CL, Shields JA, Cater J, et al. Plaque radiotherapy for retinoblastoma, long term tumor control and treatment complications in 208 tumors. Ophthalmology. 2001;108:2116-21.
38. Munier F, Gaillard MC, Balmer A, et al. Intravitreal chemotherapy for vitreous disease in retinoblastoma revisited: from prohibition to conditional indications. Br J Ophthalmol. 2012;96:1078-83.
39. Leahey AM. Systemic chemotherapy: a pediatric oncology perspective. In: Ramasubramanian A, Shields CL (eds). Retinoblastoma. Jaypee Brothers Medical Publishers: New Delhi, India, 2012:81-5.
40. Gombos DS, Kelly A, Coen PG, et al. Retinoblastoma treated with primary chemotherapy alone: The significance of tumor size, location and age. Br J Ophthalmol. 2002;86:80-3.
41. Manjandavida FP, Honavar SG, Reddy VA, Khanna R. Management and outcome of retinoblastoma with vitreous seeds. Ophthalmology. 2014;121(2):517-24.
42. Abramson DH, Frank CM, Dunkel IJ. A phase I/II study of subconjunctival carboplatin for intraocular retinoblastoma. Ophthalmology. 1999;106:1947-50.
43. Shome D, Honavar SG, Reddy VA. The role of periocular carboplatin as an adjunctive therapy in advanced intraocular retinoblastoma. Proceedings of the Annual Meeting of the American Academy of Ophthalmology 2005 October 15 - 18; Chicago, IL, USA.
44. Carcaboso AM, Chiappetta DA, Opezzo JA, et al. Episcleral implants for topotecan delivery to the posterior segment of the eye. Invest Ophthalmol Vis Sci. 2010; 51:2126-34.
45. Chantada GL, Fandino AC, Carcaboso AM, et al. A phase I study of periocular topotecan in children with intraocular retinoblastoma. Invest Ophthalmol Vis Sci. 2009;50:1492-6.
46. Yamane T, Kaneko A, Mohri M. The technique of ophthalmic arterial infusion therapy for patients with intraocular retinoblastoma. Int J Clin Oncol. 2004;9:69-73.
47. Gobin YP, Dunkel IJ, Marr BP, et al. Intra-arterial chemotherapy for the management of retinoblastoma: four-year experience. Arch Ophthalmol. 2011;129:732-7.
48. Shields CL, Bianciotto CG, Jabbour P, et al. Intra-arterial chemotherapy for retinoblastoma: report No. 2, treatment complications. Arch Ophthalmol. 2011; 129:1407-15.
49. Eagle RC Jr, Shields CL, Bianciotto C, et al. Histopathologic observations after intra-arterial chemotherapy for retinoblastoma. Arch Ophthalmol. 2011;129:1416-50.
50. Manjandavida FP, Shields CL. The role of intravitreal chemotherapy for retinoblastoma. Indian J Ophthalmol. 2015;63(2):141-5. doi: 10.4103/0301-4738.154390.
51. Shields CL, Manjandavida FP, Arepalli S, Kaliki S, Lally SE, Shields JA. Intravitreal melphalan for persistent or recurrent retinoblastoma vitreous seeds: preliminary results. JAMA Ophthalmol. 2014;132(3):319-25.

52. Ueda M, Tanabe J, Inomata M, et al. Study on conservative treatment of retinoblastoma—effect of intravitreal injection of melphalan on the rabbit retina. Nippon Ganka Gakkai Zasshi. 1995;99:1230-5.
53. Ghassemi F, Shields CL. Intravitreal melphalan for refractory or recurrent vitreous seeding from retinoblastoma. Arch Ophthalmol. 2012;130:1268-71.
54. Shields CL, Shields JA, De Potter P, et al. Plaque radiotherapy in the management of retinoblastoma. Use as a primary and secondary treatment. Ophthalmology. 1993; 100:216-24.
55. Choi SY, Kim MS, Yoo S, et al. Long term follow-up results of external beam radiotherapy as primary treatment for retinoblastoma. J Korean Med Sci. 2010;25: 546-56.
56. Abramson DH, Frank CM. Second non-ocular tumors in survivors of bilateral retinoblastoma; a possible age effect on radiation-related risk. Ophthalmology. 1998;105:573-80.
57. Wilson TW, Chan HS, Moselhy GM, et al. Penetration of chemotherapy into vitreous is increased by cryotherapy and cyclosporine in rabbits. Arch Ophthalmol. 1996;114:1390-5.
58. Shields CL, Santos MC, Diniz W, et al. Thermotherapy for retinoblastoma. Arch Ophthalmol. 1999;117:885-93.
59. Gupta R, Vemuganti GK, Reddy VA, Honavar SG. Histopathologic risk factors in retinoblastoma in India. Arch Pathol Lab Med. 2009;133:1210-4.
60. Eagle RC Jr. High-risk features and tumor differentiation in retinoblastoma: a retrospective histopathologic study. Arch Pathol Lab Med. 2009;133:1203-9.
61. Honavar SG, Singh AD, Shields CL, et al. Post-enucleation adjuvant therapy in high- risk retinoblastoma. Arch Ophthalmol. 2002;120:923-31.
62. Honavar SG, Singh AD. Management of advanced retinoblastoma. Ophthalmol Clin North Am. 2005;18:65-73.

Chapter 16

Endovascular Interventions in Ophthalmic Disorders

Hima Pendharkar

INTRODUCTION

Imaging is indispensable in patients presenting with symptoms referable to the ophthalmic system. A thorough clinical evaluation narrows down the differential diagnoses for a given patient. Cross sectional imaging with either CT and/or MRI with dedicated protocols is then performed to localize the lesion. Contrast administration is essential for complete evaluation of the lesion. Vascular lesions form a significant part of the spectrum of lesions identified on cross sectional imaging. CT angiogram or MR angiogram helps characterize the lesions well. However, the role of cerebral angiography remains indispensable in certain cases. Also with the advent of endovascular techniques many a lesions of this spectrum can be treated in a non-invasive way.

A Brief About the Cerebral Angiogram

With all the technical advances does diagnostic angiography have a role? Definitely the most essential information that an angiogram provides is the hemodynamics of a given lesion—which is extremely essential in planning therapy. Based on the diagnostic angiogram if required embolization can be done at the same sitting.

Preprocedural Work Up

Preprocedural investigations include the hemogram, coagulation profile, the total and differential leukocyte counts, erythrocyte sedimentation rate (ESR), platelets, renal function tests, electrolyte status, HIV/HBsAg status. Further tests can be tailored according to the patient's condition. The patient's drug history is required with special reference to any known drug allergies.

Cerebral Angiogram

The procedure is carried out on a single plane or biplane digital subtraction angiogram (DSA machine). Arterial access is gained via the femoral route followed by placement of the sheath in situ. This is followed under fluoroscopic guidance by the placement of the diagnostic catheter in the cerebral vessels. Selective arterial injections are taken using a non-ionic contrast medium.

Bilateral internal carotid arteries (ICA), bilateral external carotid arteries (ECA) and the dominant vertebral artery (VA) are evaluated with standard projections. At times additional projections, 3D acquisitions, selective arterial injections (may include microcatheter injection) and magnified views are also taken.

Endovascular Intervention

After the cerebral angiogram a multidisciplinary approach as regards the best therapy—interventional management versus surgical treatment—to be offered to the patient is essential in the interest of the patient. If the lesion is amenable to endovascular management the patient and/or his relatives are explained the procedure that is being planned, its advantages, limitations and the attendant complications that might happen. An informed consent is a must before proceeding with the planned therapy.

The choice of anesthesia depends on the procedure. While most diagnostic procedures are done under local anesthesia, therapeutic procedures need general anesthesia.

For proceeding with intervention, the diagnostic catheter is exchanged for a guiding catheter. Then via the guiding catheter the microcatheter is introduced and with the use of microwires and under continuous fluoroscopy it is navigated to the desired vessel. Superselective injections follow. The details of the lesion's angio-architecture can now be studied. This is followed by delivery or placement of the embolizing agent or stents or coils as the case may be. It is essential to remember that each procedure is a tailored one.

Check angiograms are done as and when needed during the procedure. From the outset it is important to rule out any dangerous intracranial anastomoses that might exist between the external carotid and the internal carotid system or vertebrobasilar system to prevent any inadvertent passage of embolizing material to the intracranial circulation. Also some anastomoses can open up after partial embolization and hence we need to be on the lookout for them throughout the procedure.

Once the procedure is over, final check angiograms are done to document the final status of the lesion—the success or otherwise of the procedure. Also it is essential to document the cerebral circulation immediate post procedure. This then decides the further follow up therapy needed.

A vast array of embolizing materials is available and once again the lesion in question dictates the correct choice. Adequate knowledge of the material to be used, its mechanism of action, complications and their management is essential when handling these materials. The materials in commonest use are solid embolics such as polyvinyl alcohol particles, embospheres and gelfoam. The liquid embolics include n-BCA i.e. n-Butyl cyanoacrylate, Onyx/PHIL/Squid, etc. There is an array of platinum microcoils for embolization: Guglielmi detachable coils (GDC), hilal microcoils, fibered platinum coils, the Berenstein liquid coils, detachable (latex) and nondetachable balloons (silicone), etc. Stents are also used in aneurysm treatment with flow diverter devices being the latest addition to the armamentarium. Each one needs a set of compatible delivery system. Also indispensable are various retrieval devices such as snares to retrieve broken fragments of catheters and coils. Closure devices are also used to achieve post-procedural puncture site hemostasis.

Post-procedure Care

After the given procedure is over the patient needs appropriate post procedural care which varies according to the procedure and the patient's clinical status.

While a patient who has undergone an uncomplicated cerebral angiogram can be monitored in the ward, a patient who has undergone endovascular coiling of an acutely ruptured aneurysm needs absolute ICU monitoring.

Depending on these, once the acute post procedure period is over and the clinical situation has improved, the patient can be discharged with appropriate instructions to be followed and guidance for seeking further medical advice as and when required.

Endovascular Therapy in Neuro-ophthalmic Lesions

Various vascular lesions that can present with ophthalmic symptoms and can be treated by endovascular means include aneurysms of posterior communicating artery (PCOM), superior cerebellar artery (SCA), cavernous carotid artery (CCA), ophthalmic artery (OA); arterio venous fisulae (AVF) which include carotid cavernous fistula (CCF), dural arteriovenous fistula (DAVF); arteriovenous malformations (AVMs) in the occipital region, other conditions such as idiopathic intracranial hypertension (IIH); stroke presenting with transient ischemic attack to name a few.

The role of CT and MRI remains complimentary though undisputed in the diagnosis of these lesions. Following examples illustrate the role of not only cerebral angiography but endovascular intervention in management of vascular lesions involving the optic pathways.

CASE 1: IDIOPATHIC INTRACRANIAL HYPERTENSION

History

A 19-year-old female presented with visual blurring since one year and neck pain since 45 days.

On examination she had bilateral papilledema; the left eye showed no waveform on visual evoked potential; waveform on the right eye was slightly prolonged.

Imaging Findings

MRI brain showed bilateral prominent perioptic nerve sheaths, kinking of optic nerves and scleral buckling. The sella was partially empty (Figs 16.1A to C). The lateral ventricles were slit like. These features were suggestive of raised intracranial pressure. MR venogram showed a narrowing at the junction of right transverse sinus and sigmoid sinus (Fig. 16.1D).

Cerebral Angiogram Findings

She underwent a cerebral angiogram which revealed a normal circulation and confirmed the tight stenosis at the right transverse sinus and sigmoid sinus junction (Fig. 16.1E).

Endovascular Management

Sinus pressure monitoring across the stenosis revealed a pressure gradient of 16 mm Hg. A 8 mm × 40 mm Protege stent was placed across the stenosis. Post stenting check angiogram revealed complete opening of the stenosis (Figs 16.1F and G) and the immediate normalization of the pressure gradient. She was put on

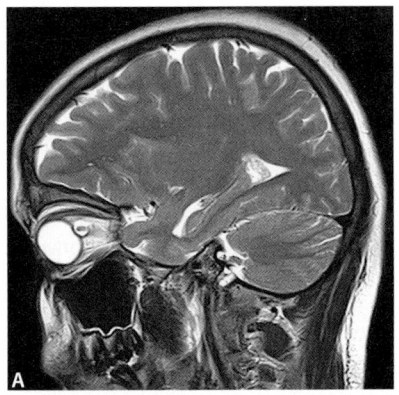 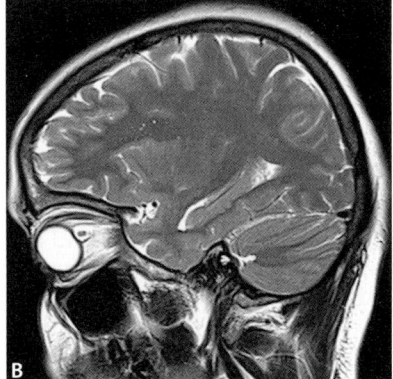

Figs 16.1A and B: Right and left parasagittal T2 WI respectively demonstrate the dilated perioptic nerve sheath bilaterally and also posterior scleral buckling

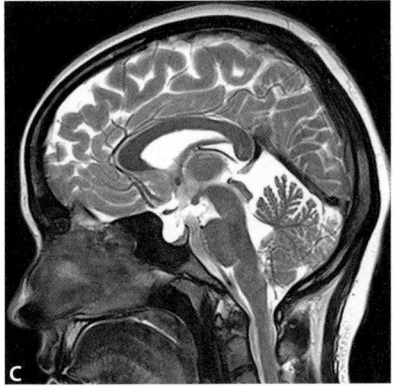 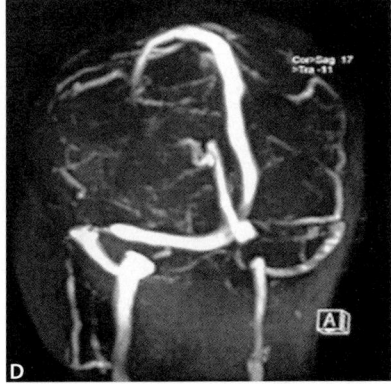

Fig. 16.1C: T2W sagittal image shows a partial empty sella

Fig. 16.1D: Right oblique view of MR venogram demonstrates the narrowing at the junction of right transverse sinus and sigmoid sinus

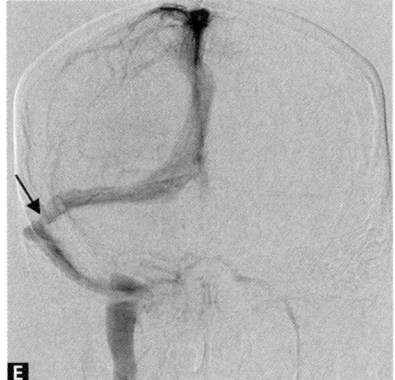 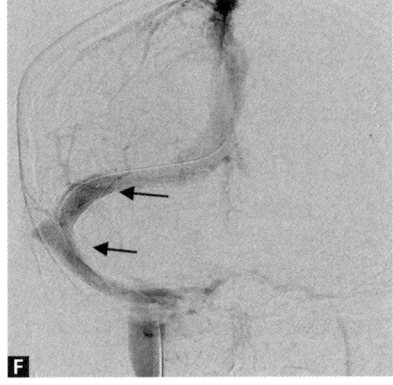

Fig. 16.1E: DSA image in the late venous phase shows the area of narrowing (arrow) at the junction of the right transverse and sigmoid sinus. Pressure monitoring was done across this stenotic segment

Fig. 16.1F: Status post stenting DSA image shows the stent (between arrows) deployed across the stenotic segment with complete opening of the stenosis. Sinus pressure difference significantly improved post stenting

dual antiplatelets for 3 months and then continued on tablet aspirin 150 mg once daily indefinitely.

At follow up the patient showed symptomatic relief with improvement in her vision.

Serial Perimetry

Perimetry was done at presentation which showed severe field defect in the left eye, enlarged blind spot and patchy field defects in the right eye. Follow up perimetry at one month and three months showed significant resolution in the field defects (Figs 16.1H to M).

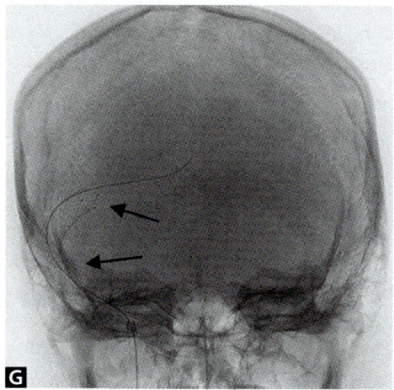

Fig. 16.1G: Unsubtracted image shows completely opened stent in situ

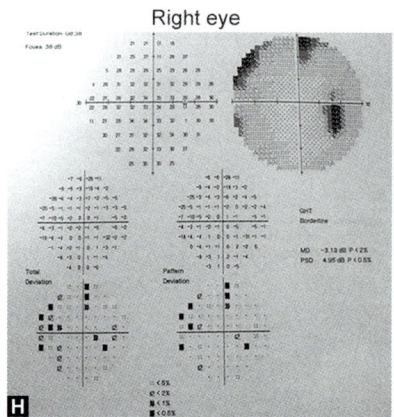

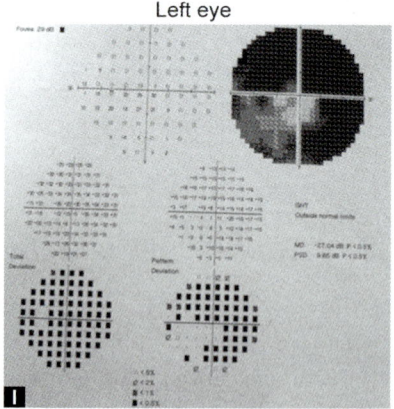

Fig. 16.1H: Right eye perimetry at presentation shows in an enlarged blind spot. Patchy areas of field defect are noted in the superonasal and superotemporal quadrants

Fig. 16.1I: Left eye perimetry at presentation shows severe field defects involving all four quadrants with relative sparing of central field

Endovascular Interventions in Ophthalmic Disorders

Right eye

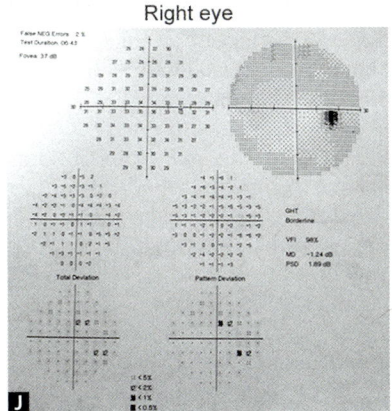

Left eye

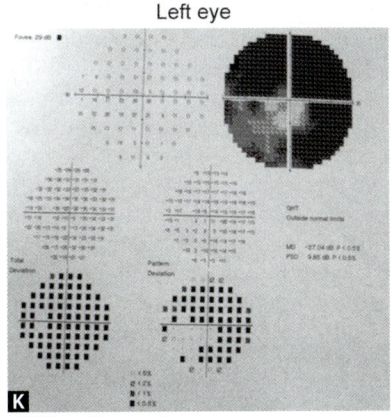

Fig. 16.1J: Right eye perimetry at 1 month post stenting shows reduction in the size of the blind spot and resolution of prior field defects

Fig. 16.1K: Left eye perimetry at 1 month post stenting shows significant improvement in the visual fields except for the superior temporal

Right

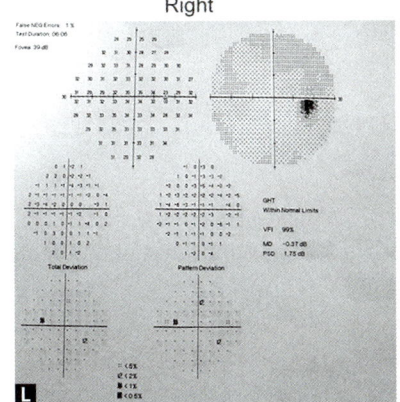

Left

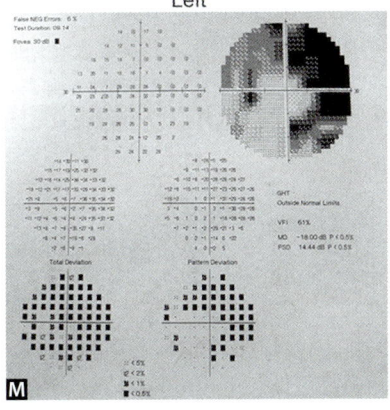

Fig. 16.1L: Right eye perimetry at 3 months post stenting remains status quo compared to last perimetry

Fig. 16.1M: Left eye perimetry at 3 months post stenting shows further improvement in the visual fields as compared to the last perimetry

Discussion

Idiopathic intracranial hypertension (IIH) is defined as a headache syndrome characterized by raised CSF pressure in the absence of an intracranial mass lesion or ventricular dilation; normal CSF composition; normal results of neurologic examination except for papilledema and occasional CN VI palsy; and a normal level of consciousness.[1] It is seen most commonly in obese young women; female to male ratios range from 4:1 to 15:1.[2-6]

Headache is the most common symptom occurring in 68-98% of patients.[3,4,7] Visual symptoms include disturbance of vision, diplopia, sparkles or the sensation of flashes of light. Occasionally, patients present with visual loss; central vision is usually spared until late in the course of the illness.[8]

The hallmark of IIH is papilledema which may be bilateral, asymmetrical, or even unilateral. Direct transmission of the elevated CSF pressure results in distension of the perioptic subarachnoid space and ballooning of the optic papilla causing it to protrude physically into the posterior aspect of the globe.[1,9-11] The long-standing effect of pulsatile CSF under high pressure also leads to downward herniation of arachnoid through a defect in the diaphragma sellae.[12,13]

The pathophysiology underlying the raised intracranial pressure remains unclear, though hypotheses have developed around the main determinants of CSF pressure. Most patients with IIH respond to maximal medical therapy. Failure of or noncompliance with medical treatment, new or worsening visual field deficits, intractable or fulminant headache are indications for intervention—surgical or endovascular. Surgical treatment includes CSF shunt insertion, optic nerve sheath fenestration or subtemporal decompression.[14]

Endovascular management of IIH involves stenting of the sinus which demonstrates narrowing with a pressure gradient across the stenosed segment. A pressure gradient of 8 mm Hg has evolved during the years as an arbitrary cutoff between normal and abnormal.[15] Dilatation and stenting of the lateral venous sinuses have produced clinical improvement in some patients with idiopathic intracranial hypertension who have high venous sinus pressures at manometry.[15,16] Authors in their experience state that just one normally functioning transverse sinus precludes the development of IIH by removing the Starling-like resistor, normalizes venous pressures, gives symptomatic relief, and can save or restore vision.[15] Post stenting these patients have to continue antiplatelet agents such as aspirin indefinitely.

CASE 2: INTRACRANIAL DURAL ARTERIOVENOUS FISTULA

History

A 52-year-old male presented with seizures since one week and blurring of vision since 2 months. On examination the patient was unconscious and had bilateral severe papilledema.

Imaging Findings

Non-contrast computed tomography (NCCT) at admission showed multiple hyperdense serpiginous channels in bilateral cerebral hemispheres. On contrast-enhanced computed tomography (CECT), there was intense enhancement of these channels (Figs 16.2A and B) suggesting a vascular lesion.

Cerebral Angiogram Finding

Cerebral angiogram revealed an intracranial dural arteriovenous fistula (DAVF) at the mid part of the left transverse sinus fed by multiple arteries (Figs 16.2C to G).

Endovascular Management

The patient was taken for transarterial embolization of the DAVF using Onyx. The left middle meningeal artery was catheterized (Fig. 16.2H) and about 3.5 mL of Onyx was injected till the fistula was completely obliterated. The onyx cast is seen in situ (Fig. 16.2I). Post embolization check angiograms revealed no residual arterial feeder suggestive of complete obliteration of the fistula (Figs 16.2J to L).

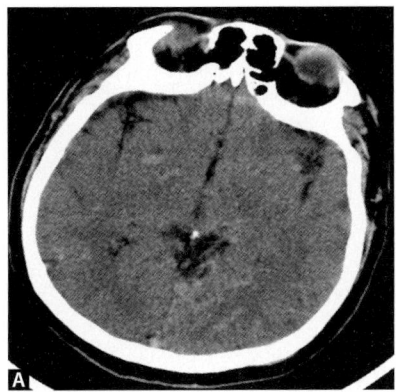

Fig. 16.2A: NCCT shows abnormal hyperdense serpiginous channels along the cortex and subcortical region in the entire parenchyma

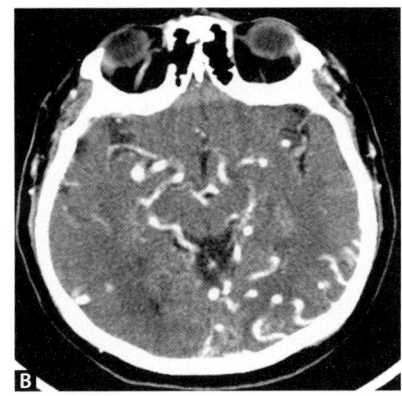

Fig. 16.2B: CECT at a lower level shows intensely enhancing serpiginous channels that represent abnormal veins suggesting venous congestion

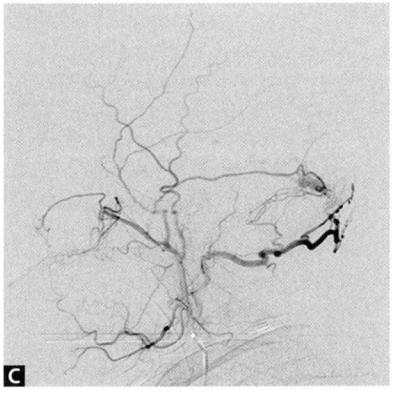

Fig. 16.2C: Left ECA lateral view injection demonstrates the supply to the fistula from the left middle meningeal artery. Supply was also noted from the occipital artery

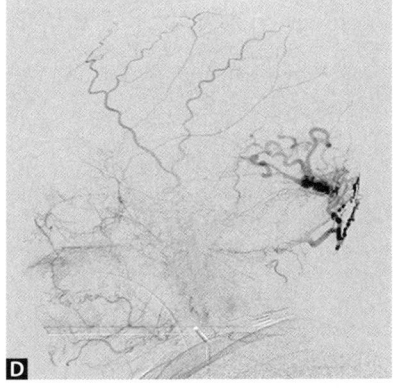

Fig. 16.2D: Left ECA lateral view in later arterial phase demonstrates the contrast reflux in the dilated abnormal cortical veins in the occipital region

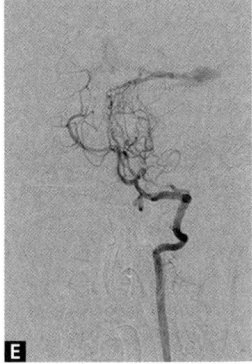

Fig. 16.2E: Left vertebral artery AP view demonstrates abnormal arteries coursing to the mid third of the left transverse sinus

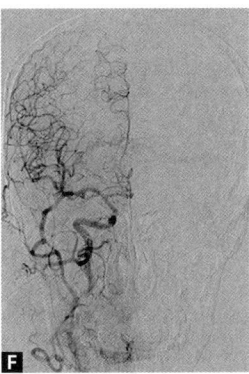

Fig. 16.2F: Right ICA AP view demonstrates dural feeders coursing to the mid third of the left transverse sinus

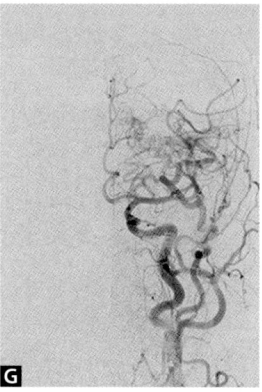
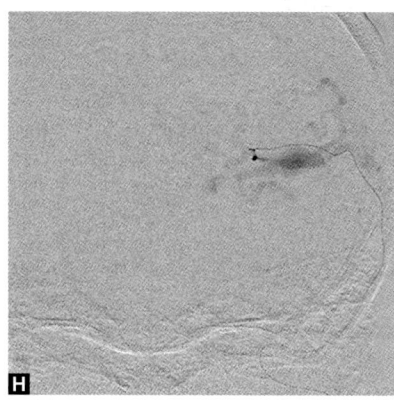

Fig. 16.2G: Left ICA AP view demonstrates abnormal arterial feeders coursing to the same region where feeders from left VA and left ICA are communicating with the transverse sinus. These features represent a dural arteriovenous fistula

Fig. 16.2H: Selective microcatheter injection demonstrates the fistula by direct filling of the venous sinus and reflux to the cortical vein

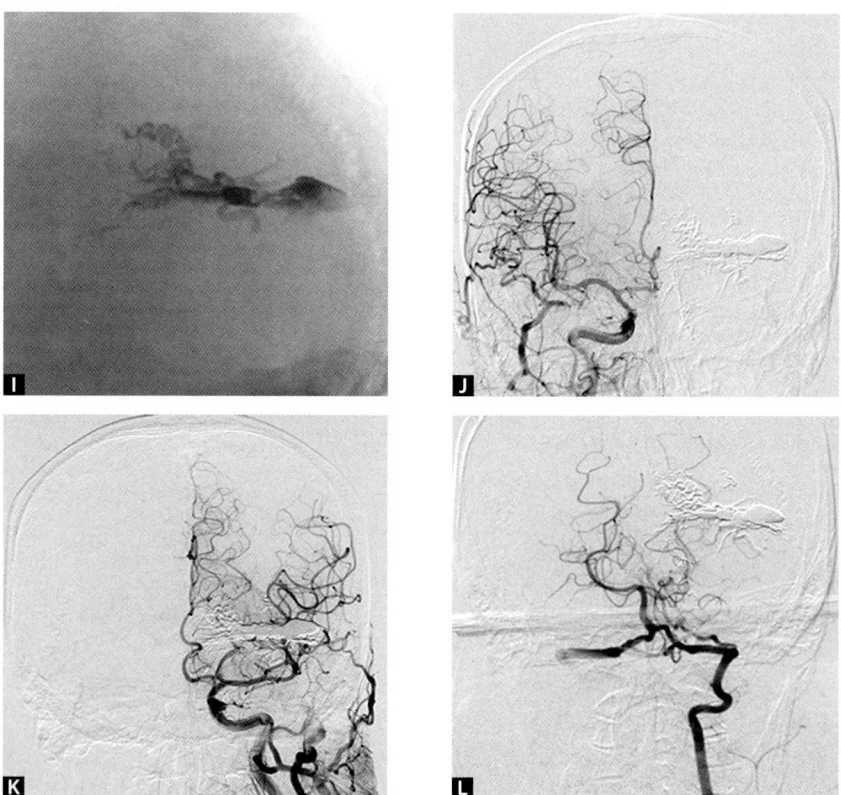

Figs 16.2I to L: Status post embolization by Onyx, AP unsubtracted view demonstrates the onyx cast in the abnormal fistulous segment of the left transverse sinus and few cortical veins. Status post embolization—right ICA AP view—left ICA AP view, left vertebral AP view—all show only arterial filling in the respective territories. There is no filling of the fistula suggesting complete obliteration

Discussion

Intracranial DAVFs are abnormal arteriovenous connections within the dura and represent 10%–15% of all intracranial vascular malformations.[17] DAVFs differ from AVMs in that there is no nidus between the artery and vein. Specific factors are known to predispose to fistula formation such as sinus thrombosis, trauma, and surgery.[18-21]

DAVFs can occur anywhere within the dura but develop most frequently near the venous sinuses. Arterial supply is usually from branches of dural arteries sometimes from osseous branches and rarely pial vessels may be involved. Venous drainage may occur into the dural sinuses, into osteodural veins, retrogradely via leptomeningeal veins into cortical, cerebral, cerebellar or perimedullary veins or any combination of these.[22]

The clinical presentation of DAVFs is highly varied and is primarily determined by the location of the fistula and the subsequent pattern of venous drainage. DAVFs can present with features of raised intracranial pressure, seizures, intracranial hemorrhage, dementia, etc. Continued increase in intracranial pressure leads to progressive visual symptoms such as visual blurring; optic atrophy occurs if fistula is left untreated.

The treatment goal for any patient presenting with hemorrhage, symptoms of cortical venous hypertension or significant ocular pathologic findings is complete obliteration of the fistula. Previously, transvenous embolization was the mode of treatment; occasionally glue and PVA particles were also injected. However with technological advances transarterial embolization has become the treatment of choice in most of the cases. Various liquid embolics such as Onyx, PHIL or Squid may be injected to obliterate the fistula. Amongst the three, the experience with onyx is the largest.

Onyx is a copolymer suspended in a solvent—dimethyl sulfoxide (DMSO).[23] The microcatheter is first flushed with DMSO which disperses in arterial blood flow; the copolymer Onyx is injected through the same microcatheter at the point of fistula and is deposited onto the arterial walls. In practice, the progress of the embolus formation can be controlled. The treatment of DAVFs by using Onyx by an arterial approach is effective and safe and allows the complete occlusion of the arteriovenous shunt in a single session in most cases.[23-25]

CASE 3: CAVERNOUS INTERNAL CAROTID ARTERY ANEURYSMS

History

A 52-year-female presented with right sided complete ptosis since 3 months. She complained of occasional headache. On examination, she had complete third nerve palsy on the right.

Imaging Findings

Magnetic resonance imaging (MRI) brain revealed right cavernous ICA aneurysm measuring about 11 mm × 12 mm and left ICA ophthalmic segment aneurysm measuring about 5 mm × 10 mm.

Cerebral Angiogram Findings

Cerebral angiogram revealed four aneurysms: saccular aneurysm of right cavernous ICA measuring 11 mm × 12 mm and directed laterally (arrow); right ICA ophthalmic segment aneurysm measuring 4.1 mm × 2.8 mm directed anteriorly (dotted arrow); right M1 segment aneurysm just at the MCA origin measuring approximately 2.2 mm × 4.7 mm directed superiorly and medially (broken arrow) (Fig. 16.3A). The left ICA ophthalmic segment aneurysm was measuring approximately 7.8 mm × 10 mm and was directed anteriorly and laterally (arrow) (Fig. 16.3B).

Endovascular Management

Two large coils of appropriate size were placed in the right cavernous ICA aneurysm. Then following the standard technique of deployment a pipeline flow diverter device (between two arrows) measuring 5 mm × 35 mm was placed across the neck of the cavernous aneurysm and across the right ophthalmic segment aneurysm (Fig. 16.3C). The right proximal M1 aneurysm was then coiled using appropriate sized coils. Subsequently the left ophthalmic segment aneurysm was also treated with pipeline flow diverter device measuring 4.25 mm × 2.5 cm (between two dotted arrows, Fig. 16.3D). Both the pipeline devices were deployed successfully. Check angiograms on either side showed normal forward flow in bilateral ICAs. Patient was started on dual anti-platelets for three months followed by single antiplatelet indefinitely.

A follow up angiogram at one year demonstrated the complete occlusion of the right cavernous ICA aneurysm and the right ophthalmic segment aneurysm; the right proximal M1 segment aneurysm remains completely occluded (Fig. 16.3E) while the left cavernous ICA aneurysm has partially reduced in size (Fig. 16.3F). Follow up angiogram after another 6 months is planned to look for the resolution of the left cavernous ICA aneurysm.

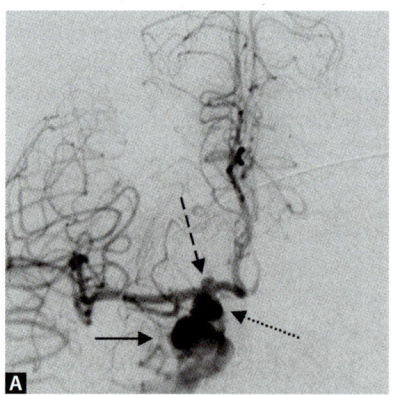
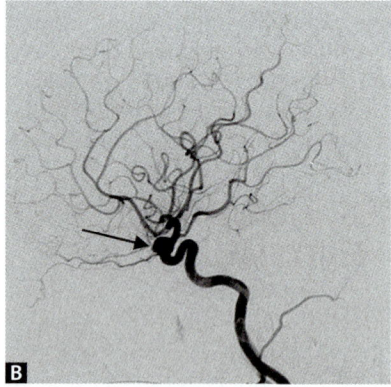

Fig. 16.3A: Right ICA tilted AP view reveals three aneurysms: saccular aneurysm of right cavernous ICA measuring 11 mm x 12 mm and directed laterally (arrow); right ICA ophthalmic segment aneurysm measuring 4.1 mm x 2.8 mm directed anteriorly (dotted arrow); right M1 segment aneurysm just at the MCA origin measuring approximately 2.2 mm x 4.7 mm directed superiorly and medially (broken arrow)

Fig. 16.3B: Left ICA lateral view demonstrates ophthalmic segment aneurysm measuring approximately 7.8 mm x 10 mm, directed anteriorly and laterally (arrow)

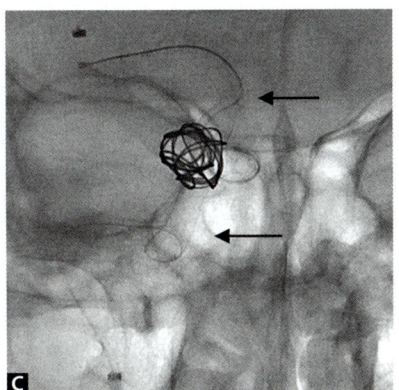 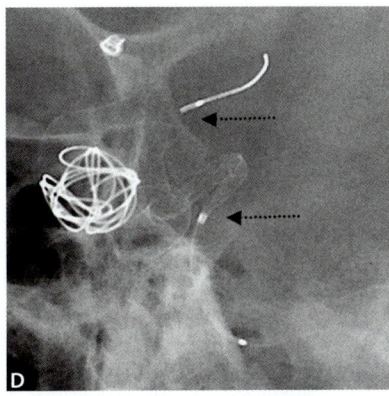

Fig. 16.3C: Unsubtracted image shows two large coils in the cavernous ICA aneurysm, Pipeline flow diverter device (between two arrows) across the neck of the cavernous aneurysm

Fig. 16.3D: Unsubtracted inverted image shows the pipeline flow diverter (between two dotted arrows) across the left ophthalmic artery aneurysm. The small coil mass distally is in the right M1 aneurysm, which was coiled prior to the left flow diverter placement

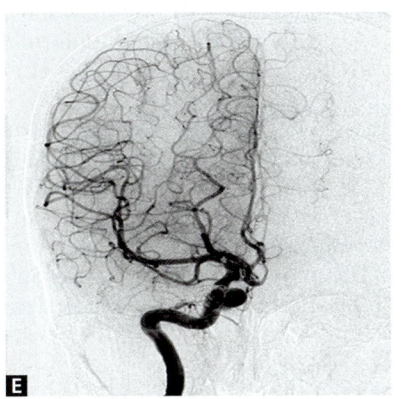 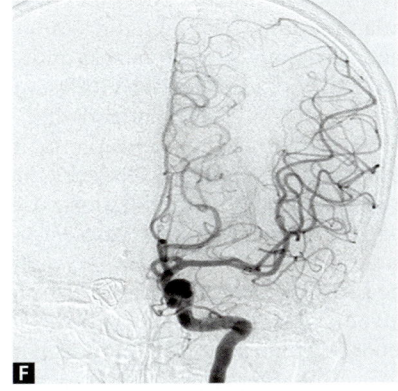

Fig. 16.3E: Right ICA AP view: check angiogram after one year demonstrated the complete occlusion of the right cavernous ICA aneurysm and the right ophthalmic segment aneurysm; the right proximal M1 segment aneurysm remains completely occluded

Fig. 16.3F: Left ICA AP view: check angiogram after one year shows the left cavernous ICA aneurysm has partially reduced in size

Discussion

Cavernous aneurysms represent 4% of all intracranial aneurysms; are usually dysplastic in nature and have a difficult morphology.[26]

When cavernous aneurysms reach a giant size, they usually present with either pain or visual symptoms. Pain is usually facial or retro-orbital in location. Diplopia is the most common visual symptom and results from paresis of the third, fourth or sixth cranial nerves. Involvement of any of the divisions of the fifth cranial nerve can result in analgesia or hypalgesia in that territory. Any combination of cranial nerves in the cavernous sinus can become affected and the degree of symptoms is highly variable. Occasionally, they can present with rupture resulting in a carotico-cavernous fistula (CCF) or rarely subarachnoid hemorrhage (SAH).

Treatment is essential to prevent compressive cranial neuropathy, the risk of rupture with the creation of a CCF, progressively worsening headache or erosion of the sphenoid sinus. Achieving complete aneurysm occlusion by using endovascular "reconstructive" techniques is difficult. "Deconstructive" ICA sacrifice for cavernous ICA aneurysms with or without bypass achieves high rates of complete aneurysm occlusion. However, ICA sacrifice is associated with several potential disadvantages because many of these patients have contralateral mirror ICA aneurysms and ipsilateral ICA occlusion limits therapeutic options for those contralateral aneurysms in the future.[27] The present day treatment for giant aneurysms of the cavernous ICA is best done with flow diverters. Flow diverters (FD) are stent-like devices which allow endoluminal reconstruction rather than endosaccular filling. They take the advantage of changing the parent artery/aneurysm sac interface thus altering the hemodynamics to induce intra aneurysmal thrombosis. Subsequent neointimal overgrowth covers the stent reconstructing the parent artery and eliminating the aneurysm/parent vessel interface. This process usually spares the origins of perforators. With time the aneurysm shrinks and collapses around the device construct relieving symptoms from mass effect. FDs take advantage of hemodynamics, thrombosis, inflammation, healing, and endothelial regrowth to achieve endoluminal reconstruction and aneurysm obliteration. Present day flow diverters that are available include Pipeline, FRED, Surpass to name a few.

Puffer et al. demonstrated that FDs are an effective treatment technique for cavernous aneurysms not only for achieving aneurysm closure but also for resolution of presenting clinical symptoms.[28] They reported resolution of 90% of cranial neuropathies, either pre-existing or developing soon after treatment, over time in all except one patient. Szikora et al. state that symptom resolution in these patients is related to decreased pulsation of the aneurysm and to regression of the sac which follows successful exclusion of the aneurysm with flow diversion.[29] Advantage with using a flow diverter is that it preserves the parent artery while achieving high complete aneurysm occlusion rates.

CASE 4: CAROTID CAVERNOUS FISTULA

History

A 32-year-old male patient met with a road traffic accident and underwent surgery for evacuation of extra dural hematoma (EDH). Three months after the accident he presented with left sided proptosis (nonpulsatile) associated with watering from the eye.

On examination, he had left axial proptosis, chemosis and scleral congestion. The left pupil was dilated. Vision was 6/6 in both eyes and there were no visual field cuts. He however had significant restriction of left eye movements due to proptosis.

Imaging

Contrast CT brain demonstrated prominent left cavernous sinus and a dilated left superior ophthalmic vein (SOV).

Cerebral Angiogram

Cerebral angiogram demonstrated a left direct CCF draining predominantly via the SOV to the facial vein (Figs 16.4A and B).

Endovascular Management

A microcatheter was placed across the fistulous site into the left cavernous sinus and coils were deployed till the rent was closed (Figs 16.4C and D). Note the clinical picture secondary to the CCF pre- and post-procedure (Figs 16.4 E and F).

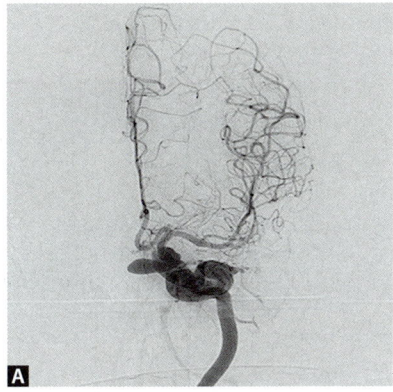

Fig. 16.4A: Left ICA AP view shows filling of the cavernous sinus and the superior ophthalmic vein in the arterial phase suggestive of a carotico-cavernous fistula

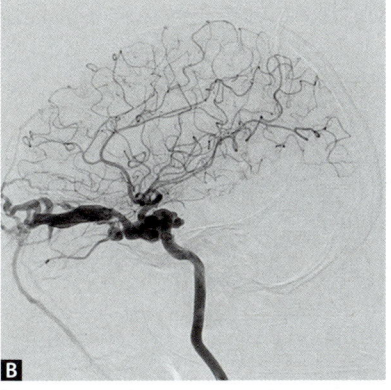

Fig. 16.4B: Left ICA lateral view demonstrates the filling of the cavernous sinus and anterior venous drainage to the superior ophthalmic vein and then via angular vein to the facial vein

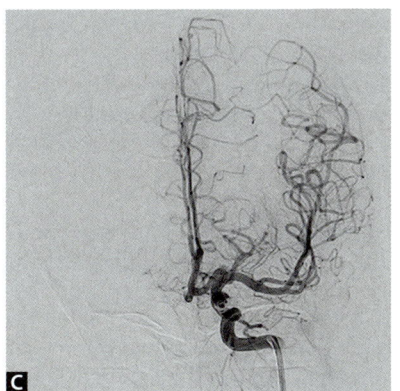

Fig. 16.4C: Postembolization left ICA AP view: The left superior ophthalmic vein is no longer filling suggesting complete closure of the fistula

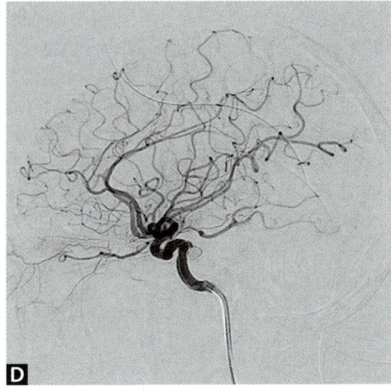

Fig. 16.4D: Postembolization left ICA lateral view: The cavernous sinus and superior ophthalmic vein are no longer filling. Forward intracranial flow is maintained. Coil mass is noted at the posterior genu of the cavernous ICA where it is obliterating the fistulous point

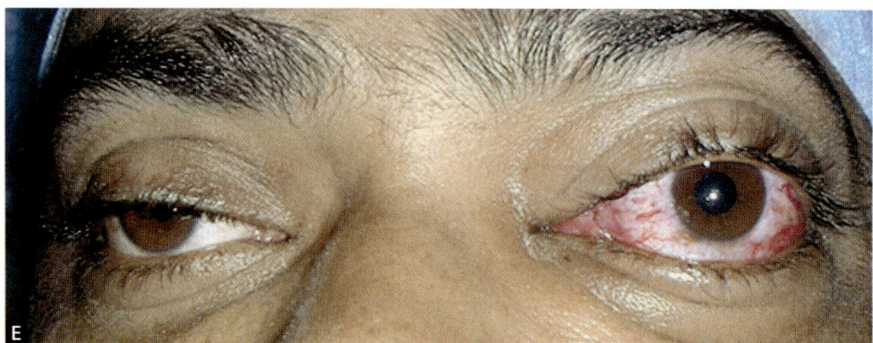

Fig. 16.4E: Clinical photograph of the patient at the time of diagnostic angiogram

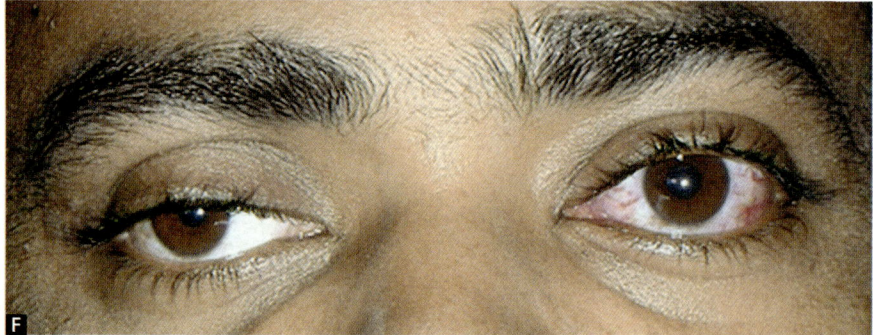

Fig. 16.4F: Clinical photograph one day after embolization shows significant resolution of all signs

Discussion

CCFs can be classified pathogenetically into: (1) Traumatic fistulas or spontaneous; (2) Hemodynamically into high-flow or low-flow fistulas and (3) Angiographically into direct or indirect (dural) fistulas.[30]

Traumatic CCFs, i.e. type A usually occur in young men and are formed by a tear in the cavernous portion of the ICA resulting in a high-pressure high-flow anomalous interconnection between the main arterial trunk and the cavernous sinus.[31] Direct fistulas are also formed secondary to ruptured aneurysms mostly in middle-aged and elderly women (Figs 16.5A to D).

Spontaneous CCFs/indirect CCFs are slow flow fistulas and are usually idiopathic. These can be angiographically divided into types B, C or D. Various implicated conditions for their development include pregnancy, sinusitis, trauma, surgical procedures, and cavernous sinus thrombosis.[28,29] They tend to appear in middle-aged women, and generally present with insidiously progressive proptosis, or a "red eye"— signs and symptoms that are usually less severe than those seen in direct fistulas.[28]

Endovascular management remains the mainstay of treating these fistulas; the goal of treatment is to eliminate the fistula and maintain the patency of the ICA.[32] Traditionally, type A CCF has been treated by inflating balloons in the cavernous sinus and across the rent. However, given the risks associated with balloons such as early deflation, rupture or delayed migration leading to recurrence of the fistula, detachable coils of various make are the present day choice for treatment. Complete packing of the fistula can thus be achieved.

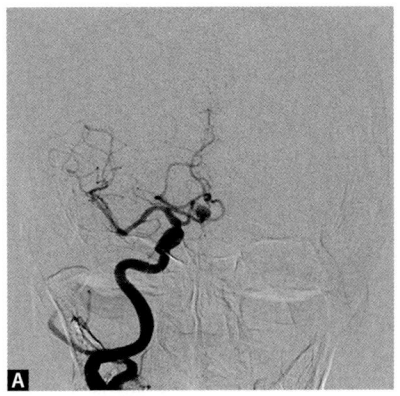 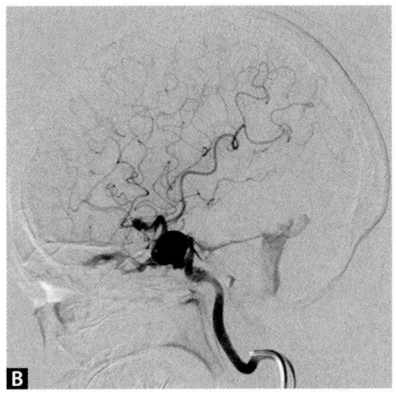

Fig. 16.5A: Right ICA AP view demonstrates a superiorly directed saccular anterior communicating artery aneurysm filling from the right, measuring about 4 mm x 3.5 mm

Fig. 16.5B: Left ICA lateral view shows a large cavernous ICA aneurysm measuring about 1.5 x 1.2 cm, it has ruptured causing a direct carotico-cavernous fistula which drains anteriorly to the superior ophthalmic vein and posteriorly to the superior petrosal sinus

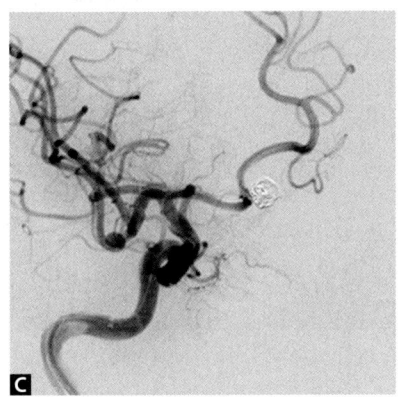 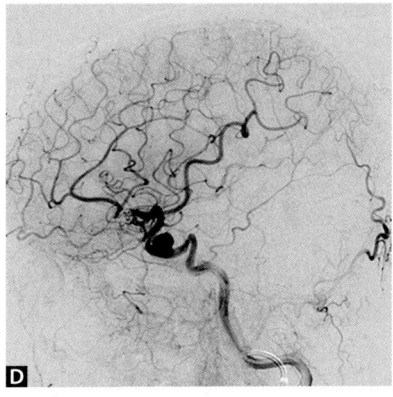

Fig. 16.5C: Right ICA oblique view demonstrates complete exclusion of the anterior communicating artery aneurysm post coiling, which was done after two days of diagnostic angiogram

Fig. 16.5D: Left ICA lateral view demonstrates spontaneous closure of the carotico-cavernous fistula; the cavernous ICA aneurysm is now better demonstrated

Spontaneous slow flow fistulas can be treated according to the angio architechture and venous drainage. The commonest venous access routes described are through the inferior petrosal sinus, facial vein, cut down of the superior ophthalmic vein (Figs 16.6A to D). Transvenous coiling achieves a complete packing of the cavernous sinus thus giving long-term obliteration of the fistula. The case demonstrates an indirect CCF accessed after SOV cut down (Figs 16.6A to F). The clinical picture taken post-procedure (Fig. 16.6G) demonstrates the site of cut down and significant resolution of clinical findings as compared to the pre-procedure picture (Fig. 16.6H).

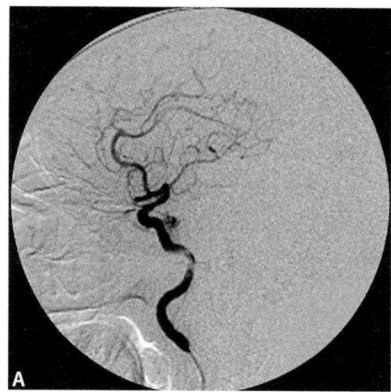

Fig. 16.6A: RICA lateral view demonstrates the subtle blush in the cavernous sinus from dural branches of cavernous ICA

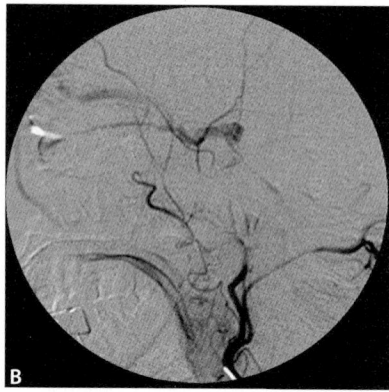

Fig. 16.6B: RECA lateral view demonstrates the filling of the superior ophthalmic vein. No other venous structures were noted filling. The only access to treat the fistula was via the superior ophthalmic vein, after angular vein cut down

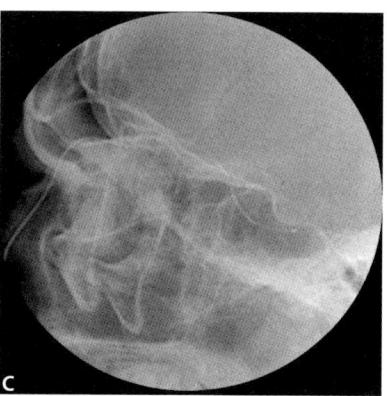

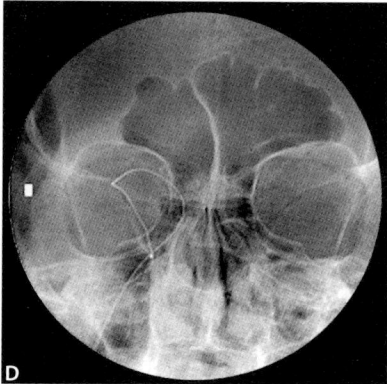

Figs 16.6C and D: Skull lateral and AP view respectively shows the microcatheter in the cavernous sinus via the superior ophthalmic vein

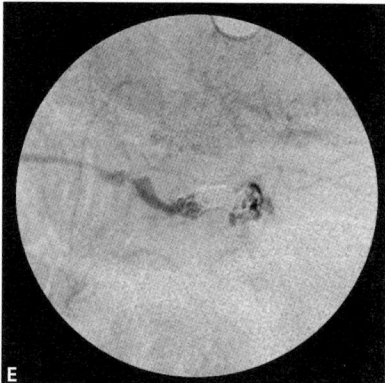

Fig. 16.6E: Right ICA capillary phase shows the residual filling of the superior ophthalmic vein, multiple coils are noted in the cavernous sinus

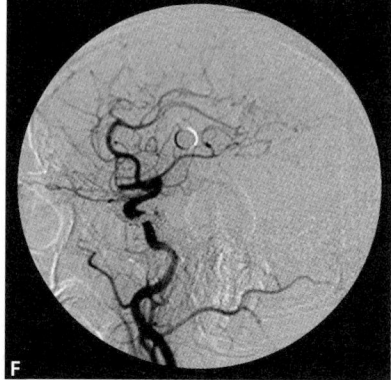

Fig. 16.6F: Right ICA lateral view, check angiogram post coiling demonstrates complete closure of the fistula, no filling of the superior ophthalmic vein is seen

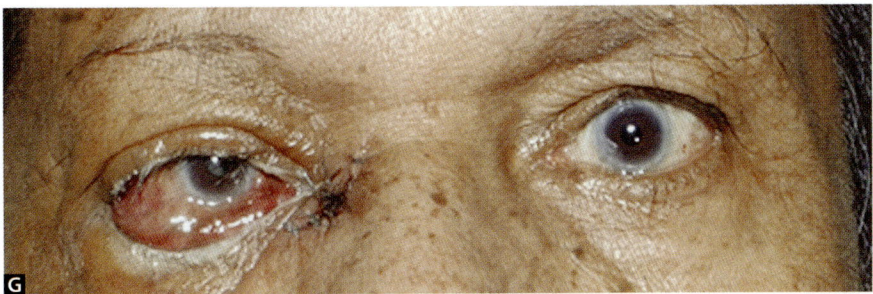

Fig. 16.6G: Clinical photograph one day after coiling shows the sutures at the site of angular vein cut down. Note the significant reduction in the chemosis of the right lower lid compared to the the preprocedure photograph in Figure 6H

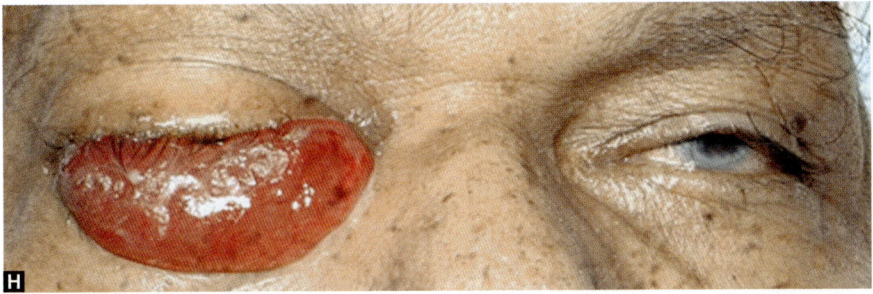

Fig. 16.6H: Preprocedure clinical photograph demonstrates chemosis and eversion of the lower eyelid with complete obliteration of the right palpebral fissure

CASE 5: POSTERIOR COMMUNICATING ARTERY ANEURYSM

History

A 55-year-old lady presented with acute onset closure of left eyelid since one week. On examination she had complete left third nerve palsy.

Imaging Findings

MRI brain revealed a left posterior communicating artery aneurysm of about 4 mm × 2 mm in size. There was no parenchymal lesion.

Cerebral Angiogram Findings

Diagnostic cerebral angiogram revealed a small saccular aneurysm measuring 4 mm × 3 mm at the origin of the posterior communicating artery region. It had a small neck and was directed laterally (Figs 16.7A and B).

Endovascular Management

The aneurysm was coiled using detachable coils of appropriate size till complete occlusion of the aneurysm was achieved (Figs 16.7C and D).

Discussion

Aneurysms in the region of the posterior communicating artery constitute about 50% of internal carotid artery (ICA) aneurysms or 25% of all intracranial

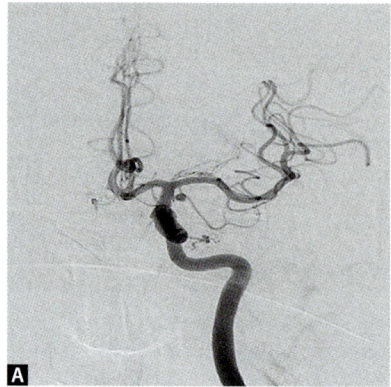
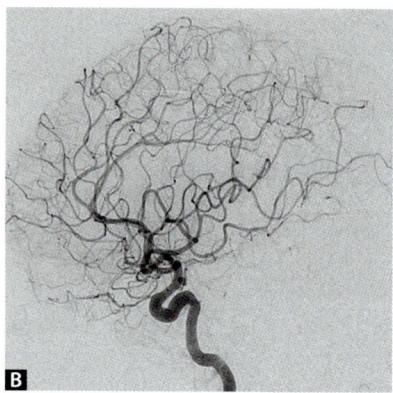

Fig. 16.7A and B: Left ICA AP and lateral views (arrow) demonstrate a small saccular aneurysm arising in the region of the posterior communicating artery. The aneurysm has a small neck and is directed laterally

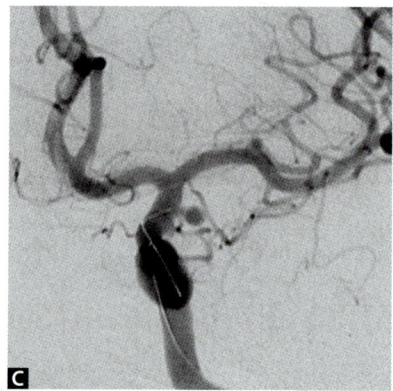
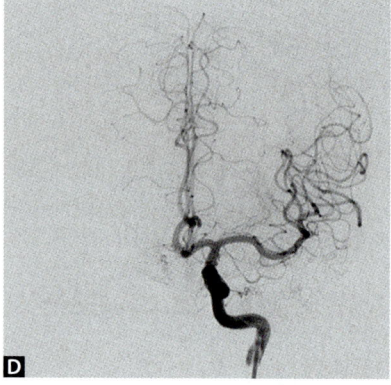

Fig. 16.7C: Demonstrates the advancement of the microwire towards the aneurysm sac. A microcatheter is passed over this wire into the sac and coils are then deployed

Fig. 16.7D: Status post coiling, left ICA AP view demonstrates the complete obliteration of the aneurysm sac. Compare to ICA AP view in the first image

aneurysms.[33,34] The oculomotor nerve lies lateral to the posterior communicating artery in most cases.[35] Direct compression of the oculomotor nerve by the aneurysmal mass is thought to be the main mechanism of nerve injury. In one study, a partial optic neuropathy (ONP) at presentation was the only statistically significant predictor of complete recovery with endovascular therapy (complete recovery in 50% of patients with partial ONP versus only 21% complete recovery in patients with complete ONP).[36] Rupture of posterior communicating artery aneurysm can also present with SAH.

CASE 6: OCCIPITAL ARTERIOVENOUS MALFORMATION

History

A 36-year-old male presented with history of seizures and occasional occipital headache since 3 months. On examination he had left homonymous hemianopia.

Imaging Findings

Non-contrast computed tomography (NCCT) demonstrated abnormal parenchymal hyperdensity in the right occipital region which on contrast enhanced CT (CECT) showed intense enhancement suggestive of a vascular malformation (Figs 16.8A and B).

On MRI, T2W axial (Fig. 16.8C) and T2W sagittal (Fig. 16.8D) images showed abnormal serpiginous flow voids in the right occipital lobe. Contrast enhanced MR angiogram (Fig. 16.8E) revealed hypertrophied occipital branch of the right middle cerebral artery and occipital branches from right posterior cerebral artery supplying an AVM with the nidus located in the right occipital lobe.

Cerebral Angiogram Findings

The cerebral angiogram revealed an AVM nidus measuring about 3.5 × 3.0 cm in the right occipital lobe. It had feeders from the occipital branch of right middle cerebral artery (MCA) (Figs 16.8F and G) and occipital branches of right PCA (Figs 16.8H and I). The venous drainage was to the mid third of the right transverse sinus.

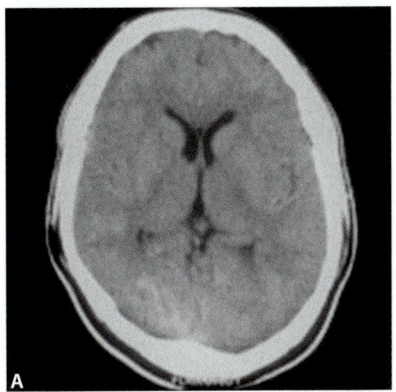

Fig. 16.8A: NCCT axial view demonstrates subtle hyperdense areas in the right occipital lobe

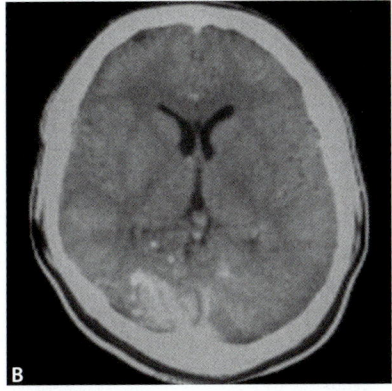

Fig. 16.8B: CECT axial view at the same level demonstrates enhancing serpiginous structures suggestive of a vascular malformation

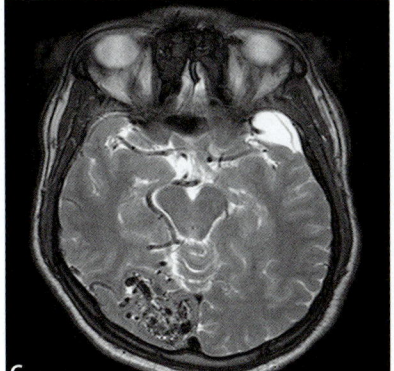

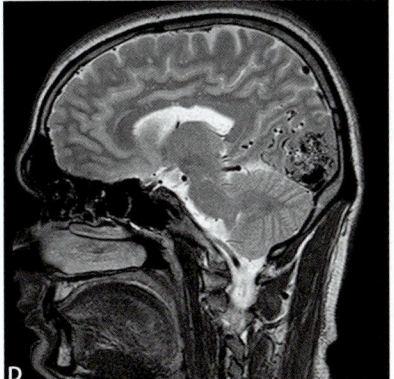

Figs 16.8C and D: T2W axial and sagittal images demonstrate abnormal flow voids in the right occipital lobe parenchyma. An incidental left anterior temporal arachnoid cyst is noted

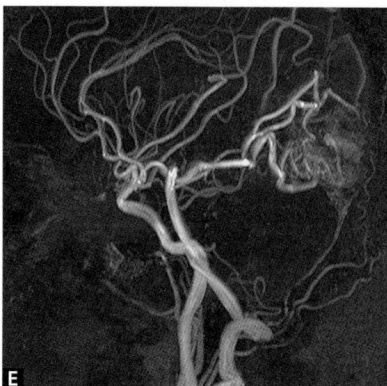

Fig. 16.8E: Contrast MR angiogram shows the hypertrophied feeding artery coursing towards the AVM nidus

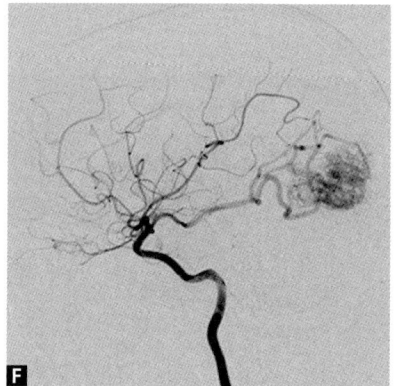 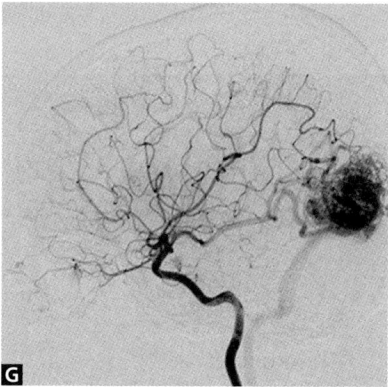

Figs 16.8F and G: Right ICA lateral view early arterial phase and a little later in the arterial phase respectively demonstrate the occipital branch of the right PCA, filling via PCom is hypertrophied and feeding the AVM nidus in the occipital lobe. The occipital branch of the right MCA is slightly hypertrophied. The AVM drains to the right transverse sinus which is seen in filling in the arterial phase. A nidus with an early draining vein is hallmark of an arteriovenous malformation

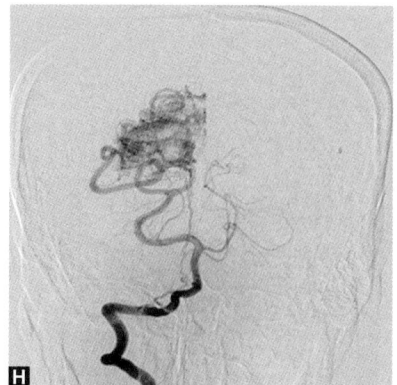 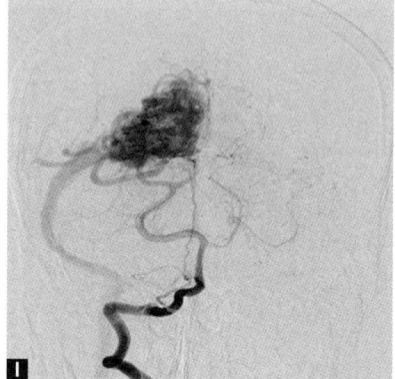

Figs 16.8H and I: Right vertebral artery AP view early arterial phase and a little later in the arterial phase demonstrate the hypertrophied occipital branches of the right PCA feeding the AVM which drains to the right transverse sinus in the arterial phase

Endovascular Management

Embolization using onyx can be carried out in this case.

Discussion

Arteriovenous malformations of the brain are congenital vascular lesions that account for approximately 2% of all hemorrhagic strokes.[37,38] The various presentations of an AVM include hemorrhage, headache, seizures or focal neurological deficits. Studies on natural history suggest that previously ruptured, large, and infratentorially and deeply located AVMs have the highest risk of future hemorrhage.[39] This risk is highest during the first few years after diagnosis and decreases thereafter but remains significant for decades.

Computed tomography without contrast is usually done as the first imaging when intracranial hemorrhage is suspected. In addition to the hemorrhage, calcification and abnormal slightly hyperdense serpiginous channels can also be seen. These serpiginous channels show enhancement after contrast administration. MRI shows an inhomogeneous signal void on PD and T2-weighted sequences commonly with hemosiderin suggesting prior hemorrhage. Contrast enhanced MR angiography shows the hypertrophied feeders and the draining veins. However DSA remains the gold standard for the diagnosis of cerebral AVMs. Not only does it give a detailed mapping of the angioarchitecture but also provides information about the hemodynamics of a given lesion. Treatment strategies are based on detailed analysis of the angioarchitecture. A multispeciality team approaches the case and decides surgical and/or endovascular and/or radiosurgical treatment for the best possible outcome in a given case. With the advent of various liquid embolic agents as stated previously and with appropriate selection complete obliteration of certain AVMs is possible. However embolization is mostly carried out as an adjunct to surgical excision or prior to radiosurgery.

CONCLUSION

There are a multitude of neurovascular lesions that can involve the optic pathways. A detailed history and complete clinical examination are essential to narrow down the differential diagnostic possibilities. A judicious use of various complimentary imaging techniques helps identify the lesion in a given case. With fast developing technology these lesions can be treated by endovascular means in a noninvasive way with good outcomes. Future developments will expand the scope of endovascular techniques.

REFERENCES

1. Soler D, Cox T, Bullock P, Calver DM, Robinson RO. Diagnosis and management of benign intracranial hypertension. Arch Dis Child. 1998;78:89-94.
2. Duncan J, Corbett J, Wall M. The incidence of pseudotumour cerebri: population studies in Iowa and Louisiana. Arch Neurol. 1988;45:875-77.
3. Radhakrishnan K, Thacker AK, Bohlaga NH, Maloo JC, Gerryo SE. Epidemiology of idiopathic intracranial hypertension: a prospective and case-control study. J Neurol Sci. 1993;116:18-28.
4. Kesler A, Gadoth N. Epidemiology of idiopathic intracranial hypertension in Israel. J Neuroophthalmol. 2001;21:12-14.

5. Mezaal M, Saadah M. Idiopathic intracranial hypertension in Dubai: nature and prognosis. Acta Neurol Scand. 2005;112:298-302.
6. Galvin J, Van Stavern G. Clinical characterisation of idiopathic intracranial hypertension at the Detroit medical centre. J Neurol Sci. 2004;223:157-60.
7. Wall M, George D. Idiopathic intracranial hypertension: a prospective study of 50 patients. Brain. 1991;114:155-80.
8. Rowe F, Sarkies N. Assessment of visual function in idiopathic intracranial hypertension: a prospective study. Eye. 1998;12:111-18.
9. Brodsky MC, Vaphiades M. Magnetic resonance imaging in pseudotumor cerebri. Ophthalmology. 1998;105:1686-93.
10. Jinkins JR, Athale S, Xiong L, Yuh WTC, Rothman MI, Nguyen PT. MRI of optic papilla protrusion in patients with high intracranial pressure. AJNR Am J Neuroradiol. 1996; 17:665-8.
11. Gass A, Barker GJ, Riordan-Eva P, et al. MRI of the optic nerve in benign intracranial hypertension. Neuroradiology 1996;38:769-73.
12. Zagardo MT, Cali WS, Kelman SE, Rothman MI. Reversible empty sella in idiopathic intracranial hypertension: an indicator of successful therapy? AJNR Am J Neuroradiol. 1996;17:1953-6.
13. Geoge AE. Idiopathic intracranial hypertension: pathogenesis and the role of MR imaging. Radiology. 1989;170:21-2.
14. Corbett JJ, Thompson HS. The rational management of idiopathic intracranial hypertension. Arch Neurol. 1989;46:1049-51.
15. Ahmed RM, Wilkinson M, Parker GD, Thurtell MJ, Macdonald J, McCluskey PJ, et al. Transverse Sinus Stenting for Idiopathic Intracranial Hypertension: A Review of 52 Patients and of Model Predictions. AJNR. 2011;32:1408-14.
16. Ahmed R, Friedman DI, Halmagyi GM. Stenting of the Transverse Sinuses in Idiopathic Intracranial Hypertension. J Neuro-Ophthalmol. 2011;31:374-80.
17. Newton TH, Cronqvist S. Involvement of dural arteries in intracranial arteriovenous malformation. Radiology. 1969;93:1071-8.
18. Chaudhary M, Sachdev V, Cho S. Dural arteriovenous malformations of the major venous sinuses and acquired lesion. Am J Neuroradiol. 1982;3:13-9.
19. Houser OW, Campbell JK, Campbell RJ, Sundt TM Jr. Arteriovenous malformation affecting the transverse dural venous sinus—an acquired lesion. Mayo Clin Proc 1979;54(10):651-61.
20. Kuhner A, Krastel A, Stoll W. Arteriovenous malformations of the transverse dural sinus. J Neurosurg. 1976;45(1):12-19.
21. Obrador S, Soto M, Silvela J. Clinical syndromes of arteriovenous malformations of the transverse sigmoid sinus. J Neurol Neurosurg Psychiatry. 1975;38(5):436-51.
22. Miller TR, Gandhi D. Intracranial dural arteriovenous fistulae: Clinical presentation & management strategies. Stroke. 2015;46:2017-25.
23. Mounayer C, Hammami N, Piotin M, et al. Nidal embolization of brain arteriovenous malformations using Onyx in 94 patients. Am J Neuroradiol. 2007;28:518-23.
24. Cognard C, Januel AC, Silva NA Jr, et al. Endovascular treatment of intracranial dural arteriovenous fistulas with cortical venous drainage: new management using Onyx. AJNR Am J Neuroradiol. 2008;29:235-41.
25. Trivelato FP, Abud DG, Ulhoa AC, et al. Dural arteriovenous fistulas with direct cortical venous drainage treated with Onyx: a case series. Arq Neuropsiquiatr. 2010; 68:613-18.
26. Linskey M, Shekhar L, Hirsch W, Yonas H, Horton J. Aneurysms of the intracavernous carotid artery: natural history and indications for treatment. Neurosurgery. 1990;26: 933-8.

27. van der Schaaf IC, Brilstra EH, Buskens E, et al. Endovascular treatment of aneurysms in the cavernous sinus: a systematic review on balloon occlusion of the parent vessel and embolization with coils. Stroke. 2002;33:313-8.
28. Puffer RC, Piano M, Lanzino G, Valvassori L, Kallmes DF, Quilici L, et al. Treatment of Cavernous Sinus Aneurysms with Flow Diversion: Results in 44 Patients. AJNR Am J Neuroradiol. 2014;35:948-95.
29. Szikora I, Marosfoi M, Salomvary B, et al. Resolution of mass effect and compression symptoms following endoluminal flow diversion for the treatment of intracranial aneurysms. AJNRAmJ Neuroradiol. 2013;34:935-9.
30. Barrow DL, Spector RH, Braun, Landman JA, Tindall SC, Tindall GT. Classification and treatment of spontaneous carotid-cavernous sinus fistulas. J Neurosurgery. 1985;62:248-56.
31. Halbach VV, Higashida RT, Larsen DW, et al. Treatment of dural arteriovenous fistulas. In: Maciunas RJ, (Ed), Endovascular neurologic intervention. Park Ridge: American association of neurologic surgeons. 1955;217-46.
32. Lewis A I, Tomsick T A, Tew J M Jr. Management of 100 consecutive direct carotid-cavernous fistulas: Results of treatment with detachable balloons. Neurosurgery. 1995;36(2):239-45.
33. Fein JM. Internal carotid posterior communicating artery aneurysms. In: Fein JM, Flamm ES, eds. Cerebrovascular Surgery, vol. III. Berlin: Springer-Verlag. 1985:841-60.
34. Ojemann RG, Heros RC, Crowell RM. Internal carotid artery aneurysms. In: Surgical Management of Cerebrovascular Disease, 2nd edn. Baltimore: Williams and Wilkins; 1988:179-98.
35. Zhang WG, Zhang SX, Wu BH. A study on the sectional anatomy of the oculomotor nerve and its related blood vessels with plastination and MRI. Surg Radiol Anat. 2002;24:277-84.
36. Chalouhi N, Theofanis T, Jabbour P, Dumont AS, Gonzalez LF, Starke RM, et al. Endovascular Treatment of Posterior Communicating Artery Aneurysms with Oculomotor Nerve Palsy: Clinical Outcomes and Predictors of Nerve Recovery; AJNR. 2013;828-32.
37. Choi JH, Mohr JP: Brain arteriovenous malformations in adults. Lancet Neurol. 2005;4:299-308.
38. Friedlander RM. Arteriovenous malformations of the brain. N Engl J Med. 2007;35: 2704-12.
39. Hernesniemi JA, Dashti R, Juvela S, Väärt K, Niemelä M, Laakso A. Natural history of brain arteriovenous malformations: a long-term follow-up study of risk of hemorrhage in 238 patients. Neurosurgery. 2008;63(5):823-9.

Chapter 17

Nystagmus

Mihir Kothari

Nystagmus is vast and intricate subject. It is described under following heads:
1. Definition and current classification of nystagmus
2. Clinical pathophysiology of nystagmus
3. Relevant special examinations in nystagmus
4. Graphic recording of nystagmus
5. Abnormal head posture
6. Investigations
7. Optical management
8. Pharmacological management
9. Surgical management
10. Visual/social function questionnaire 14 for nystagmus.

DEFINITION

Nystagmus is a rhythmical, involuntary and repetitive to and fro movement/oscillations of the eyes.[1,2]

Current classification of nystagmus is based on Classification of Eye Movement Abnormalities and Strabismus (CEMAS),[3] National Eye Institute, USA, 2001.

Physiological Nystagmus

1. **Vestibular nystagmus:** It comes up with head rotation (utilized in rotation test for vision assessment of young infants). Visual dampening should occur in 5–10 seconds after stopping the rotation. If it does not, it means that there exists significant visual impairment.[4] Calorie testings (Hot and cold) are utilized by ENT surgeons as Vestibular function tests.
2. **Optokinetic nystagmus (OKN):** It comes up with fixation on a repetitive moving target. OKN are used for:
   a. Assessment of vision in young infants and uncooperative adults.[4,5]
   b. Reversal of OKN is seen in infantile esotropia syndrome[5] and congenital nystagmus (now called infantile nystagmus syndrome).[6]
   c. Asymmetry/disjugacy/Absent vertical OKN is diagnostic of neurological/neurometabolic lesion and warrants neuroimaging in children with nystagmus.[7]

   There are many smart phone, android/Apple apps with clinical OKN testing. Many are free and very useful viz. Eye handbook.
3. **Eccentric gaze nystagmus:** Comes up as transient nystagmus on extremes of gazes.

Pathologic Nystagmus (Table 17.1)

TABLE 17.1: Showing different types of pathological nystagmus

1. Infantile nystagmus syndrome (INS)
2. Fusion maldevelopment nystagmus syndrome (FMNS)
3. Spasmus nutans syndrome (SNS)
4. Vestibular nystagmus
    a. Peripheral vestibular imbalance
    b. Central vestibular imbalance
    c. Central vestibular instability
5. Gaze-holding deficiency nystagmus
    a. Eccentric gaze nystagmus
    b. Rebound nystagmus
    c. Gaze-instability nystagmus ("Run-Away")
6. Vision loss nystagmus
    a. Pre-chiasmal
    b. Chiasmal
    c. Post-chiasmal
7. Other pendular nystagmus and nystagmus associated with disease of central myelin
    a. Multiple sclerosis, pelizaeus-merzbacher, cockayne's peroxisomal disorders, toluene abuse.
    b. Pendular nystagmus associated with tremor of the palate.
    c. Pendular vergence nystagmus associated with whipple's disease.
8. Ocular bobbing (typical and atypical)
9. Lid nystagmus

Three common forms of nystagmus are detailed below.[3]

Infantile Nystagmus Syndrome (CEMAS)

Earlier it was known as congenital nystagmus or "motor and sensory" nystagmus.
Diagnostic criteria:
Infantile onset, ocular motor recordings show diagnostic (accelerating) slow phases.
Common associated findings:
Conjugate, horizontal-torsional, increases with fixation attempt, progression from pendular to jerk, family history often positive, constant, conjugate, with or without associated sensory system deficits (e.g. albinism, achromatopsia), associated strabismus or refractive error, decreases with convergence, null and neutral zones present, associated head posture or head shaking, may exhibit a "latent" component, "reversal" with OKN stimulus or (a) periodicity to the oscillation. Candidates on chromosome X and 6 may decrease with induced convergence, increased fusion, extraocular muscle surgery, contact lenses and sedation.
General comments:
Waveforms may change in early infancy, head posture usually evident by 4 years of age. Vision prognosis is dependent on integrity of sensory system.

Infantile nystagmus is an involuntary, bilateral, conjugate, and rhythmic oscillation of the eyes which is present at birth or develops within the first 6 months of life. It may be associated with an afferent visual defect or without visual or neurological impairment.

Louis F Dell'Osso Criteria of Infantile Nystagmus Syndrome.[8]
The criteria of diagnosis of infantile nystagmus are summarized in Table 17.2.

Fusion Maldevelopment Nystagmus Syndrome (FMNS)

It was earlier known as latent manifest nystagmus.

TABLE 17.2: Showing diagnostic criteria of infantile nystagmus

Clinical observations	Ocular motor findings
Binocular with similar amplitude in both eyes	Increasing-velocity slow phases (some linear) (Fig. 17.1)
Usually horizontal (vertical, diagonal, or elliptical rare and *small components missed*)	Distinctive waveforms with foveation periods and breaking saccades (Fig. 17.2)
"Pendular" or "jerk" appearance (often *misdiagnosed*)	Many INS waveforms cannot be differentiated, nor can their direction be determined (Fig. 17.3), clinically (*misdiagnosed* as nystagmus type or jerk direction)
Apparent jerk direction not always correct (often misdiagnosed)	"Horizontal" INS actually has a torsional component (Fig. 17.4) and subclinical SSN
Asymmetric aperiodic alternation possible (baclofen ineffective)	Gaze-modulated, not gaze-evoked, nystagmus
Provoked or increased by "fixation attempt" and stress	Normal smooth pursuit, optokinetic, and vestibulo-ocular systems (each causing a shift in the INS "null") (Fig. 17.5)
Abolished in sleep or inattention to visual tasks	Reversal of the IN with alternate cover due to INS "null" shift (INS with a latent component *misdiagnosed*, "FMNS")
Diminished (damped) by gaze-angle or convergence nulls	Two head postures due to the INS "null" shift in INS with a latent component (*misdiagnosed* as INS with "two nulls")
Reversal with cover (often *misdiagnosed* as FMNS)	Reversal of the IN during optokinetic stimulation (*misinterpreted* as "inversion" of the optokinetic reflex)
Apparent "inversion" of the optokinetic reflex (*misinterpreted*)	Reversal of the IN during smooth pursuit (*misinterpreted* as "reversal" of smooth pursuit)
Apparent "reversal" of smooth pursuit (*misinterpreted*)	Associated head oscillation not *compensatory* due to normal vestibuloocular reflex
Associated head oscillation (*misinterpreted as compensatory*)	Head turns or tilts provide waveforms with the best foveation quality
Associated head turn and/or tilt	Convergence damping improves foveation over a broader range of gaze angles
No oscillopsia except under rare conditions	Tenotomy portion of EOM surgery improves foveation over a broader range of gaze angles
Patients complain of being "slow to see"	Target acquisition time much longer than saccadic reaction time, reducing visual function

Note: Null—the null zone is defined as that position of gaze where nystagmus intensity (amplitude x frequency) is least.

Criteria of diagnosis
Infantile onset, associated strabismus, ocular motor recordings show two types of slow phases may be linear and decelerating (Fig. 17.6) plus high-frequency, low amplitude pendular nystagmus (dual-jerk waveform), jerk in direction of fixing eye.

Common associated findings:
Conjugate, horizontal, uniplanar, usually not associated with sensory system deficits (e.g. albinism, achromatopsia), may change with exaggerated

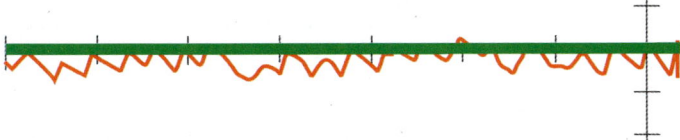

Fig. 17.1: Increasing-velocity slow phases

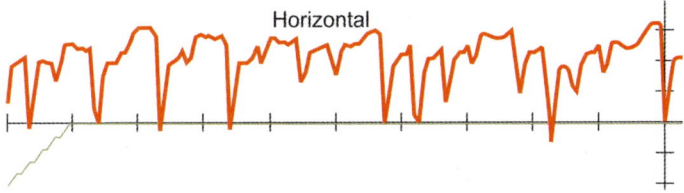

Fig. 17.2: Distinctive waveforms with foveation periods and breaking saccades

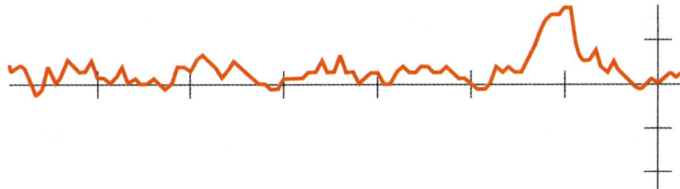

Fig. 17.3: INS waveforms that cannot be differentiated or characterized

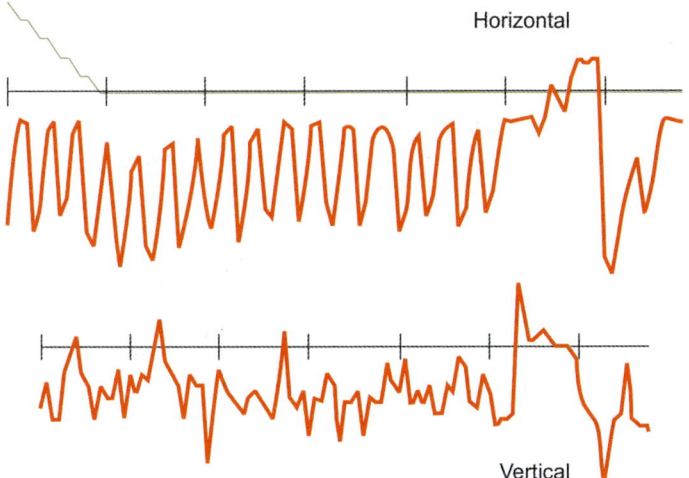

Fig. 17.4: "Horizontal" INS actually has a torsional component (large vertical) in a patient with optic atrophy

convergence ("blockage"), head posture associated with fixing eye in adduction, no headshaking, may exhibit "reversal" with OKN stimulus, no (a)periodicity to the oscillation. Dissociated strabismus may be present. It decreases with increased fusion (binocular function).
Comments: Intensity decreases with age.

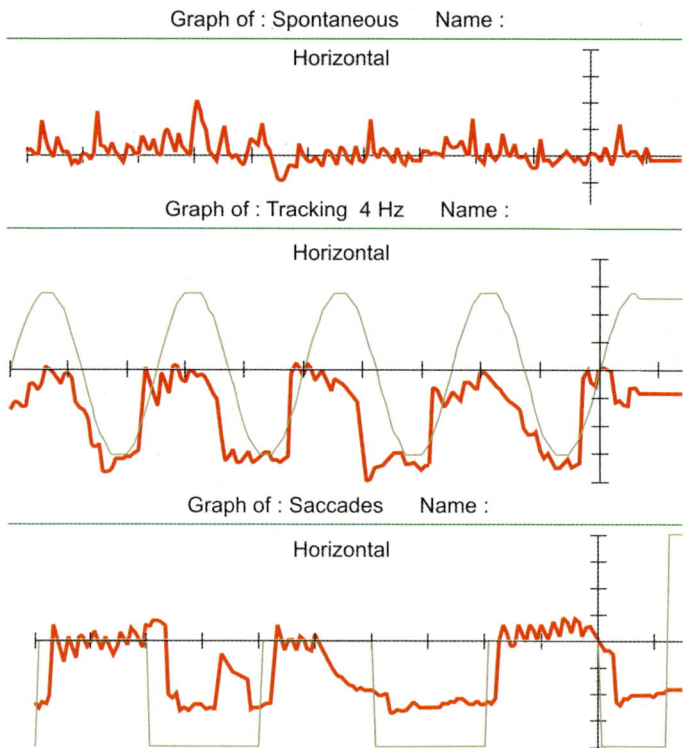

Fig. 17.5: VNG of a child with oculocutaneous albinism showing spontaneous, pursuit and saccadic records

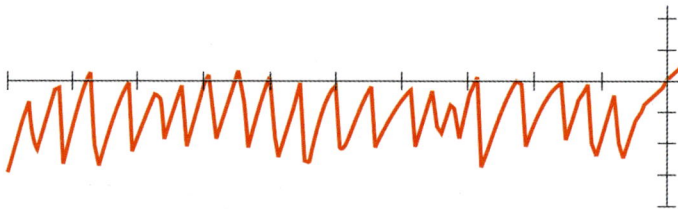

Fig. 17.6: VNG of a man with exotropia and fusion mal development nystagmus syndrome (FMNS) showing decelerating slow phases

Spasmus Nutans Syndrome (SNS)
Criteria of diagnosis
Infantile onset, variable conjugacy, small frequency, low amplitude oscillation, abnormal head posture and head oscillation, improves ("disappears") during childhood, normal MRI/CT scan of visual pathways. Ocular motility recordings show high frequency of >10 Hz (Fig. 17.7), asymmetric, variable conjugacy, pendular oscillations.
Common associated findings:
Dysconjugate, asymmetric, multiplanar, family history of strabismus, may be greater in one (abducting) eye, constant, head posture/oscillation (horizontal

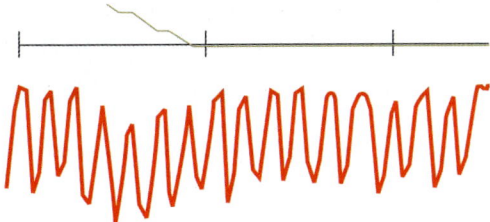

Fig. 17.7: VNG waveforms of a spasmus nutans syndrome

or vertical), usually no associated sensory system deficits may have associated, strabismus and amblyopia, may increase with convergence, head bobbing, head posture may be compensatory. Normal fundus exam decreases with increased fusion (binocular function).

General comments: Usually spontaneously remits in 2–8 years.

Pathophysiology of Nystagmus[9]

Infantile nystagmus syndrome is due to:
1. A high gain instability in the slow eye movement control system.
2. The time constant of the neural integrator is lengthened by a velocity feedback signal and, when the sign of the feedback signal is reversed, the small post-saccadic drift velocities are amplified by the unstable velocity feedback loop, leading to exponentially growing slow phases.
3. Excessive gain in an internal efference copy loop in the smooth pursuit system around a leaky neural integrator.
4. The behavior of burst cell firing, in the form of a saccadic termination abnormality, could account for the variety of CN waveforms.

Acquired Nystagmus

The pathophysiology of acquired nystagmus can be attributed to disturbances of the three mechanisms that normally ensure steady gaze—visual fixation, the vestibulo-ocular reflex, and the mechanism that makes it possible to hold the eyes at an eccentric eye position (e.g. far right gaze).

Knowledge of the nystagmus characteristics can often give clues to the location of the lesion, pathogenesis, and underlying mechanism. Frequently there are multiple mechanisms at work causing the nystagmus.

Procedure of critical examinations in nystagmus is shown in Table 17.3.[10]

Graphic Recording of the Nystagmus

Nystagmus should be recorded in 9 cardinal positions as shown in Figure 17.8.
- Side of the arrow indicates the direction of fast, i.e. corrective phase (direction of nystagmus)
- Number of arrows indicate the frequency (per second beats)
- Length of arrow indicates the amplitude (subjective)
- Type of arrow indicates the trajectory
- Two sided arrows indicate pendular nystagmus
- Alternate direction of arrow indicate periodic alternating nystagmus (PAN).

TABLE 17.3: Showing technique of examination and interpretation of nystagmus

Examination	Technique	Interpretation	Diagnostic utility/relevance
Vision under partial fogging	+4D lens in front of the eye to be occluded after the full optical correction	Prevents latent nystagmus to become manifest	Necessary to assess monocular vision in FMNS/LN
Near vision versus distance vision and convergence dampening	Use logMAR vision assessment for both near and distance testing	In 10% patients there is a true convergence dampening that lead to better vision for near	These patients are highly benefitted by base in prisms or MR recessions (artificial divergence surgery)
Vision in preferred head position	Monocular occlusion and subject reads the optotypes	Reads with head posture. Reads with eye in adduction	Look for null zone. Look for FMNS
Gaze dependant acuity	Best corrected binocular visual acuity is measured with straight ahead posture and then progressively with face turned/tilted/chin up and down 10, 20 and 30 degrees eccentric	Significant change in vision is noted in INS with change of gaze	Very good clinical parameter to assess visual functions in nystagmus
OKN	Smart phone app (viz. eye hand book) OKN drum	Abnormal vertical OKN (absent in up and/or down gaze) indicates neurological anomaly	The patient will need MRI brain
Abnormal head posture (Static/dynamic)	Ask the child to read at distance or resolve a target. Use a goniometer (simple protractor with scale or an android app to measure	Face turn or chin up or down or mixed or pure head tilt	Indicates eccentric Null, (associated with) better vision. Absence of AHP is more likely with sensory defects
Cover test	Apply a cover in front of one eye and alternate		Will reveal any squint or latent nystagmus
Head nodding	Ask the patient to read or resolve	Associated with spasmus nutans where holding the head increases nystagmus. No increase in nystagmus on holding head if INS with or without sensory defects	Only in spasmus nutans, it is compensatory and 180 degrees out of phase with nystagmus that lead to improved vision
Pupil	Direct reaction to light, RAPD and near distance dissociation	Sluggish reaction/ RAPD indicates anterior visual pathway disease	Warrants further investigation–ERG/MRI

Contd...

Contd...

Optic disc evaluation	Pallor/hypoplasia		Warrants further investigation–ERG/MRI
Prism test 1	Keep prisms with apex towards the head posture in front of both/dominant eye	Improvement in head posture	Helps to measure the effect of surgery on face turn and attendant squint/induction of squint
Prism test 2	Keep prism bar apex in to induce convergence	Dampening of nystagmus and improvement in distance visual acuity	Helps to measure the maximum improvement in visual acuity with artificial divergence surgery. Also helps to calculate the amount of bimedial recession

Abbreviations: FMNS, fusion maldevelopment nystagmus syndrome; LN, latent nystagmus (Old terminology).

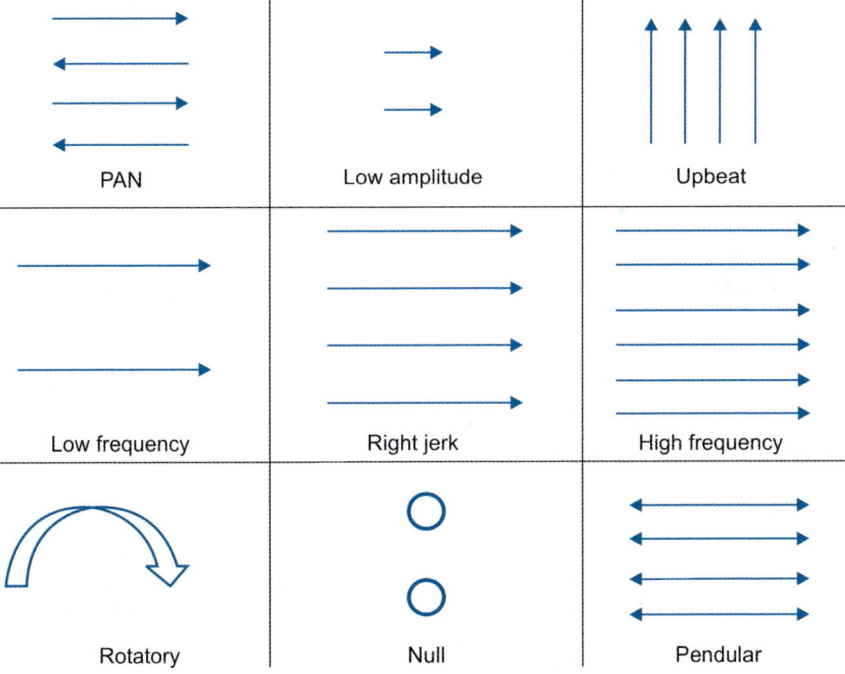

Fig. 17.8: Graphic recording of nystagmus

Abnormal Head Posture (AHP)

In most patients with infantile nystagmus, the head position corresponds roughly to the null zone. However, an anomalous head posture may be present in patients with INS for reasons other than nystagmus, e.g. uncorrected astigmatism, incomitant squint, muscular torticollis, etc. Nevertheless, presence of AHP in a patient with INS has better visual prognosis than no AHP (no null or central null or severe sensory defect that preclude any benefit by maintaining AHP).[11] Horizontal torticollis is seen in 26% alternating head turn in 13% periodic alternating nystagmus (PAN); aperiodic alternating nystagmus (APAN); fusion maldevelopment nystagmus syndrome (FMNS) with fixation switch, vertical abnormal posture in 15%, mixed head position in 2% and pure head tilt is very rare.[12]

The examination algorithm for evaluation of abnormal head posture/torticollis in patient with and without nystagmus is shown in Figure 17.9.

Broad points for the examination of patient with nystagmus are listed in Table 17.4.

Video Nystagmography (VNG) Eye Movement Recording

VNG: Nystagmus eye movements can be recorded at a very high (500–Hz) sampling rate using either an infrared limbus reflection goggle system or a high speed remote video eye tracker.

How does it help in improving the patient care?

1. It provides the correct classification of nystagmus (Table 17.5) and hence the treatment.[13,14]

About 40–60% patients with nystagmus have associated squint. 35% patients having squint and nystagmus have FMNS.[13] The best only method to differentiate INS from FMNS is eye movement recordings.

2. VNG helps to evaluate the evolution of nystagmus.[15]

Many INS waveforms begin as pendular nystagmus. Growth and development of the visual sensory system evoke evolution of waveforms during early infancy from pendular to jerk-type nystagmus by development of corrective fast phases as well as breaking saccades in slow phases producing the so called 'mature' waveforms associated with better vision.

3. Objective assessment of visual functions of a patient with nystagmus.

Using the eye movement recordings one can calculate ANAF/NAFX (foveation time calculation-foveation eye position and eye velocity criteria).[16,17]

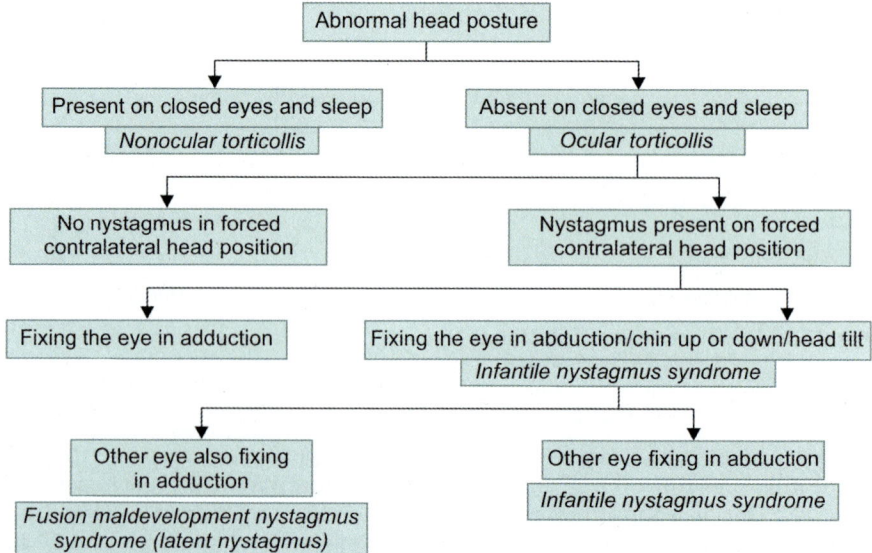

Fig. 17.9: Examination algorithm for evaluation of abnormal head posture

TABLE 17.4: Showing common investigations for patients with nystagmus.

Name of the investigation	Indications	Inferences
Video nystagmography/ eye movement recording	Preferably in every patient of nystagmus to objectively assess → nystagmus with strabismus (to differentiate INS from FMNS)	• Type of nystagmus (classify accurately) • Potential for vision improvement with treatment (NAFX/ANAF) • Objective documentation of response to treatment • Null point evaluation • Identifies vertical components in seemingly horizontal nystagmus • To understand the natural history of the disease and progression/regression in individual patient
OCT	Retinal dystrophy/mal development	• Foveal hypoplasia • Schisis cavity • Accumulation of deposits • Retinal/choroidal thinning
ERG	Sensory nystagmus	• Achromatopisa • CSNB • LCA • Other atypical retinal dystrophies
MRI Brain	Neurological disorder	• Space occupying lesions • Demyelinations • Perinatal damage • Congenital malformations/infections
Red free fundus photography (autofluorescence)	Macular dystrophy	Accumulation of lipofuscin in various macular dystrophies

Abbreviations: NAFX, expanded nystagmus acuity function; ANAF, automated nystagmus acuity function.

TABLE 17.5: Classification of nystagmus

Waveform on VNG	Description	How does it help?
(pendular waveform)	Pendular nystagmus (worse vision than jerk types)	Vision of the patient is likely to be poor as there are no corrective saccades
(jerk with accelerating slow phase)	Jerk with accelerating slow phase	Seen with INS (infantile nystagmus syndrome) with or without sensory defects
(jerk with decelerating slow phase)	Jerk with decelerating slow phase (best visual prognosis)	Seen with FMNS (latent nystagmus). Correct the squint and nystagmus is significantly reduced
(jerk with linear slow phase)	Jerk with linear slow phase	Associated with vestibular or neurological nystagmus

Abbreviations: VNG, Video nystagmography; FMNS, Fusion maldevelopment nystagmus syndrome.

Automated nystagmus acuity function (ANAF)/expanded nystagmus acuity function (NAFX) represents the foveation time which is the period of time during which the eyes are within 30 minutes of arc of the target and moving at less than 4° per second (Fig. 17.10).
4. It can identify patients who need MRI or ERG (Fig. 17.11).
   A patient having disjugate nystagmus or pure vertical nystagmus needs MRI. A patient having large vertical component in the setting of a horizontal nystagmus often needs an ERG/MRI due to an associated sensory defect.
5. Objective evaluation of treatment outcomes:
   VNG can help to assess the effects of various treatment modalities on the ocular motility (Figs 17.12 to 17.15).
6. VNG can help to detect null point as well as convergence dampening (Fig. 17.16).

What is the cause of nystagmus in neurological or retinal disorders?[16,17]

Detailed and routine ERG/MRI and OCT in patients with nystagmus may reveal that as many as 90% patients with nystagmus have associated neurological or retinal diseases. However, the sensory defect is not the cause of nystagmus in them rather an association.[16]

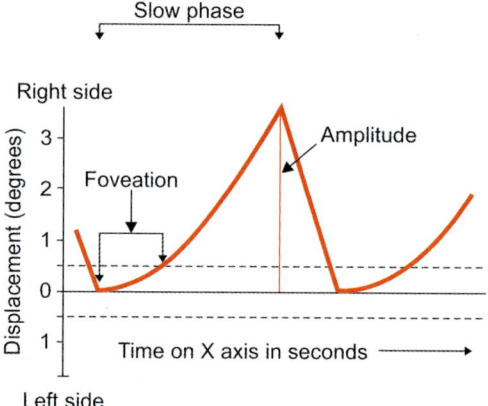

Fig. 17.10: Graphic depiction of the wavelet analysis to determine the foveation time

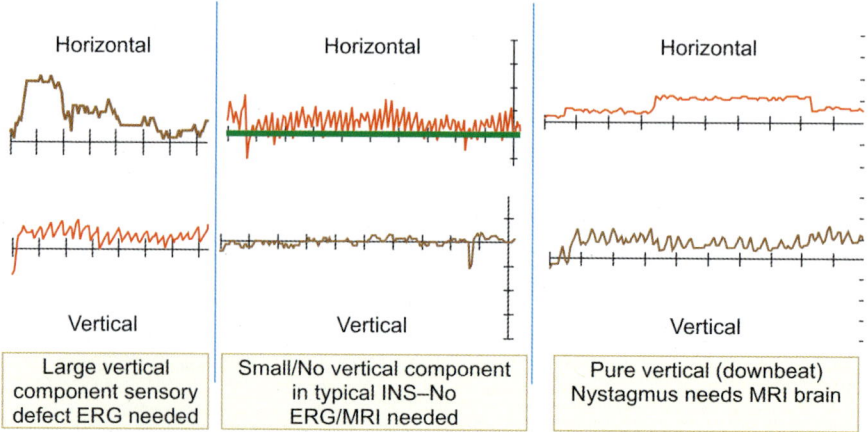

Fig. 17.11: VNG can help to identify a patient who needs MRI or ERG

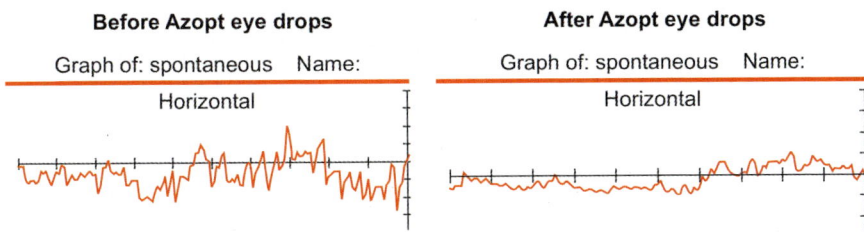

Fig. 17.12: VNG of a patient showing significant improvement with the use of topical brinzolamide eye drops

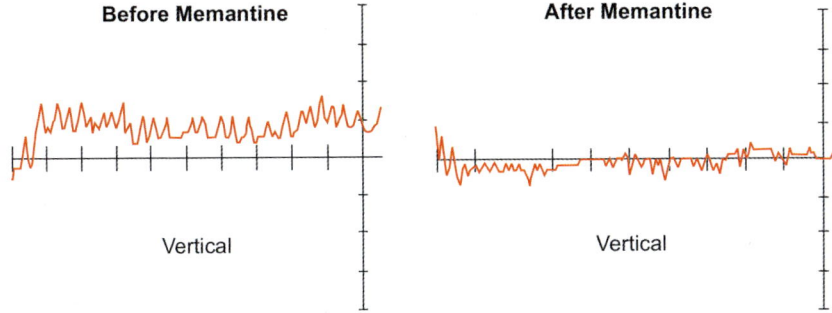

Fig. 17.13: VNG of a patient showing significant improvement in the vertical nystagmus with the use of oral memantine associated with abolition of oscillopsia

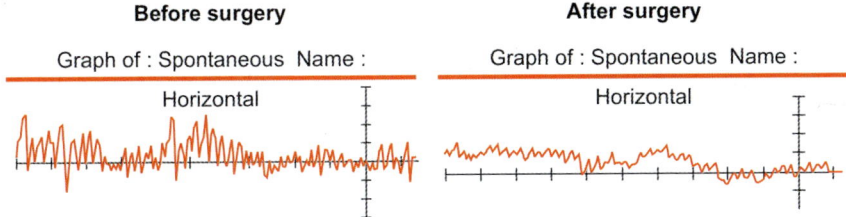

Fig. 17.14: VNG showing the effect of the correction of exotropia in a patient with associated fusion maldevelopment nystagmus

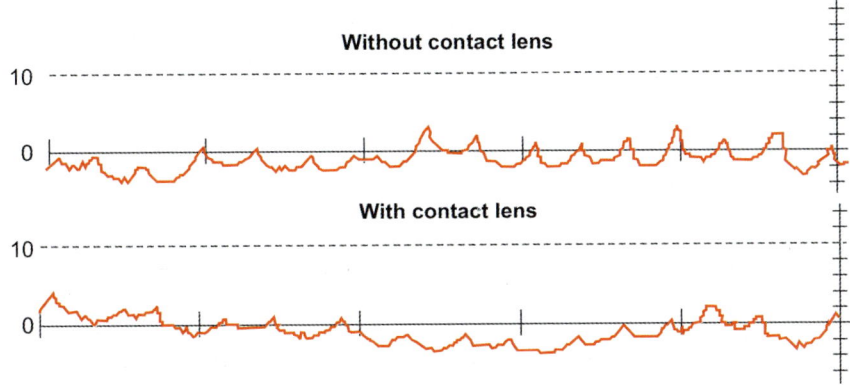

Fig. 17.15: VNG showing the effect of the plano bandage contact lens in INS in a patient experiencing 1 line logMAR improvement

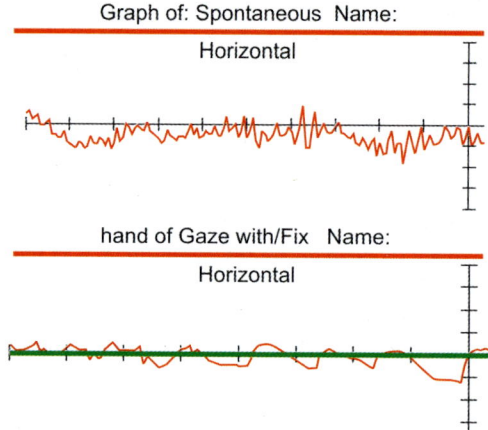

Fig. 17.16: VNG showing the convergence dampening (Gaze with Fix) in a patient with INS

If neurological cause is suspected in nystagmus a MRI brain should be ordered (Table 17.6).

TABLE 17.6: Indication of MRI in nystagmus

	Symptoms or signs that warrant investigations	Disease suspected
See saw nystagmus[17]	All patients need MRI	Chiasmal pathology
Pendular nystagmus with →	Optic atrophy, relative afferent pupillary defect and/or visual field loss[23]	Chiasmal Glioma
Pendular nystagmus with →	Wasting despite a normal appetite, excessive food intake, diabetes insipidus, euphoric affect, headache or lethargy[24]	Hypothalamic tumors
Spasmus nutans:[25] "minimal" head nodding, the small-amplitude and the high-frequency of the oscillations, and the asymmetry of the nystagmus is typical for spasmus nutans. A head turn and tilt is common in congenital nystagmus, but it also occurs in about 2/3rd of patients with spasmus nutans."	Age of onset <4 months or >2 years, significant vertical component, any systemic/ocular signs of neurological deficit. Cafe-au-lait spots/stigmatas of Neurofibromatosis	Gliomas/subacute necrotizing encephalopathy
Vertical nystagmus	Vertical pendular Down beat Upbeat	1. Brainstem and cerebellar disease 2. Craniocervical junction/cerebellar disease 3. Anticonvulsants 4. Cerebellar/pontomedullary abnormalities

Contd...

Contd...

Asymmetric horizontal nystagmus		Non localizing may need ERG also
Abnormal (absent in upgaze and/or downgaze) vertical OKN[7]		Non localizing

Hertle's criteria for neurological work up.[18]

Criteria for neurological work-up in patients with nystagmus are as follows:
1. History
    a. Onset of nystagmus after 6–9 months of age
    b. History of severe prematurely or developmental or genetic diseases
    c. Abnormal pregnancy, labor or delivery
    d. Abnormal and/or delayed growth
    e. Exposure to toxins or drugs
2. Ophthalmic examination
    a. Abnormal vision of the eye(s) (e.g. photophobia, delayed visual behavior)
    b. Abnormal structural examination of the eye(s) (e.g. foveal or optic nerve dysplasia)
    c. Nystagmus pattern vertical, asymmetric, dysconjugate or associated with other ocular motor disorders (e.g. decreased pursuit, abnormal saccades, and paretic gaze).
3. General pediatric examination
    a. Pediatrician is concerned with growth, development or patient has manifest hard, soft, focal or diffuse neurologic signs
    b. Localizing signs of acquired nystagmus[19] are tabulated in Table 17.7.

TABLE 17.7: Showing localizing signs in acquired nystagmus

Location	Movement disorder
Diencephalon	See-saw nystagmus
Mesencephalon	Convergence retraction nystagmus
Myoclonic triangle (ipsilateral red nucleus and inferior olive and contralateral dentate nucleus)	Oculopalatal myoclonus
Anterior vermis of cerebellum and intrinsic medullary disease	Upbeat type 1 (large amplitude in primary position, type in upgaze) Upbeat type 2 (small amplitude in primary position, type in downgaze, 1 in upgaze)
Superior vestibular nucleus	Periodic alternating nystagmus
Cerebellar hemispheres	Rebound nystagmus
Cervicomedullary junction	Downbeat nystagmus

An ERG is indicated when abnormal ocular condition associated with nystagmus.[29] They are listed in Table 17.8.

TABLE 17.8: Order ERG if abnormal ocular conditions are associated with nystagmus

Diseases	Features	ERG abnormalities
Leber's congenital amaurosis (LCA)	Paradoxical pupil reaction (pupil constrict when room lights are switched off), oculo digital sign +, enophthalmos	ERG—extinguished (rule out mental retardation, SNHL, cardiomyopathy, medullary cystic renal disease, cerebellar vermis hypoplasia)
Achromatopsia	Pronounced paradoxical pupil reaction, light sensitivity, dyschromatopsia	Photopic ERG attenuated. scotopic ERG normal
Congenital stationary night blindness	Paradoxical pupil reaction, nyctalopia	Negative wave ERG (attenuated 'a' wave)
Joubert syndrome	Developmentally delayed infants, breathing problems	Attenuated or non-recordable ERG, MRI brain, cerebellar vermis hypoplasia
Peroxisomal disorders	High, bulging forehead, hepatomegaly, renal cysts, sensorineural hearing loss, hypotonia, retinal dystrophy'	ERG extinguished

Nystagmus can be the initial sign of life-threatening neurological or vision threatening retinal diseases/vestibular diseases. Appropriate investigations should be done to rule them out.

MANAGEMENT

Optical Management of Nystagmus[10]
Optical management of nystagmus is shown in Table 17.9.

TABLE 17.9: Optical management of nystagmus

Type of defect	Correction measure	Remark
Refractive error	Full correction	
Contact lenses	Soft, bandage or powered/semisoft clear or tinted contact lenses can be prescribed	There may or may not be significant improvement in visual acuity, foveation and light sensitivity[20]
Convergence dampening	Base out prism	Typically 7PD base out with -1DS in non-presbyopic
Accommodation failure	Bifocals	Patients with aniridia, albinism, cerebral vision impairment, foveal hypoplasia, etc... may have significant defects in accommodation
Head postures	Prisms with apex in the direction of the head (will move the eye to center)	Good for small (<20 PD) postures. More useful for the vertical torticollis
Nystagmus/refractive error and light sensitivity	Contact lenses	CL Material does not matter, Correct the refractive error and use painted contact lenses for aniridia or albinism
Low vision	Optical and non-optical aids	
Light sensitivity	Photogray/tinted lenses	In spectacles or contact lenses
Oscillopsia	Apex of prism towards head posture (e.g. apex up for down beat nystagmus)	with image stabilization (high–contact lens with high + spectacles)

Pharmacological Treatment of Nystagmus[21-23]

Pharmacological treatment of nystagmus is summarized in Table 17.10.
Brinzolamide eye drops for nystagmus.[24-26]

Topical brinzolamide (1%) eye drops thrice a day is noted to improve foveation by 50%, with a 50% broadening of the null zone (Fig. 17.17). Its effect may be equivalent to systemic acetazolamide or eye muscle surgery but intermediate between those of soft contact lenses or convergence. Topical brinzolamide and contact lenses had equivalent LFD (longest foveation domain) improvement and were less effective than convergence. 80% patients on the drops may experience improvement in best corrected vision corresponding to a one-line improvement on the Snellen chart. Visible reduction in nystagmus takes place in 27% and reduced AHP in 22%.

Nearly 30% patients would experience no change. Topical brinzolamide may be contraindicated in congenital or acquired pathologies of corneal endothelium. The effect comes within one week and lasts as long as the drops are continued (Fig. 17.18). There may be an additive effect of the drops when used after the tenotomy and reattachment procedure (Fig. 17.19).

The surgical procedures in nystagmus:[27-32]
The aims of surgery are:

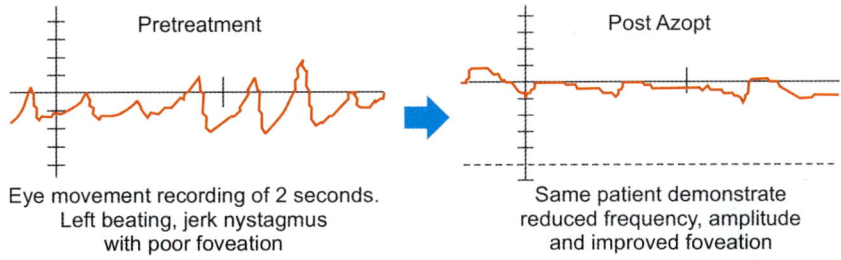

Fig. 17.17: VNG showing significant improvement in the foveation even after one year of continued use of Azopt eye drops

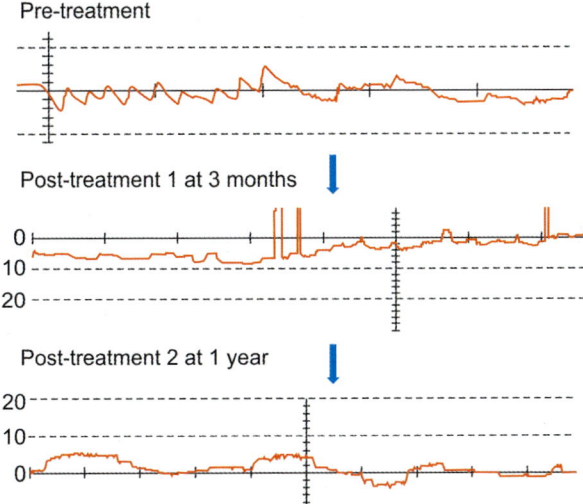

Fig. 17.18: Marked improvement after 1 year treatment with Azopt

TABLE 17.10: Etiolgy, clinical characteristics, pharmacological treatment of different types of nystagmus

	Downbeat nystagmus (DBN)	Upbeat nystagmus (UBN)	Acquired pendular nystagmus (APN)	Periodic alternating nystagmus (PAN)	Infantile (congenital) nystagmus
Direction of nystagmus (quick phase)	Downward, may be diagonal with lateral gaze	Upward	Mainly horizontal, may have vertical and/or torsional components	Horizontal	Mainly horizontal; may have torsional and small vertical components
Waveform (slow phase)	Jerk, constant, increasing, or decreasing slow-phase velocity	Jerk, constant, increasing, or decreasing slow phase velocity	Pendular, sinusoidal slow-phase	Jerk, mostly constant slow-phase velocity	Accelerating slow phases; Foveation periods when the eye is transiently still
Special features	Increased intensity during lateral and downward gaze; sometimes influenced by convergence	Increased intensity during upward gaze; may convert to DBN on convergence	Associated with other oscillations (e.g., palate) and with hypertrophic degeneration of the inferior olive	Changes direction every 90–120 s	Null zone, in which nystagmus is minimal; often suppressed with convergence
Sites of lesion	Cerebellum (bilateral flocullar hypofunction); rarely lower brainstem lesions	Medial medulla, pontomesencephalic junction, rarely cerebellum	Pontomedullary, probably affecting components of neural integrator for gaze holding	Cerebellum (nodulus, uvula)	Uncertain; some cases are associated with afferent visual system anomalies
Etiology	Cerebellar tumors, degenerations, Chiari malformations, and stroke; idiopathic; often associated with bilateral vestibulopathy and neuropathy	Brain stem or cerebellar stroke and tumors; Wernicke's encephalopathy	Multiple sclerosis, oculopalatal tremor due to brainstem or cerebellar stroke involving Guillain-Mollaret triangle	Cerebellar degeneration, craniocervical anomalies, multiple sclerosis, cerebellar tumors and stroke	Uncertain; may be associated with afferent visual system anomalies; hereditary in some patients (e.g. FRMD7 mutations)

Contd...

Contd...

Treatment (dose, frequency)	1. 4-aminopyridine (5–10 mg, tid) 2. 3,4-diaminopyridine (10–20 mg, tid) 3. Baclofen (5–10 mg, tid) 4. Clonazepam (0.5–1 mg, bid)	Often transient, treatment often not necessary 1. Memantine (10 mg, qid) 2. 4-aminopyridine (5–10 mg, tid) 3. Baclofen (5–10 mg, tid)	1. Gabapentin (300 mg, qid) 2. Memantine (10 mg, qid)	1. Baclofen (5–10 mg, tid) 2. Memantine (5–10 mg, qid)	1. Gabapentin (300 mg qid) 2. Memantine (10 mg qid)
Side effects	1. Dizziness, paresthesias, incoordination 2. Dizziness, paresthesias, incoordination 3. Drowsiness, dizziness, lethargy 4. Drowsiness, dizziness, incoordination	1. Lethargy, dizziness, headache 2. Dizziness, paresthesias, incoordination 3. Drowsiness, dizziness, lethargy	1. Dizziness, incoordination, drowsiness 2. Lethargy, dizziness, headache	1. Drowsiness, dizziness, lethargy 2. Lethargy, dizziness, headache	1. Dizziness, incoordination, drowsiness 2. Lethargy, dizziness, headache
Seesaw nystagmus	Clonazepam (0.5–1 mg, bid)/memantine (10 mg, qid)—drowsiness, dizziness, incoordination/lethargy, dizziness, headache				
Torsional	Gabapentin (300 mg, qid)—dizziness, incoordination, drowsiness				

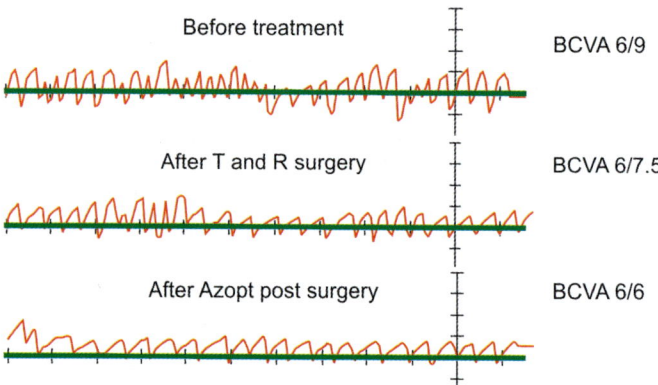

Fig. 17.19: VNG showing synergistic effect of Azopt with surgery

1. To try to improve visual acuity (usually by 1–3 logMAR lines), contrast vision, reaction time (improves by 0.3 seconds)[36c] and gaze dependent acuity by improving the foveation.
2. To transfer the nystagmus null zone from an extreme position to a frontal one, in order to improve abnormal head position and spectacle centration.
3. To correct strabismus when it is present to restore binocular fusion and stereopsis.

The protocol of the author is shown in Figure 17.20A.

Procedures, principle and benefits of surgery are listed in Table 17.11.

TABLE 17.11: Procedures, principle and benefits of surgery

Abnormality	Procedures	Principle	Benefits of surgery	Indication
Nystagmus only	Tenotomy and reattachment (large 4 muscle recessions or muscle extirpations are not preferred)	4 horizontal recti are detached and resutured at the same insertion	25% reduced intensity of nystagmus Broadening of null zone 1–3 lines (logMAR) improvement in vision in 50% patients 40% increase in NAFX in 90% patients	Nystagmus with no null, primary position null or alternating null (periodic or aperiodic) nystagmus with or without sensory/neurological defects
Convergence dampening (near vision better than distance vision)	Artificial divergence surgery	Bilateral medial rectus recession only suitable in patients with confirmed presence of fusion and stereoacuity after measuring the fusional convergence amplitudes	70–90% dampening of nystagmus, marked improvement in vision	Patients with INS and convergence dampening with near vision > distance vision

Contd...

Contd...

Combined with abnormal head posture (move the eyes in the direction of head turn/tilt/chin)	Augmented Anderson procedure	9 mm MR recession and 12/13 mm LR recession	1. 20 degrees correction of face turn 2. 2.5 degree reduction in amplitude of nystagmus 3. 1.5 Hz reduction in frequency of nystagmus	Patients with INS and moderate face turn (<25 degrees)
	Augmented Kestenbaum Anderson Procedure	Classic 5,6,7,8 recess resect augmented with degree appropriate to the face turn to move the null to the centre (20% augmented for 20 degree face turn, 30% for 30 degrees, so forth and so on)	1. 20–60 degrees correction of face turn 2. 25% reduction in amplitude and frequency of nystagmus 3. 1–3 lines (LogMAR) improvement in vision	Patients with INS with moderate to severe face turn
	Oblique/torsional Kestenbaum Anderson procedure	Inferior oblique advance or recess and superior oblique anterior fibres tenotomy or advancement (Harada Ito)	1. Correction of head tilt—approximately 5 degrees per mm of surgery	Head tilts
	Elevator weakening or depressor weakening	IO myectomy with SR recession 5mm for chin down or SO tenectomy with IR recession 4 mm for chin up	1. Correction of the head posture	Chin up or down
Combined squint and nystagmus	FMNS with Squint (diagnosis in VNG/EMR)	Correct the squint only	1. Correction of squint and recovery of fusion and stereopsis 2. Conversion of Manifest nystagmus to a latent nystagmus 3. Improvement in vision	VNG/EMR needed for any patient with squint and nystagmus to identify this type
	INS with Squint	Correct the squint and add T and R	Benefits of both – squint and nystagmys surgery	

Contd...

Contd...

| Combined squint, abnormal head posture and nystagmus | FMNS/INS with squint and abnormal head posture | Squint surgery on non-dominant eye and head posture surgery on dominant eye | Benefits of squint surgery, nystagmus surgery and correction of abnormal head postures ++ | Use prisms to correct the head posture in front of dominant eye and then correct the squint with prisms in front of non dominant eye and then calculate the amount of surgery |

Abbreviations: T and R, Tenotomy and reattachment of horizontal muscles

The author performs vertical off sets of horizontal recti for small (up to 10–15 degrees) head tilts associated with face turns. For larger head tilts, oblique/torsional Kestenbaum Anderson procedure have given excellent results (Figs 17.20B).[33,34]

Surgical Protocol of Dr Richard Hertle[18] is also popular. The readers can find the details of operation elsewhere,

Surgical Treatment of Nystagmus

1. **Induced convergence damping (artificial divergence)**
   It is indicated for establishing binocular function (stereopsis) with measurable foveation improvement with prism adapt with 7 base out each eye, not Fresnell.
   Operation 1: Bilateral medial rectus recess 3.0 and bilateral lateral rectus tenotomy with reattachment.
2. **Eccentric horizontal null position**
   Measurable or clinically observable eccentric gaze null with head posture in opposite direction.
   Preparation: Rule out aperiodic or periodic infantile subtype, no changing posture over 10 minutes of observation.
   Operation 2: Recess lateral rectus 10.0 in the abducted eye and medial rectus 7.0 in the adducted eye with tenotomies and reattachment of the other horizontal recti for turns up to 20 degrees or recess lateral rectus 10.0 mm in the abducted eye and medial rectus 7.0 mm in the adducted eye.
   Operation 3: Torsional head posture
   Indication: Torsional head posture alone, rule out aperiodic or periodic infantile subtype, no changing posture over 10 minutes of observation.
   Technique: Horizontal transposition of vertical recti one full tendon width, (take the vertical recti off, move the eyes in the direction of the head posture, reattach the vertical recti).
   Operation 4: Chin up head posture
   Indication: Chin-up head posture alone, nystagmus changes intensity in upgaze. Rule out aperiodic or periodic infantile subtype, no changing posture over 10 minutes of observation.
   Technique: Bilateral superior oblique 5.0 mm tenectomy nasal to the superior rectus plus bilateral inferior rectus 4 mm recessions.
   Operation 5: Chin down head posture

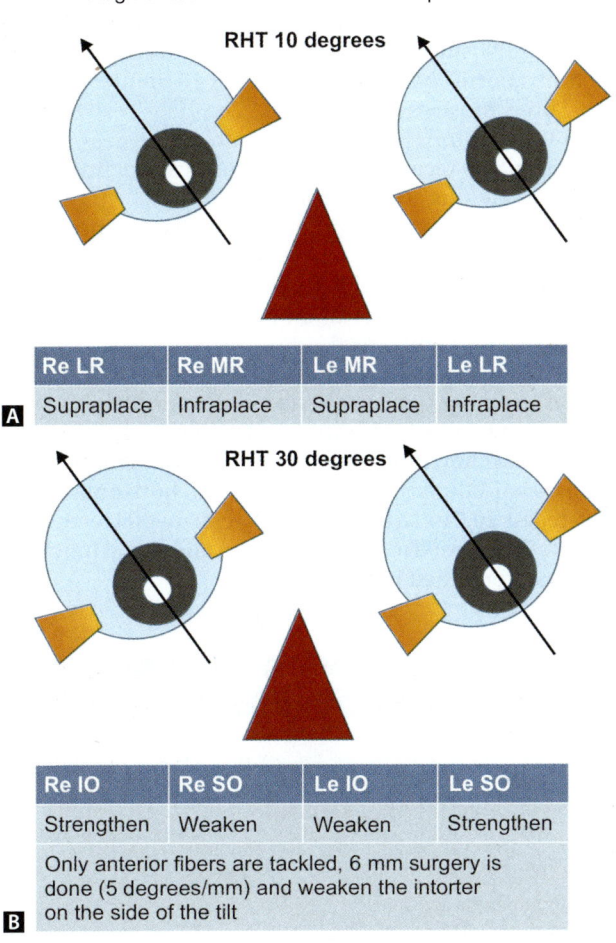

Figs 17.20A and B: (A) Vertical offsets of horizontal muscle for right head tilt of 10 degrees; (B) Oblique Kestenbaum Anderson procedure for right head tilt of 30 degrees

Indication: Chin-down head posture alone, nystagmus changes intensity in down gaze. Rule out aperiodic or periodic infantile subtype, no changing posture over 10 minutes of observation.
Technique: Bilateral inferior oblique myectomy plus bilateral superior rectus 4.0 mm recessions.
Operation 6: Head posture, nystagmus and strabismus.
Indication: Rule out aperiodic or periodic infantile subtype or esotropia with fusion maldevelopment and adduction null, i.e., no changing posture over 10 minutes of observation. Determine fixing eye (eye driving the head posture)
Technique: Straighten the head with prism correction over the preferred eye, neutralize the resulting strabismic deviation with prism over the non-preferred eye. Perform bilateral recess/resect on each eyes respective measured prism correction or bilateral recess plus tenotomy with reattachment on the remaining two horizontal recti.

Operation 7: Multiplanar head posture
Indication: Combination chin up/down and face turn. Rule out aperiodic or periodic infantile subtype or esotropia with fusion maldevelopment and adduction null, i.e., no changing posture over 10 minutes of observation.
Technique: Three muscles of each eye. Combine respective oblique plus vertical recti (above) for chin up/down with 10.0 recess of lateral rectus of abducting eye and 7.0 recess of medial rectus of adducting eye.

Operation 8: Nystagmus and strabismus
Indication: Nystagmus and horizontal strabismus with no head posture treat refractive errors.
Technique: Recess/resect all four horizontal recti for the total deviation or bilateral recess for the total deviation plus tenotomy with reattachment on the remaining two horizontal recti.

Operation 9: Nystagmus alone (about 15%) with or without periodicity and no strabismus, static anomalous head posture or fusion with convergence damping. Rule out strabismus, static head posture or convergence damping
Technique: Bilateral horizontal recti tenotomy with reattachment and, if the patient desires additional damping, bilateral horizontal rectus recession (lateral recti recess 10.0 to 12.0 mm and bilateral medial recess 8.0 to 10.0 mm).

A questionnaire is designed to study the visual and social functions of the child with nystagmus and appended in Annexure 1.

ANNEXURE 1

Visual function Questionnaire-14	Nil	Mild problem	Medium problem	Severe problem
Do you/your child have any difficulty, even with glasses…..				
1. Reading small print—e.g. food label, phone book				
2. Reading a book or newspaper				
3. Reading a large print book or recognising numbers on TV				
4. Recognising people when they are close to you				
5. Seeing steps, stairs, or curbs				
6. Reading traffic signs, street signs, or shop signs				
7. Doing fine handwork—e.g. sewing, knitting, crafts				
8. Filling in forms				
9. Playing games—e.g. cards, dominoes, board games				
10. Taking part in sport				
11. Cooking				
12. Watching television				
13. Driving during the day—omitted from child questionnaire				
14. Driving at night—omitted from child questionnaire				

REFERENCES

1. Sarvananthan N, Surendran M, Roberts EO, Jain S, Thomas S, Shah N, et al. The prevalence of nystagmus: the Leicestershire nystagmus survey. Invest Ophthalmol Vis Sci. 2009;50(11):5201-6.
2. Spielmann A. Clinical rationale for manifest congenital nystagmus surgery. J AAPOS. 2000;4(2):67-74.
3. https://nei.nih.gov/sites/default/files/nei-pdfs/cemas.pdf accessed on 4/7/17.
4. Hyvärinen I, lindstedt E, (EDs). Early visual development—normal and abnormal. Acta opthalmol (copenh). 1983;(suppl 157):1-122.
5. Shin YJ, Park KH, Hwang JM, Wee WR, Lee JH, Lee IB. Objective measurement of visual acuity by optokinetic response determination in patients with ocular diseases. Am J Ophthalmol. 2006;141(2):327-32.
6. Halmagyi GM, Gresty MA, Leech J. Reversed Optokinetic Nystagmus (OKN): Mechanism and Clinical Significance. Ann Neurol. 1980;7(5):429-35.
7. Garbutt S, Harris CM. Abnormal vertical optokinetic nystagmus in infants and children. Br J Ophthalmol. 2000;84(5):451-5.
8. Hertle RW, Dell'Osso LF. Clinical and ocular motor analysis of congenital nystagmus in infancy. J AAPOS. 1999;3:70-9.
9. Abadi RV. Mechanisms underlying nystagmus. J R Soc Med. 2002;95(5):231-4.
10. Hertle RW. Examination and refractive management of patients with nystagmus. Surv Ophthalmol. 2000;45(3):215-22.
11. Relationships between visual acuity and anomalous head posture in patients with congenital nystagmus. J pediatr Ophthalmol Strabismus. 2003;40:259-64.
12. Spielmann A. "clinical rationale for manifest congenital nystagmus surgery," Journal of Aapos. 2000; 4(2):67-74.
13. Motor and sensory characteristics of infantile nystagmus. Br J Ophthalmol. 2002;86:1152-60.
14. Dell'osso LF. Congenital, latent and manifest latent nystagmus: similarities, differences and relation to strabismus. Jpn J Ophthalmol. 1985;29:351-68.
15. Hertle RW, Maldanado VK, Maybodi M, Yang D. Clinical and ocular motor analysis of the infantile nystagmus syndrome in the first 6 months of life. Br J Ophthalmol. 2002;86(6):670-5.
16. Nystagmus in Infancy and Childhood: Current Concepts in Mechanisms, Diagnoses, and Management, Richard W. Hertle and Louis F. Dell'Osso. Oxford university press, UK. 2010.
17. Nystagmus in infancy and childhood. In: Brodsky MC, Baker RS, Hamed LM, editors. Pediatric neuro-ophthalmology. New York: Springer; 1996. p. 302-47.
18. https://www.google.co.in/url?sa=t&rct=j&q=&esrc=s&source=web&cd=1&cad=rja&uact=8&ved=0ahUKEwj4rYXLzevNAhUGsY8KHS33De8QFgguMAA&url=http%3A%2F%2Fwww.privateeyeclinic.com%2Fpublectandaud%2FSQUINTCLUB08%2FNystagmus_workshop_%255BHertle%2520et%2520al%255D.pdf&usg=AFQjCNFKB_jfvxoGDM4N-xVh-NJXRB86Hg Accessed on 11/7/2016.
19. Wertenbaker C, Henkind P, Keltner JL, Miller NR, Burde RM. Downbeat nystagmus. Surv Ophthalmol. 1981;25(4):263-9.
20. Infantile nystagmus syndrome: broadening the high-foveation-quality field with contact lenses. Clinical Ophthalmology. 2008;2(3):585-9.
21. Thurtell MJ, Rucker JC, Tomsak RL, et al. Medical treatment of acquired nystagmus. Expert Rev Ophthalmol. 2011;6:307-14.
22. Mehta AR, Kennard C. The pharmacological treatment of acquired nystagmus. Pract Neurol. 2012;12(3):147-53.
23. Strupp M, Thurtell MJ, Shaikh AG, et al. Pharmacotherapy of vestibular and ocular motor disorders, including nystagmus. J Neurol. 2011;258:1207-22.

24. Hertle RW, Yang D, Adkinson T, Reed M. Topical brinzolamide (Azopt) versus placebo in the treatment of infantile nystagmus syndrome (INS). Br J Ophthalmol. 2015;99(4):471-6. doi: 10.1136/bjophthalmol-2014-305915. Epub 2014 Oct 21.
25. Dell'osso LF, Hertle RW, Leigh RJ, Jacobs JB, King S, Yaniglos S. Effects of topical brinzolamide on infantile nystagmus syndrome waveforms: eyedrops for nystagmus. J Neuroophthalmol. 2011;31(3):228-33.
26. Gokyigit B, Demet Aygıt E, Akar S, Gunes H, Demirok A. The effects of topical carbonic anhydrase inhibitor for treatment of nystagmus. http://www.comtecmed.com/cophy/2013/Uploads/Editor/Gokyigit2.pdf Accessed on 12/7/16.
27. Dell'Osso LF, Hertle RW, Williams RW, Jacobs JB. A new surgery for congenital nystagmus: effects of tenotomy on an achiasmatic canine and the role of extraocular proprioception. J AAPOS. 1999;3(3):166-82.
28. ElKamshoushy A, Shawky D, ElMassry A, ElBaha S, Abdel Wahab MM, Sprunger D. Improved visual acuity and recognition time in nystagmus patients following four-muscle recession or Kestenbaum-Anderson procedures. J AAPOS. 2012;16(1):36-40.
29. Hertle RW, Dell'Osso LF, FitzGibbon EJ, Yang D, Mellow SD. Horizontal rectus muscle tenotomy in children with infantile nystagmus syndrome: a pilot study. J AAPOS. 2004;8(6):539-48.
30. Hertle RW, Dell'Osso LF, FitzGibbon EJ, Thompson D, Yang D, Mellow SD. Horizontal rectus tenotomy in patients with congenital nystagmus: results in 10 adults. Ophthalmology. 2003;110(11):2097-105.
31. Spielmann A. Clinical rationale for manifest congenital nystagmus surgery. J AAPOS. 2000;4(2):67-74.
32. Gupta R, Sharma P, Menon V. A prospective clinical evaluation of augmented Anderson procedure for idiopathic infantile nystagmus. J AAPOS. 2006;10(4):312-7.
33. Prakash P, Arya AV, Sharma P, Chandra VM. Torsional Kestenbaum in congenital nystagmus with torticollis. Indian J Ophthalmol. 1990;38(2):70-3.
34. Lee J. Surgical management of nystagmus. Journal of the Royal Society of Medicine. 2002;95(5):238-41.

Chapter 18

Cystinosis

Shefali Vyas

INTRODUCTION

Embryonic organogenesis of the kidney and eye has been studied since 19th century but the recent evolution of molecular technologies has advanced our understanding of mechanics of various genes regulating the development of eye and the kidney tubules. Recent knowledge in understanding the genetic pathways for renal tubular acidosis have triggered a renewed interest in variety of congenital and acquired oculo renal disorders.

The classic Fanconi syndrome was first described by Abderhalden[1] in 1903 in a patient with cystinosis. Fanconi syndrome is characterized by proximal renal tubular dysfunction causing polyuria and wasting of solutes like bicarbonate, glucose, phosphate, uric acid, low molecular weight proteins, sodium and amino acids in the urine. The genetic causes of Fanconi could be primary due to missense mutation in Na phosphate cotransporter (NaPi-II) of the proximal tubular apical membrane. The human Na-HCO_3-cotransporter (NBC1) gene encodes two sodium-bicarbonate cotransport proteins, pancreatic type (pNBC1) and kidney type (kNBC1). Both kNBC-1 and pNBC-1 transporters are present in the corneal endothelium, trabecular meshwork, ciliary epithelium, and lens epithelium. This rare mutations in the human NBC1 gene in exons common to both pNBC1 and kNBC1 results in severe ocular and renal manifestations which include blindness, band keratopathy, glaucoma, cataracts, and proximal renal tubular acidosis.[2]

The secondary genetic causes of Fanconi include multitude of conditions like cystinosis, tyrosinemia, Wilson's disease, Lowe's syndrome, galactosemia, hereditary fructose intolerance but most common of them all is cystinosis. The most common cause of acquired Fanconi is drugs induced RTA. Today in this chapter we will focus on cystinosis and its ocular manifestations.

Genetics

Cystinosis is a rare autosomal recessive disorder caused by mutation in cystinosis gene (CTNS) and maps to chromosome 17p13, a 367 amino acid integral membrane protein that transports cystine out of the lysosome. In patients many mutations (>100) have been described in the first 10 exons and in the promotor of the cystinosis gene, with the clinical phenotype segregating with specific defects. Cystinosis is a metabolic disease, characterized by an accumulation of cystine, a disulfide of the amino acid cysteine, in different organs and tissues, leading to potentially severe organ dysfunction. These effects are especially seen in the eye and the kidney but other organs are also involved like the muscles, thyroid and even testes and pancreas may be affected.[3,4] Three forms of cystinosis have been described: the infantile (nephropathic) form (MIM #219800), the late-onset (juvenile) form (MIM #219900); and the adult (benign) form (MIM #219750). Nephropathic cystinosis, which is by far the most common and also the most severe of all the three, is estimated to affect 1 of every 100,000 to 200,000 children.

CLINICAL MANIFESTATIONS

Renal

Children with cystinosis are born asymptomatic and usually start having clinical symptoms by 6 months of age. They present with failure to thrive, polyuria, dehydration, vomiting and sometimes rickets from hypophosphatemia. They can also have carnitine deficiency due to urinary losses of carnitine. If untreated they can progress to end stage renal disease by first decade of life. The availability of cystine depleting agent cysteamine has greatly improved the life expectancy and reduction in end organ damage. So it is imperative that the patients are diagnosed early to ensure appropriate treatment with cysteamine is started as soon as possible.

EXTRARENAL MANIFESTATIONS

Growth Retardation

This is noted early within the first 2 years of life. Aggressive management with fluid and electrolyte corrections, early treatment with cysteamine and sometimes Growth hormone therapy is needed to treat the failure to thrive and growth problems. Hypophosphatemic rickets due to excessive phosphate losses can cause osteodystrophy. Phosphate repletion and vitamin D supplementation with orthopedic involvement for braces and splints is required to ensure proper limb growth and avoidance of osteodystrophy. Patients may need gastrostomy tube for feeding and medications to provide nutrition and access for fluid electrolyte management.

Endocrine

There are anecdotal reports of insulin dependant diabetes in patient on peritoneal dialysis and in one patient post-transplant on high doses of corticosteroids. Thyroid problems have been reported in the form of hypothyroidism and usually seen after first decade of life. Thyroid functions have to be monitored closely for early detection and treatment.

Myopathy

Muscle weakness is seen in the beginning due to hypokalemia and carnitine deficiency. Carnitine levels need to monitored and replaced. In the second decade of life progressive distal muscle weakness and swallowing difficulties have been described.

Neurology

Most children have normal neurological functions but may develop mild decline. Increased risk of Chiari I malformation have been described. More severe neurological problems have been described after 2nd decade in life.[3]

Gonads

Delayed puberty and infertility has been reported in males. Testesterone replacement therapy allows for pubertal development in males but does not affect infertility. Females have delayed puberty but successful pregnancies have been reported in females.

The other two forms of cystinosis are milder—the intermediate of juvenile form usually diagnosed later in adolescence with less severe renal manifestations. The adult onset is characterized by the presence of corneal crystals and photophobia and less often renal disease and hence has been also termed "ocular" or non-nephropathic cystinosis.

PATHOGENESIS

Cystine is end product of protein degradation in the lysosomes of cells and is normally transported through the lysosomal membrane to the cytosol where it is reutilized after its transformation to cysteine. The defect in the gene that encodes cystinosin, the protein that transports cystine across the lysosomal membrane causes accumulation of cystine which is poorly soluble and forms crystals as its concentration increases.

Herein are two pictures with cystine deposits in the eye and renal interstitium: the first picture shows classic refractile crystals in the cornea (Fig. 18.1) and the second picture shows H and E stain of renal biopsy with birefringent crystals of cystine in the renal interstitium (Fig. 18.2).

The exact mechanism causing cellular dysfunction is not known.[5] A proposed mechanism is cysteinylation of protein kinase delta by accumulated cystine resulting in increased apoptosis of the cystine-laden renal proximal tubular cell, which causes tubular dysfunction. It has also been shown that cystine accumulation in proximal tubular cells in vitro is associated with ATP depletion

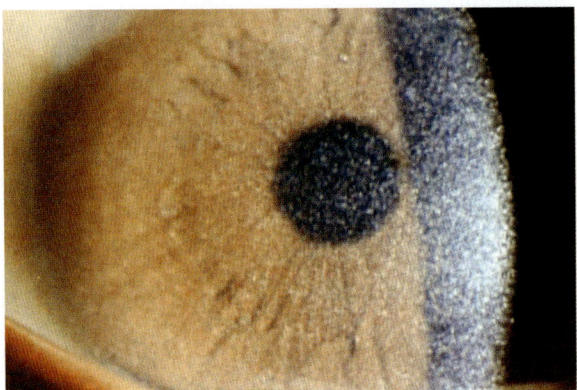

Fig. 18.1: Crystals are seen the cornea in a patient with cystinosis

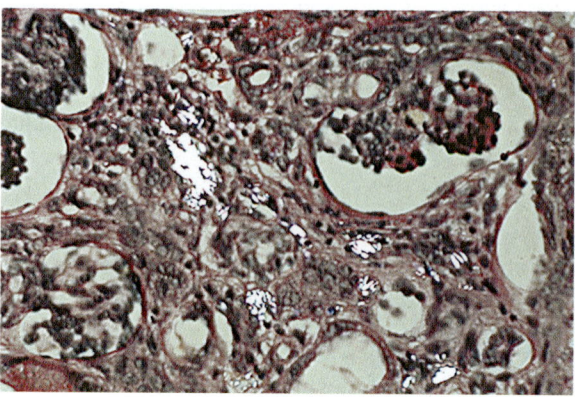

Fig. 18.2: Nephropathic cystinosis is marked by the depositoin of birefrigerant interstitial crystals in the kidney. The H and E stain of renal biopsy here shows birefringent crystals of cystine in the renal interstitium

and inhibition of Na⁺ dependent transporters. A study using a cystinosin knockout mice model showed decreased expression of megalin, cubilin, and sodium transporters at the apical surface of proximal tubular cells. Inhibition of adenylate cyclase activity by cystine in rat brain is prevented by cysteamine. In addition, cellular cystine accumulation may inhibit pyruvate kinase and creatine kinase activity in rat brain or pig retina. Cystine depletes the glutathione cell pool, thereby favoring oxidative stress and apoptosis.

Pathogenesis Involving the Eye

Crystal accumulation in the conjunctiva and cornea were initially described by Bürki in 1941 and is the pathognomonic ophthalmic manifestation of cystinosis. Tsilou et al. in their paper have described at length the various ophthalmic manifestations with review of literature.[6] They note that the corneal crystals are myriad needle-shaped, highly reflectile opacities easily seen by slitlamp examination and appear to be present in the corneal epithelium, stroma and endothelium (As shown in the picture). These can easily be differentiated from other crystalline keratopathies due to their characteristic appearance and distribution.

The accumulation of crystals in the cornea begins in infancy and is definitely evident by 16 months of age. Deposition begins in the anterior periphery and proceeds posteriorly and centripetally. By approximately 7 years of age, the entire peripheral stroma and endothelium accumulates crystals. By approximately 20 years of age, crystals can be seen in the entire corneal stroma. Crystal deposition advances more rapidly in the periphery. Increased density of cystine crystals results in a hazy cornea that is easily recognizable with the naked eye in older, untreated cystinosis patients.

DIAGNOSIS AND MANAGEMENT

Early diagnosis of cystinosis is important to start therapy with cysteamine and prevent end organ damage. Currently, as per the cystinosis consensus research group 50% patients worldwide are diagnosed after 1 year of age.

The following three tests can confirm diagnosis of cystinosis:
1. Measurement of leukocyte cystine levels (LCL)
2. Demonstration of corneal cystine crystals by the slit lamp examination and
3. Genetic analysis of the CTNS gene.

Cystine crystals in the cornea are present by 18 months of age. Measuring LCL requires dedicated laboratories, levels are >2 nmol 1/2 cystine/mg protein in affected patients, whereas normal subjects have LCL <0.2 nmol 1/2 cystine/mg protein.

Prenatal diagnosis in the first trimester can be reliably performed by molecular methods measuring 35S-labeled cystine incorporation into fibroblasts cultured from amniotic fluid cells or chorionic villi.

TREATMENT

The early therapy for these children is optimizing electrolytes and nutrition and so sometimes gastrostomy tube is needed to provide optimal nutrition for growth and for replacement of various electrolytes. Additional therapies may be needed like thyroxine for hypothyroidism, insulin for diabetes, growth hormone for growth failure and carnitor for carnitine deficiency.

It is crucial to start cystine depleting therapy with cysteamine as no curative cure is currently available but cysteamine does improve the overall prognosis. The amino-thiol cysteamine depletes lysosomal cystine content by a disulfide-exchange reaction with cystine. Therapy with cysteamine should be started early and continued even after renal transplantation as the extrarenal damage will continue to progress. The most widely used cysteamine preparation is cysteamine bitartrate (Cystagon), which needs to be given every 6 hours. Leucocyte cystine level (LCL) is used as a biomarker to monitor the effectiveness of cystine depletion, but no definitive demonstration of this approach is available at the tissue level. Cysteamine was approved for clinical use in the USA and Europe in the 1990s, based on its demonstrated efficacy in reducing LCL and the decline of renal function. Recently, a delayed-release cysteamine bitartrate was approved in the USA and Europe in 2013 (Procysbi). Using a microspheronized enteric-coated formulation of cysteamine bitartrate, the pharmaco kinetic characteristics have been modified to allow 12 hours dosing and improve compliance and has reportedly decreased gastrointestinal side effects.

Ophthalmic Treatment

Topical treatment with cysteamine hydrochloride eye drops is needed 6–10 times per day as oral cysteamine has no effect on corneal cystine crystals (patients are usually instructed to use it every waking hour). Most patients, however, apply cysteamine eye drops less frequently (four to six times per day), in part because they cause eye burning, due to the low pH of the solution. In addition, the free thiol can oxidize to cystamine at room temperature, so it is recommended to store frozen aliquots. A commercial 0.44% cysteamine ophthalmic solution (Cystaran) has recently been approved for clinical use in the USA. A 0.55% gel formulation (Cystadrops) has also been developed and preliminary results note superior efficacy. Very rarely, patients not treated with cysteamine eye drops develop corneal lesions severe enough to require a corneal transplant. Cystine crystals can reappear in the transplanted cornea due to invading host cells, if topical cysteamine treatment is not used.

Gene Therapy

Studies are in the works wherein hematopoietic stem cell (HSC) transplantation in a mouse model of cystinosis has been used to test adult bone marrow stem cells as vehicles to bring wild-type CTNS to tissues.[7] Currently research is focused in developing an autologous HSC transplantation strategy whereby the patient's own stem cells are gene-modified ex vivo using a lentiviral vector and re-injected into the patient to introduce a functional CTNS copy in tissues. This is exciting as it may pave road to cure for cystinosis in future.

SUMMARY

The overall prognosis of children with cystinosis has improved with cystine depleting therapy and there is ongoing research to find cure with gene therapy. It is critical to identify and treat these patients early to prevent end organ damage. The role of ophthalmologists to treat and monitor the ocular manifestations of this rare disorder is important part of the multidisciplinary care needed for patients with cystinosis.

REFERENCES

1. Abderhalden E. Familiare cystindiathese. Z Physiol Chem. 1903;38:557-61.
2. Usui T, Hara M, Satoh H, Moriyama N, Kagaya H, Amano S, et al. Molecular basis of ocular abnormalities associated with proximal renal tubular acidosis. J Clin Invest. 2001;108:107-15.
3. Niaudet P. Cystinosis. https:// www.uptodate.com, May 2016.
4. Middleton R, Bradbury M, Webb N, et al. Cystinosis. A clinicopathological conference. "From toddlers to twenties and beyond" Adult-Paediatric Nephrology Interface Meeting, Manchester 2001. Nephrol Dial Transplant. 2003;18:2492.
5. Gahl WA, Thoene JG, Schneider JA. Cystinosis. N Engl J Med. 2002;347:111.
6. Tsilou E, Zhou M, Gahl W, Seiving P, Chan C. Opthalmic manifestations and histopathology of infantile nephropathic cystinosis: Report of a case and review of the literature. Surv Opthalmol. 2007;52(1):97-105.
7. Emma F, Nesterova G, Langman C, Labbé A, Cherqui S, Goodyer P, et al. Nephropathic cystinosis: an international consensus document. Nephrol Dial Transplant. 2014;29: 87-94.

Chapter 19

Behçet's Disease

Upender Wali

HISTORICAL ASPECT

The disease or syndrome is named after Benediktos Adamantiades, a Greek ophthalmologist and Hulusi Behçet, a Turkish dermatologist who in separate publications on their patients reported the findings of recurrent iritis as well as oral and genital ulcers. The description of the disease is reported by Hippocrates as forms of fever, ulcerations, watery ophthalmes, pains, fungus growth on eyelids, anthraxes and herpes.[1] Professor Hulusi Behçet first described the triad of symptoms of recurrent oral ulcers, recurrent genital ulcers and iritis amongst Turkish patients in 1937.[2] The disease is now accepted as a systemic vasculitis.

Definition

Behçet's disease (BD), also referred as Adamantiades-Behçet's disease is an idiopathic, chronic, relapsing inflammatory multisystem disorder, characterized by recurrent oral and genital aphthous ulcers, ocular inflammations,[2] and skin lesions mainly in the form of erythema nodosum and acneiform eruptions. There is no specific diagnostic test for BD and the diagnosis relies mainly on its typical clinical features. Behçet's disease is the leading cause of endogenous uveitis and acquired blindness in Turkey and Japan.

Epidemiology

Due to its widespread importance globally, the epidemiology of BD can be divided into different categories mainly geography, gender, age and heredity.
Geographic and ethnic distribution: Behçet's disease has worldwide distribution but is more common in Eastern Mediterranean and Eastern Asian countries. The hot bed being northern hemisphere latitudes of 30 and 45 degrees spanning Japan and Western Europe.[3] Interestingly, this corresponds to the old silk route used by Marcopolo. The disease is uncommon in the American continents, Oceania and sub-Saharan Africa. Behçet's disease has its highest prevalence in Turkey (80–420 cases per 100,000 populations).[4,5] Prevalence of BD from other countries in given in Table 19.1.
Gender: Reports from Mediterranean Basin and Far-East show preponderance of males.[6] Stratigos et al. have reported worse overall prognosis for males in

the Mediterranean region, middle and Far-East.[7] However, recent evidence suggests a varied distribution between the sexes (Table 19.2). Larger series show equal involvement of genders with male patients having a more severe course and more frequent involvement of vital organs. One explanation why earlier disease was more common in males is that in previous years women in many conservative countries would have been reluctant to visit physicians for the signs that constitute BD.

Age: The mean age of onset of BD is 25–35 years world-wide (young adult group), the range being 2 months to 72 years. Onset of the disease in early childhood or at advanced age is rare. Most pediatric cases of BD are diagnosed in late childhood.[8-10] Majority of cases are sporadic.

Heredity and sexual transmission: No consistent inheritance pattern exists in BD though several familial cases and a pair of monozygotic brothers have been reported within the criteria of this disease.[11-13] Behçet's Disease is associated with HLA-B51. The global distribution of this antigen among healthy control populations roughly corresponds to the overall distribution of the disease.[14] Behçet's disease and HLA-B51, a subtype of HLA-B5, show influence of genetics on the risk of development of uveitis in BD,[15] a disease more common in areas in which HLA-B51 gene is prevalent in the gene pool, e.g. Asia and Middle East. The association of HLA-B51 is a specific relative risk for the subgroup. In Japanese and Middle-East descent, the relative risk is 4–6.

TABLE 19.1: Prevalence of Behçet's disease in world populations

Country	Prevalence per 1000 inhabitants
Turkey	80–420
Iran	16–100
Japan	8–10
Germany	2.26
USA	0.4

TABLE 19.2: Sex ratio of Behçet's disease in different countries

Country	M:F ratio (Males > Females)
Japan	2:1
Lebanon	11:1
Greece	7.9:1
Egypt	5.3:1
Israel	3.8:1
Turkey	3.4:1
Iran	1.2:1
	F:M ratio (Females > Males)
Germany	1:0.9
Brazil	1:0.7
USA	1:0.2

Clinical Features

Behçet's disease is classically a bilateral non-granulomatous panuveitis and retinal vasculitis. Minority of patients, especially females may have isolated anterior uveitis. The disease may remain unilateral for many years in some patients.[16] Behçet's disease is a blinding disease and usually bilateral.[17] The second eye is generally affected within one year of the disease onset in the first eye, although the gap may be as long as seven years. The frequency of different clinical features in BD is laid down in Table 19.3.

Diagnostic Criteria

The first such criteria were suggested in 1969. Since then different criteria followed, the most notable being from Japan[18] and one suggested by the International Study Group for Behçet's disease (ISGB) in 1990.[19] The major difference between the two groups is that the Japanese classification emphasizes ocular symptoms while the ISGB stresses the importance of oral aphthae. The current diagnostic or classification criteria do not allow diagnosis of Behçet's uveitis based on ocular findings alone.

A useful and easy epidemiological classification of BD is outlined as below:

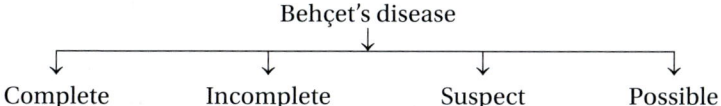

Complete type: It includes all four major criteria of Japanese classification system (recurrent oral ulceration, genital ulceration, uveitis and skin lesions). It is common in men.
Incomplete type: Three major criteria which can occur at different times, or typical ocular inflammatory disease that is recurrent, plus one major criterion.
Suspect type: Two major symptoms, no ocular symptoms.
Possible type: One major criterion or symptom.

The Japanese committee also identified four special clinical types of BD, depending on the predominant manifestations; namely neuro-Behçet's, ocular

TABLE 19.3: Frequency of clinical features in Behçet's disease

Clinical features	Frequency (%)
Oral ulcers	98–99
Genital ulcers	80–87
Skin disease	69–90
Ocular disease	68–79
Arthritis	44–59
Cutaneous pathergy	40
Vasculitis	25
Strokes, palsies and confusional states	25
Thrombophlebitis	24–30
Cardiac disease	17
CNS disease	14–18

Behcet's, intestinal Behcet's and vasculo-Behcet's. However, the modified diagnostic criteria for BD include features which are a blend of the Japanese criteria and the ISGB criteria.[18] These are given below:

Modified Diagnostic Criteria
1. Painful oral aphthous ulcers which have recurred at least three times in a year.
2. Inflammatory eye disease (uveitis, retinal vasculitis)
3. Recurrent genital ulceration.
4. Skin lesions (erythema nodosum, folliculitis/pseudofolliculitis, acneiform nodules, papulopustular lesions)
5. Positive pathergy test (pustule formation after 24-48 hours at the site of a sterile needle prick). This test is positive in 40% cases only.

Nondiagnostic Criteria
1. Major vascular complications: aneurysms of pulmonary artery or systemic arterial system, coronary artery disease, cardiomyopathy, valvular disease, venous thrombosis of superficial and deep veins, vena cava, portohepatic veins and cerebral sinuses.
2. Arthritis.
3. Skin lesions.
4. Gastrointestinal tract ulcers.
5. Neurological involvement of brainstem, spinal cord and meningoencephalitis.
6. Others (glomerulonephritis, epididymitis).

NONOCULAR MANIFESTATIONS

Patients with BD have recurrent inflammatory attacks in almost all organ systems involved.[20-22]

Oral aphthae are the earliest and the most frequent sign in majority of the BD patients. The aphthae are very painful, recurrent, occur in crops and cause severe discomfort. Morphologically they are discrete round or oral white mucosal ulcers with red rim, measuring 3-15 mm in diameter. The common sites are lips, gums, palate, tongue, uvula and posterior pharynx. Recurrence may be every 5-10 days or every month. They usually last for 7-10 days and heal without scarring except when they are large. Some patients do not recover fully before the next crop of ulcers appears. The other causes of aphthous ulcers include Steven-Johnson syndrome and Reiter's syndrome (these aphthae are painless, irregular, heaped up and occur commonly on tonsils and pharynx, structures which are rarely involved in BD).

Skin Lesions
1. Erythema nodosum. These are tender, painful, violaceous recurrent subcutaneous nodular lesions, most common over tibia (also occur on face, neck and buttocks). They persist for several weeks and disappear with or without scarring.
2. Acne vulgaris, folliculitis or pseudofolliculitis, papullo-pustular and pyoderma-like lesions. Acne vulgaris and folliculitis are common above the neck but may appear on thorax as well. The acne lesions are not sterile and are commonly associated with arthritis.

3. Superficial thrombophlebitis of both upper and lower extremities. It may occur after an injection, be migratory and may warn of a more widespread systemic vascular disease. Superficial thrombophlebitis, in combination with thrombosis of large veins and dural sinus thrombi constitute up to 20% of all CNS lesions in Behçet's syndrome.[20] Superficial thrombophlebitis and erythema nodosum are equally frequent, and sometimes difficult to distinguish.
4. Pathergy: It is an increased dermal hypersensitivity to needle trauma. The test is variable and only forty percent of BD patients exhibit it. The test is read positive if a sterile papullo-pustule develops following pricking of skin with a needle at 48 hours. The test is rarely positive when the systemic activity is absent. Pathergy test is not pathognomonic of BD but is included in the diagnostic criteria by some investigators.[23] Similar hyperreactivity can also be induced following trauma at other sites like joints, oral mucosa, and conjunctiva.
5. Dermatographia: It is hypersensitivity in the form of erythematous lesion following stroking of the skin. It is a form of vasculitis and occurs in 33–50% of BD patients.
6. Skin rash which can be a manifestation of a vasculitic disease.

Genital Ulcers

These ulcers are morphologically similar to oral aphthous ulcers. The common sites in males are scrotum and penis, and in females, vulva and vaginal mucosa. They frequently occur during premenstrual days.[24] Uncommon site being perianal area. The pain is variable and scarring may be a sequel. Epididymitis occurs commonly but urethritis is uncommon, this helps in differentiating BD from reactive arthritis.

Vasculitis

Vasculitis is rarely a presenting symptom. Arteries and veins of any size and caliber are affected in about 25% of Behçet's patients. It may be migratory and the most common lesions are superficial and deep thrombophlebitis of the legs. The frequencies of these lesions vary from 8%[25] to 38%.[26] The vasculitis may be complicated by occlusions, aneurysms and varices.

Vascular Occlusions

Vascular occlusion may occur in the form of superficial and deep venous thrombosis, vasculitic arterial obstructions, Budd-Chiari syndrome, or as varicose veins and aneurysms. An associated endothelial dysfunction is suspected.[27]

Aneurysms

Aneurysms have worse prognosis than occlusive lesions because of their tendency to rupture or bleed. Mortality in such cases may be as high as 60%.[28] Aneurysms may be complicated by peripheral gangrene.

Cardiac Manifestations

Cardiac manifestations include vasculitis, arterial occlusions, aneurysms granulomatous endocarditis, ventricular arrhythmias, myocarditis, myocardial fibrosis, myocardial infarctions, coronary arteritis and pericarditis. Incidence of heart lesions in BD is reported as 5%–10%[29] to 17%.[30]

Neuro-Behçet's Disease

Neuro-Behçet's disease is uncommon but life-threatening complication of BD, it is the most serious of all manifestations and may be caused by primary neural parenchymal lesions or secondary to vascular involvement. Reported frequency of CNS involvement in BD ranges from 3% to 10%.[6] The usual onset of neurological symptoms is 4–6 years after the onset of BD, but may be before or coexisting. Ten percent of patients with neuro-Behçet's show ocular involvement whereas up to 30% of patients with ocular-Behçet's have neuro-Behçet. A study from Japan has shown variable incidence of neuro-Behçet's vis-a-vis cyclosporine therapy.[31] Males are affected more than females. The varied ma-nifestations in neuro-Behçet's include benign intracranial hypertension, migraine-like headache due to widespread vasculitis, stiff neck, audiovestibular deficits like deafness, palsies, strokes, seizures, hemipareses, cerebellar ataxia, multiple sclerosis-like picture, pyramidal and extrapyramidal signs, peripheral neuropathies, confusion and hallucinations. Twenty five percent patients have psychiatric manifestations like agitation. The common sites of involvement include motor areas of CNS and pyramidal brain stem. MRI is more sensitive than CT scan in detecting lesions in patients with neuro-Behçet's disease.[23]

Three types of neuro-Behçet disease have been described. These include brain stem syndrome, meningoencephalitis (both are parenchymal lesions and carry worse prognosis with a higher rate of morbidity and mortality) and confusional states. Nonparenchymal lesions include vasculo neuro-Behçet's, mostly as dural sinus thrombosis, aneurysms and arterial occlusions. Mortality in neuro-Behçet's is reported as 10%, may be less now since reported because of the use of immunomodulatory drugs.

Neuro-ophthalmic involvement:[32]
1. Cranial nerve palsies: Commonly involved are VI and VII cranial nerves. These palsies are usually temporary.
2. Papillitis: Produces visual field defect like central scotoma.[33]
3. Papillodema: Usually due to pseudotumor cerebri caused by superior sagittal /intradural venous sinus thrombosis.[34, 35]
4. Ischemic optic neuropathy.[36]

Genitourinary Involvement

These patients may present with epididymitis, acute glomerulonephritis, IgA nephropathy and amyloidosis. Other rare disorders include renal vein thrombosis and necrotizing glomerulonephritis. Nephritis may be a manifestation of vasculitis.

Gastrointestinal Disease

It is an uncommon but life-threatening complication of BD.[37] Multiple ulcers of esophagus, stomach or intestines may develop causing diarrhea and hemorrhages. Gastrointestinal involvement is more common in the Japanese population than in the Mediterranean and the Middle-Eastern populations. Ileocecal region is the most frequently affected part of the gastrointestinal tract and may cause perforation.

Pulmonary Involvement

Majority of the lesions are vessel based. Pulmonary arteritis, aneurysmal dilatation of the pulmonary artery, pulmonary embolisms and infarctions are some of the serious implications of BD which occur secondary to superior venacaval and/or mediastinal vascular lesions. Other lesions include pulmonary hypertension, pleural effusion and cor-pulmonale. Most common symptoms include hemoptysis, dyspnea, cough, chest pain and fever. CT and MRI are often required and emergency surgery may be required for severe hemoptysis.

Joint Involvement

Arthralgias are common but true arthritis develops in about 30% to 50% of Behçet patients. These patients have arthritis at some time during their course of the disease with knee and ankle joints being the most commonly affected.[24] Joint disease may be monoarticular, oligoarticular or polyarticular. Joints of lower extremities are mainly affected and lesions tend to be symmetrical. Other joint-related disorders include ankylosing spondylitis and sacroiliatis. Attacks of arthritis are usually non-erosive. Chronic or destructive arthritis is very rare. Another variant of joint disease may be asymmetric non-deforming large joint polyarthritis, which usually is corticosteroid responsive.

Laboratory Tests

Erythrocyte sedimentation rate, C-reactive protein, full blood count (as a marker for inflammation and screening of immune system activation).

Pathergy Test
HLA testing for HLA B-51.

OCULAR MANIFESTATIONS OF BEHÇET'S DISEASE

Uveitis

The eye is the most commonly affected vital organ in BD. Uveitis is initial manifestation in 10% to 15% of the patients with ocular involvement. Uveitis is reported to be present in 50% of these patients in multidisciplinary settings, but in 90% in ophthalmology clinics.[20,38] Uveitis usually occurs within two years after the onset of oral aphthae, however, the delay between the two manifestations may be as long as 14 years. The ocular involvement in BD disease incurs serious implications because of recurrences and relapses. Recurrences are common, and if not treated, each recurrent attack damages the eye further heralding permanent ocular damage. Males suffer more severe attacks and therefore, more damage. The ocular disease may initially be unilateral; it almost always becomes bilateral in the long run. Simultaneous development of ocular and systemic manifestations is uncommon. The main pathologic process is a non-granulomatous necrotizing obliterative vasculitis in both anterior and posterior segments of the eye.[39] It is important to recognize Behçet uveitis as a distinct entity that can be diagnosed in the absence of systemic manifestations.

Anterior segment involvement may occur without posterior segment and anterior uveitis may be the only ocular manifestation in BD. Recurrent acute anterior uveitis and hypopyon are classical findings in BD. With the advent of steroids and immunomodulatory drugs, the hypopyon has become an uncommon finding now.[40] Anterior uveitis is almost always non-granulomatous and bilateral. Common symptoms being redness, periorbital pain, photophobia and blurred vision. Such symptoms may have an onset of few hours, sometimes within 2-3 hours of a perfect vision, and may resolve spontaneously. This is a diagnostic feature of BD. Slit-lamp examination shows conjunctival and/or ciliary hyperemia (ciliary injection may be disproportionately mild to the severity of anterior uveitis), endothelial keratic precipitates in the form of a fine dusting, anterior chamber cells and flare. Free movement of the cells can be seen due to aqueous currents caused by temperature difference between anterior and posterior portions of the anterior chamber.

Hypopyon (labeled as cold hypopyon) is found in only 10% to 30% of cases.[17] It is transient, migratory otherwise in a quite and white eye, and changes position with changes in the head position of the patient. It has a smooth layer and may form and dissolve rapidly, especially with corticosteroids. Sometimes it is visible only in the inferior angle as a layer of lymphocytes with a gonioscope, hence called *angle hypopyon*. Later reports show marked decrease in frequency of hypopyon from as high as 88% in seventies and eighties to as low as 9% now, due mainly to early diagnosis and aggressive treatment.[39,40] Hypopyon may be an important marker for posterior segment inflammation.

The usual course of anterior uveitis in BD is that of spontaneous resolution within 2-3 weeks, sometimes without treatment, even in severe cases. Chronic inflammation is uncommon but relapses do take place. The sequels of anterior uveitis include posterior synechiae, iris atrophy, peripheral anterior synechiae, iris bombé, secondary angle closure glaucoma and cataract.

Other less common anterior segment lesions include conjunctival ulcers,[17,41] episcleritis, scleritis, filamentary keratitis, and corneal immune rings and opacities.[42] Rarer complications include orbital inflammation, isolated optic neuritis and extraocular muscle palsies.[21,43,44]

Posterior segment involvement: These lesions tend to be persisting, smoldering and blinding. The inflammation can affect any or all portions of the uveal tract.

Acute Phase

1. The common lesion is non-granulomatous, obliterative, necrotizing retinal vasculitis affecting both arteries and veins (Fig. 19.1).[45] Retinal vasculitis is a major cause of visual loss in BD, and is difficult to treat. Recurrent branch

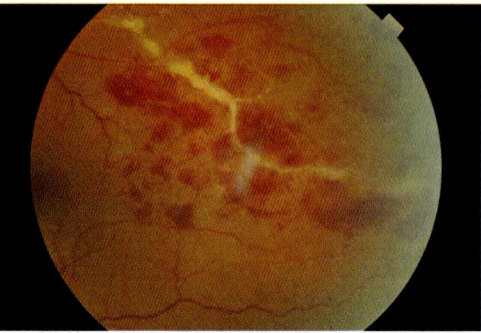

Fig. 19.1: Active vasculitis with vascular sheathing and retinal hemorrhages in a young male patient with first attack of Behçet posterior segment inflammation

retinal venous occlusions are more common in BD than in any other type of retinal vasculitis. Isolated branch artery occlusions, combined branch retinal venous and branch retinal arterial occlusions with vascular sheathing are associations of BD vasculopathies. Sheathing may not be visible in acute episode but becomes readily visible after the resolution when diffuse gliotic sheathing occurs. Capillary closure leads to retinal and macular ischemia due to non-perfusion (Figs 19.2A and B) and if extensive, causes neovascularization of the retina, disc and iris.

2. Vitritis is universal in eyes with active disease and often persistent. It tends to be diffuse and severity may range from moderate white cell deposition on vitreous fibrils to severe plasmoid reaction with sheets of inflammatory cells on vitreous collagen (Fig. 19.3). Vitreous haze is an indicator of inflammatory activity and is most severe at the onset of uveitis. In severe attacks there may be loss of fundus reflex. An important and frequent sign is posterior vitreous detachment (Fig. 19.4) which occurs early in 92% of affected eyes.[46] Sometimes exudates may form a string-of-pearls in the vitreous (Fig. 19.5). Vitreous cells are sometimes a secondary feature of vasculitis.[47]

3. Acute periphlebitis and/or thromboangiitis obliterans is hallmark of Behçet vasculitis and may be both leaky and occlusive. The lesions cause extensive intraretinal and vitreous hemorrhages. Other manifestations include engorged veins, perivascular sheathing and red-centered hemorrhages. Frosted branch angiitis is an uncommon manifestation in Behçet uveitis, but

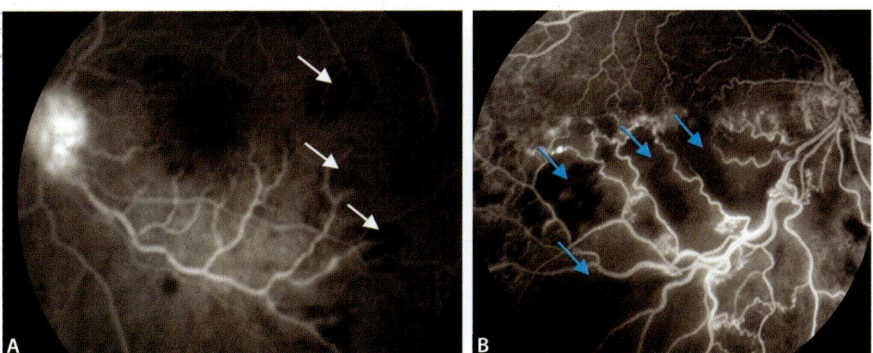

Figs 19.2A and B: (A) FA of a 27-year-old male patient showing multiple areas of non-perfusion (white arrows) and prominent vascular staining in early stage (eight months after the onset of oral ulcers); (B) FA of another patient showing extensive areas of retinal and macular ischemia (blue arrows) in late stage

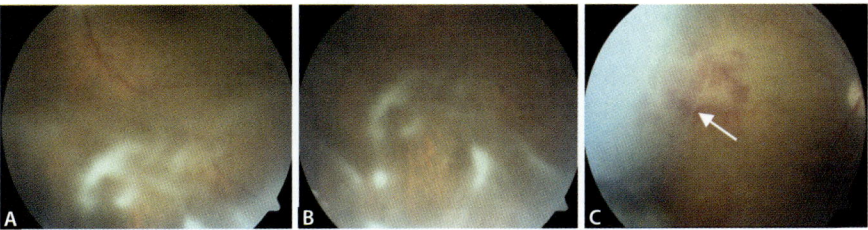

Figs 19.3A to C: Vitritis: Sheets of inflammation in the vitreous in two areas of the same eye. The visual acuity was 0.1. Note associated vasculitis (arrow) and retinal hemorrhages

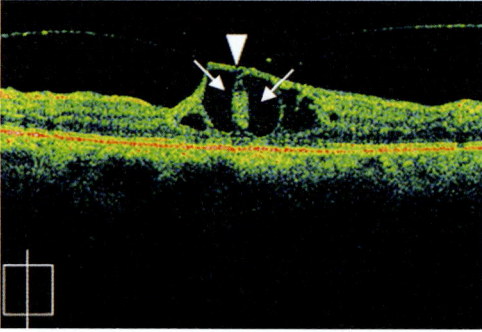

Fig. 19.4: OCT (Cirrus HD) image of a male patient with Behçet disease who had chronic recurring anterior uveitis with relatively quite posterior segment. His marked reduction in visual acuity (0.06) was attributed to cystoids macular edema (white arrows)
Note the prominent posterior hyaloids (vitreous) detachment which is still attached to the macula (arrow head)

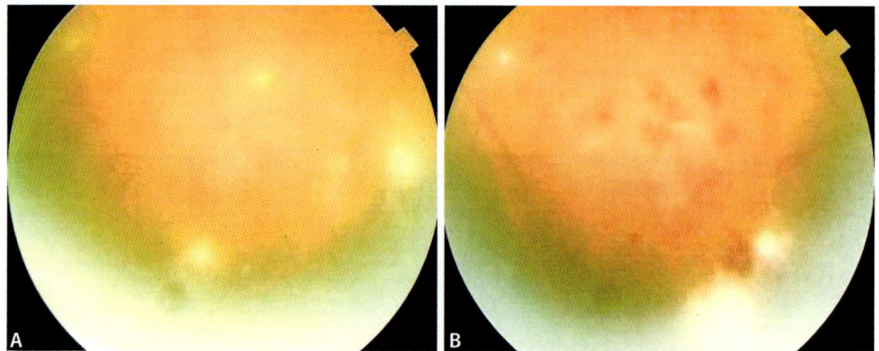

Figs 19.5A and B: Pearls of inflammatory cells in the vitreous of a patient with recurrent Behçet uveitis. Note the retinal hemorrhages in the background indicating active vasculitis. The whole vitreous is hazy due to 4 + vitritis

often seen in patients from Middle-East. It is associated with breakdown of blood-retinal barrier and may produce a fundus picture of typical angiitis with sheathing, neuroretinitis and hemorrhages all along the inflamed retinal vascular tree.[48] Isolated arteriolitis is not seen.

4. Retinitis is a cocktail manifestation of vasculitis and vitritis with clinical features overlapping with the twin inflammation. Transient inflammatory yellowish white retinal infiltrates or exudates, so called *chalky white retinitis*, are common in the active stage of Behçet posterior uveitis. Superficial necrotic retinal infiltrates denote activation and are pathognomonic of Behçet uveitis. The infiltrates may be in any number and location and resolve within few days without any visible scarring. Deeper retinal infiltrates may be associated with edema and turbidity of overlying retina, take longer to resolve, and may leave scars. Another characteristic finding is accumulation of inflammatory precipitates on the surface of inferior peripheral retina during the resolution of diffuse vitritis. They appear several days after the onset of attack and resolve within few weeks without any sequel. Cystoid

macular edema may be responsible for markedly reduced vision. Explosive cases may develop exudative retinal detachments. Such acute inflammatory signs in vitreous, retina and blood vessels usually do not get worse, rather may gradually resolve, even without treatment. Spontaneous resolution is an important diagnostic feature; however, new attacks of occlusive vasculitis of different branches, or new infiltrates may occur before complete resolution of previous signs.
5. Choroidal infarcts due to involvement of choroidal vessels and optic atrophy may occur (Fig. 19.6).
6. Late stages, due to frequent relapses there is retinal atrophy or retinal wipeout (Fig. 19.7).
7. Development of fibrous tissues produces epiretinal membrane (Fig. 19.8).
8. Neovascularization of the disc (NVD) and neovascularization elsewhere (NVE) appear.[39,40,49] NVD is more commonly due to uncontrolled intraocular inflammation. Neovascular glaucoma develops in 6% of Behçet's patients and may result in phthisis bulbi. Often it is associated with central or branch retinal venous and occasionally artery occlusion.[50]

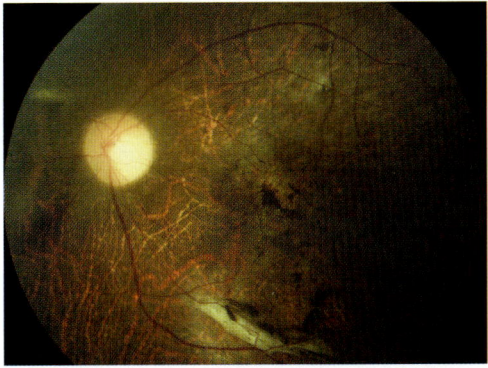

Fig. 19.6: Diffuse chorioretinal degeneration, retinal pigment epithelial changes, vascular attenuation, subretinal scarring and partial optic atrophy as an end stage sequel in a patient with Behçet disease

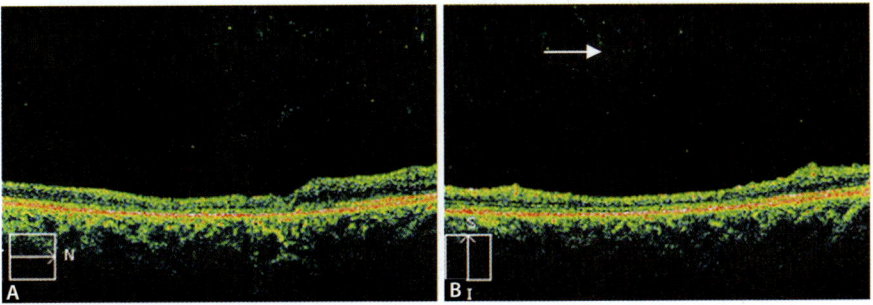

Figs 19.7A and B: OCT image of a patient who had several recurrent posterior uveitis. End stage image reveals severe retinal thinning/atrophy. Note the residual vitreous opacities (arrow) as sequel of long standing posterior uveitis

9. The natural course of Behçet's disease can be studied by a close follow up. The disease starts as benign vasculitis and end up in optic atrophy and blindness (Figs 19.9A to D).
10. Ghost vessels, subretinal scarring and retinal pigment epithelial changes are common (Fig. 19.10).
11. Macular scar (encircled) following chronic posterior uveitis is not a uncommon sequel (Fig. 19.11).
12. Optic nerve is affected in 25% of patients with BD. Optic disc hyperemia and papillitis are common findings while papilledema is uncommon.[51] Occlusive microvasculitis of the disc arterioles ultimately leads to progressive optic atrophy. Sequelae of recurrent, vision-robbing inflammatory episodes of posterior uveitis, in the long run, leads to fibrotic attenuation of both arteries and veins, which appear as occluded silver wired chords (Fig. 19.11).

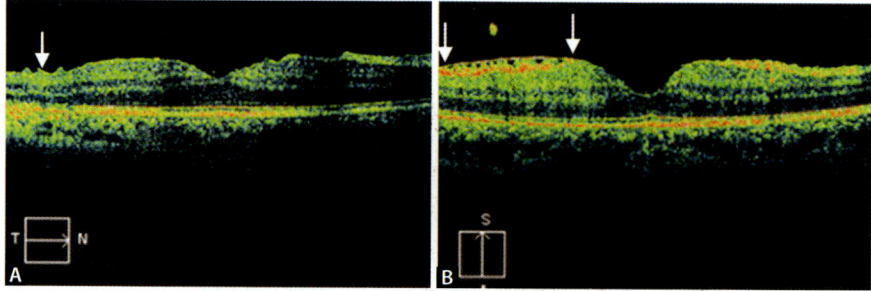

Figs 19.8A and B: Epiretinal membrane (arrows) in a patient with Behçet posterior uveitis

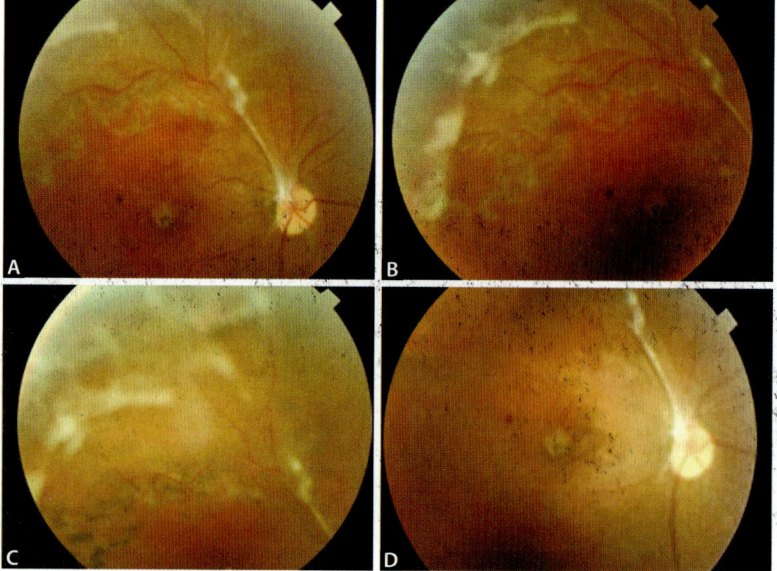

Figs 19.9A to D: Events in a 32-year-old male patient with ocular Behçet's, over a period of 24 months showing sequence of progressing tractional retinal detachment, retinal pigment epithelial changes and subretinal scarring. Note the optic disc in 10A appears normal in the beginning. The patient was lost follow up and came at a stage when optic atrophy had set in (10D)

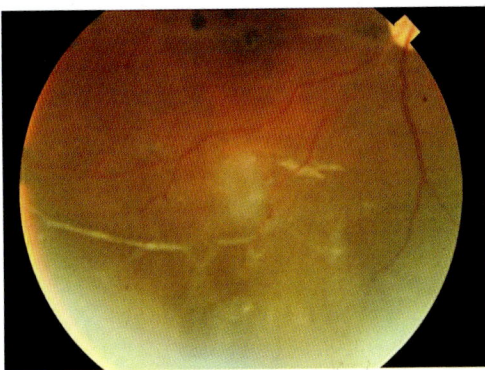

Fig. 19.10: Ghost vessels, subretinal scarring and retinal pigment epithelial changes as sequel of chronic recurrent Behçet's vasculitis and uveitis

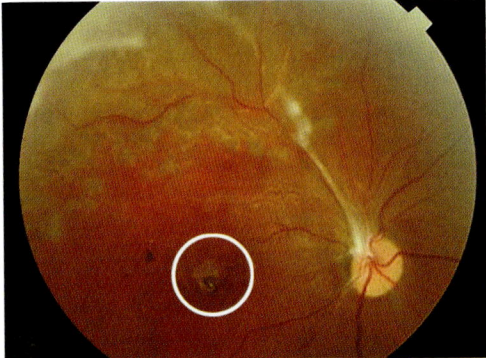

Fig. 19.11: Macular scar (encircled) following chronic posterior uveitis associated with retinal detachment in a 32 year old patient with Behçet's disease

Chorioretinal scars, gliosis, vessel attenuation, retinal pigment epithelial changes and optic atrophy are other end stage findings.

BEHÇET'S DISEASE IN CHILDREN

The information about the occurrence and course of BD in children is mostly based on case reports (Table 19.4). Neonatal BD with mother having oral and genital ulcers, and transient BD with life-threatening complications have been reported in the literature.[52,53] In Japan, the incidence of childhood BD is 1.5% of all reported cases. BD in pediatric age group is characterized by more frequent uveitis (31%) and arthritis, and less frequent genital and oral ulcers. A study from Turkey has reported lower vascular, neurological and ocular manifestations in children BD than in adult BD.[54] Most pediatric cases of BD are diagnosed in late childhood.[8,10] Treatment related complications are maximum with steroids while response to conventional immunosuppressive therapy is variable in children. The effectiveness of cyclophosphamide and chlorambucil in the treatment of sight-threatening ocular inflammation in children is controversial and is best considered on a case to case basis.

TABLE 19.4: Behçet's disease in children in a series of 36 patients (Tugal-Tutkun et al)

Gender	M:F 25:11
Mean age at onset of uveitis	13.6 years
Oral ulcers as initial symptoms	63.8%
Bilateral involvement	83.3%
Panuveitis as most common manifestation	86.2%
Retinal vasculitis	83.3%
Retinitis	68.2%
Most common complications	Cataract (46.9%), maculopathy (45.4%), optic atophy (39.4%)
Final visual acuity of < 0.1	22.7%

BEHÇET'S DISEASE IN PREGNANCY

Almost all aspects of BD, like improvement, deterioration and stability have been described in fetal and pregnancy related outcomes. Overall, such outcomes have been reported with the frequencies of spontaneous abortions, congenital malformations and perinatal deaths in babies born to mothers with BD, being not significantly different from those of healthy women with recurrent oral ulcers.[55] Miscarriages have also been reported in BD,[56] so has been Budd-Chiari syndrome during puerperium.[57]

Etiology

Etiology of BD is not fully clear yet. It is generally accepted that in immunogenetically susceptible individuals, certain environmental agents may trigger an enhanced and disregulated immune response[58,59] resulting in inflammatory vascular injury in multiple organ systems. Since immunoglobulins are not routinely found in blood vessel walls, the role of immune-complexes in the causation of vasculitis is not sure. A dysregulation of both innate and adaptive immune systems may be involved in the pathogenesis of BD.

Infectious agents: Though familial incidence and epidemiological data do suggest an infectious cause for BD, no microorganism has been identified from any lesion of BD.[60] Viral (herpes simplex, hepatitis C virus),[61] bacterial (elevated serum anti-streptococcal sanguinis antibody titers),[62] and immunoglobulin antibodies (specific to *Mycobacterium tuberculosis*) associated theories are found in the literature, but nothing conclusive has been proved so far.

Immune Mechanisms

Controversy still exists regarding the status of BD as an autoimmune disease. On one hand autoimmune mechanisms are involved in its pathogenesis while on the other hand BD lacks features of a classic autoimmune disease. Following features suggest that BD is not a classic autoimmune disease:
1. Male preponderance
2. Absence of autoantibodies and lack of its association with other autoimmune diseases
3. Lack of definite T-cell lymphocytic hypofunction
4. Hyperactivity of B-cell lymphocytes

5. Lack of association with HLA-alleles.

However, the recent review of literature shows following associations between BD and its immune mechanism:
1. Activation of T-cells during acute phase of the disease.[63]
2. Increase in number and activity of natural killer (NK) cells and neutrophils.
3. Th1 and Th2 cell-induced inflammation.[64]
4. Elevated levels of proinflammatory interleukins (ILs) in the sera.[65]
5. Circulating immune complexes in Behçet's uveitis and in ocular specimens. Such complexes have been reported to be protective and help to terminate "potentially harmful effects" of immune reactions, thereby promoting a better visual prognosis.[66]
6. Elevated levels of immunoglobulins A, E and M.
7. Elevated levels of antiphospholipid and antiendothelium antibodies in Behçet's patients with retinal vasculitis.[67]
8. Overproduction of tumor necrosis factor alpha (TNF-α), a proinflammatory cytokine in the sera of Behçet's patients. This cytokine is produced due to elevated numbers of T-lymphocytes and monocytes. In addition the TNF receptors are also found to be elevated in the peripheral blood of such patients.[68-70]

Genetic Factors

The strong association between BD and different ethnic groups from Middle-East to Far East such as Japan, Turkey, Germany and Greece, but no association with whites in USA and United Kingdom suggests a confident genetic predisposition to this disease.[71] The association of BD with major histocompatibility complex antigens was first reported in 1973. HLA-B5 phenotype and its subtype HLA Bw51 are found in significantly higher number of patients with BD.[72] The strongest allele in BD is HLA-B 5101 in Japan and Greece. These are called as *disease susceptible genes*. HLA-51 is the most consistent genetic marker of BD; however, the genetic association of BD with HLA-B51 is only 20%. A whole genome study has shown associations with 16 different loci.[20] Individuals who carry HLA-DR1 and HLA-DQw1 subtypes have been shown to be resistant to the disease.[73] An overall impression of the genetic story of BD seems to be of possibilities and hypothesis. The laboratory tests for HLA-B5, B51 are beneficial in confirming suspected cases only, not diagnostic of BD.

Pathology

Behçet's disease is primarily an inflammatory disease involving blood vessels, particularly venules. The early lesions resemble a delayed type hypersensitivity reaction, whereas late lesions resemble immune-complex type reaction. Only few reports are available on ocular immunopathology in BD, even though the disease can cause blindness.[74,75] The presence of clinical clusters indicates a dual pathogenetic pathway; one—a reactive arthritis pathway and second—a thrombophilia pathway.[20]

Histopathology

Systemic histopathology reveals leukocytoclastic and monocytic occlusive vasculitides (which lead to organ failure), perivascular infiltrates of lymphocytes and mononuclear cells, fibrinoid degeneration and necrosis of small blood vessels especially venules, demyelination of brain[76] and neutrophils, mast cells and fibrinoid necrosis in mucocutaneous lesions.

Ocular Histopathology

Uvea
In the acute phase shows infiltration of neutrophils, mast cells, lymphocytes and monocytes in iris, ciliary body and choroid. An increased collagen which is responsible for iris atrophy, posterior synechiae, inflammatory cyclitic membranes, choroidal thickening, hypotony and eventual phthisis bulbi is seen in chronic recurrent phase.

Retina
Infiltration of leukocytes and plasma cells in and around blood vessels (venules more than arterioles) occur leading to vasculitis, swelling and proliferation of retinal vascular endothelial cells causing thrombus formation, destruction of rods and cones and fibrosis of internal nuclear layer. Advanced stage shows fibrinoid, obliterated blood vessels. Overall retinal pigment epithelium remains minimally affected.

Optic Nerve
An obliterative vasculitis of the optic nerve head may be seen causing ischemic optic neuropathy which eventually leads to optic atrophy.

Immunopathology
Both cell-mediated immunity (T-cell predominance) and delayed–type hypersensitivity (type-IV) reactions have been observed in patients with early BD.[77] Late lesions resemble immune-complex—type reactions (type III). Aberrant T-helper type I lymphocytes cell function is accompanied by increased cytokine production including TNF-α, producing inflammatory symptoms. TNF-α is produced by monocytes as part of the inflammatory cascade. New etiopathological molecules like phospho-antigens, superantigens, heat-shock proteins, adenosine deaminase, nitrous oxide, endothelin and homocysteine have a possible role in the immunopathogenesis of BD.

Diagnosis
The diagnosis in BD can be established by:
1. Clinical findings based on diagnostic criteria
2. Serology
3. Pathergy test
4. HLA
5. FFA and ICG
6. Imaging (chest X-ray, CT chest, MRI brain with contrast. These investigations may be helpful as indicated by clinical presentations).
    - For diagnosis of BD, the criteria laid down by ISGB (1990)[19,78] or the Japanese Research Committee of Behçet's disease (1974) is applied worldwide. However, these were developed as classifications and not as diagnostic criteria, so, especially in early stages of the disease, the diagnosis of BD is often very difficult. Older sets of criteria, most

commonly by Mason and Barnese,[79] O'Duffy[80] and Dilsen[81] are still in use. The diagnosis of BD is structured on clinical observations only, with laboratory tests being only adjunctive for evaluation or confirmation. There is no specific diagnostic test for BD. Recurrent oral ulcers plus at least two of the following criteria are mandatory to be eligible for classification:
- Recurrent genital ulcers
- Skin lesions
- Eye lesions and
- Positive pathergy test.

Serology: Different serological factors enumerate different aspects of BD.

ANCILLARY TESTS

Fundus Fluorescein Angiography

The common findings in FFA in BD are:

Acute stages: There is diffuse leakage from retinal capillaries around fovea and optic disc which is related to deposition of immune complexes. The leakage may persist even after inflammation resolves. Retinal edema and vascular staining indicate active vasculitis.[82,83]

Late stages: FFA findings may include vascular staining, areas of capillary nonperfusion, retinal neovascularization, collateral vessels, macular ischemia, cystoid macular edema (Fig. 19.4), epiretinal membrane (Fig. 19.8) and macular hole. Hyalinization, thickening of vessel walls and perivascular fibrosis occur in chronic phase of BD.

Indocyanine Green Angiography

Choroidal abnormalities in BD were first reported by Matsuo et al. and these changes could be seen with ICGA only.[84] Common findings include disc hyperfluorescence, choroidal fuzziness, and hypofluorescent plaques. Choroidal inflammation or ischemia may be present in a minority of patients. This may be seen as hyperfluorescent zones in late phases of ICGA.[85]

Electrophysiology

It is indicated for monitoring retinal changes and help the physician to explain visual prognosis to the patient.[86]

Laser Flare Photometry

It is another very useful tool in diagnosis and monitoring Behçet's uveitis, especially during remissions when it may be difficult clinically to comment on the degree of inactivity.[87-89] Vitreous haze, disc hyperemia, blurred disc margins and macular edema are all signs of incomplete remission of the intraocular inflammation. Laser flare photometry correlates with both anterior segment and posterior segment inflammatory signs. The procedure offers an objective quantitative and a non-invasive technique to measure level of intraocular inflammation. The risk of a recurrent attack of uveitis is higher if LFP readings are more than six photons/msec.[87] The laser flare readings correlate with the degree of FFA leakage.[90]

DIFFERENTIAL DIAGNOSIS IN BEHÇET'S DISEASE

Though BD has a classical combination of physical and ocular signs and symptoms, certain atypical illnesses with uveitis can mimic it. These include:
- HLA B27/spondyloarthritides associated recurrent anterior uveitis with hypopyon: This variant is confined to anterior segment with severe recurrent iridocyclitis which is not simultaneously bilateral. The hypopyon tends to be sticky (hot) unlike cold hypopyon in BD.
- Reiter's disease: It is an incomplete form of BD. Unlike BD, Reiter's disease is not associated with vasculitis, and oral ulcers are painless.
- Sarcoidosis: It is associated with vasculitis and posterior uveitis. Sarcoid uveitis is not explosive in nature and affects only or more frequently veins (Table 19.5)
- Systemic lupus erythematosus (SLE) like BD is a multisystem disease. It is characterized by arterial occlusions, cotton wool spots, retinal and optic disc infarcts; however, unlike BD, veins are not involved in SLE, and there are no or minimal inflammatory changes in anterior chamber or vitreous.
- Periarteritis nodosa (PAN) is characterized by necrotizing vasculitis involving medium-sized arteries and arterioles but not veins. This is contrary to BD in which vasculitis is occlusive in nature and veins are involved as well. Vitritis is not a prominent feature in PAN while it forms an important component of BD. Nephropathy is common in PAN but rare in BD.
- Wegener's granulomatosis (WG) is a disease of granulomatous retinal vasculitis (contrary to non-granulomatous inflammation in BD) with concomitant glomerulonephritis, upper and lower respiratory tract infections and positive anti-neutrophilic cytoplasmic antibody (ANCA). None of these features are specific for BD.
- Ocular Whipple's disease: Ocular inflammation in Whipple's disease occurs late while in BD it is an early manifestation. Besides, PCR differentiates the two conditions.
- Viral retinitis (herpes simplex and herpes zoster) resembles BD due to its rapid, explosive, progressive and severe inflammation. However, unlike BD, viral retinitis has lesions uniformly located in the periphery and lacks systemic signs and symptoms which are so characteristic of BD. The retinal infiltrates in viral retinitis (acute retinal necrosis) often coalesce. CMV retinitis mostly affects immunocompromised patients especially with AIDS. Centrifugal spread of granular hemorrhagic retinal lesions differentiates it from BD. In idiopathic acute multifocal retinitis there is lack of anterior segment findings.
- Pars planitis is vasculitis with exudates in the area of pars plana. BD, however, is characterized by more severe occlusive retinal vasculitis with no exudates in the pars plana. Pars planitis lacks the classic sign of recurrent hypopyon.
- Multiple sclerosis: The episodic and multifocal CNS lesions, clinical and MRI features are common to both MS and BD; however, oral and genital ulcers in BD are quite distinctive. Pars planitis is more common in MS and very rare in BD. Anterior uveitis and hypopyon are common in BD and almost

TABLE 19.5: Behçet's disease versus sarcoidosis

Behçet's disease	Sarcoidosis
Both arteries and veins involved	Only veins involved
Diffuse involvement of arteries and veins	Segmental involvement of veins only
Occlusive vasculitis	Nonocclusive vasculitis
Vasculitis is common and more severe	Uncommonly seen

nonexistent in MS. Behçet's disease is more often associated with papillitis while MS is known for retrobulbar neuritis (less than half cases of MS have papillitis).

TREATMENT

The treatment of Behçet's disease is basically empiric and molded to control the symptoms, suppress the inflammation and prevent the organ damage. BD is a complex disease and no best therapeutic regimen is available yet. Two patients with similar manifestations may respond differently to the same drug or its combination. The intricacies of BD, its changing characteristics, and selecting the best possible therapeutic recipe, especially to reduce or prevent long lasting remissions is an art of medicine which requires the earned experience of treating patients with BD.

The treatment modality of Behçet's uveitis differs from country to country, depending upon the health care system and its financial implications. For example, infliximab has been approved as first line therapy in Japan while in Turkey the first line of treatment continues to be a triad of azathioprine, cyclophosphamide and low-dose corticosteroid with the second line therapy in non-responding patients being IFN-α monotherapy.

The use of systemic immunomodulatory agents alone or in combination with corticosteroids has become the gold standard for treatment in BD, and its uveitis is one of the best examples of an absolute indication for immunomodulatory therapy. However, in patients with strictly anterior uveitis, systemic therapy is not indicated. Cells in the posterior vitreous and leakage on FFA are a definite indication for immunomodulatory therapy even in the absence of other clinical signs in the posterior segment.

The introduction of biologic agents has prevented visual loss in most severe cases of Behçet's uveitis. Although there are limited controlled trials available, commendable results have been reported with interferon α and anti-TNF-α monoclonal antibody infliximab in patients with Behçet's uveitis resistant to conventional therapy (see Fig. 19.9). Interferon-α is effective in over 90% of such cases.[91-98]

European League Against Rheumatism (EULAR) is multidisciplinary evidence based expert committee that lays down following recommendations for the treatment of Behçet's disease:[99]

1. To treat the acute, explosive disease onset.
2. To prevent or to reduce number of recurrences of ocular inflammatory episodes.

The following features require more aggressive treatment:
1. Complete Behçet's disease, i.e. recurrent oral aphthae, skin lesions, recurrent genital ulcers and ocular inflammation
2. Neuro-Behçet's
3. Vascular Behçet's
4. Retinal involvement
5. Bilateral eye disease
6. Male gender[17]
7. Location in Mediterranean basin and Far-East.[17]

The commonly used drugs in BD include:
- Corticosteroids (it is not uncommon for Behçet's patients to become refractory to corticosteroids with progressive loss of vision and eventual need for additional therapeutic agents)

- Cytotoxic drugs
- Colchicine
- Ciclosporin-A (CsA)
- Tacrolimus

Noncytotoxic immunosuppressive drugs control immune-mediated ocular inflammation by selectively and reversibly targeting cellular subsets in the immune system without producing myelosuppression. Some of these drugs have been used as adjuvants either to reduce dose of immunosuppressive drugs or in the prophylaxis of recurrent inflammation. The use of immunomodulatory drugs is now mandatory in all patients with posterior segment eye involvement. The protocol accepted world-wide is to start initial therapy with corticosteroids combined with azathioprine and/or ciclosporin, and reserve interferon and infliximab for resistant cases.[90]

Corticosteroids

Though systemic and topical steroids are beneficial in controlling both anterior and posterior segment inflammations in BD, they may not prevent vision loss, and may have little effect on the late sequel of the disease.[100] Both high-dose intravenous corticosteroids (in acute severe inflammations) and low dose corticosteroids in combination with cytotoxic drugs have been recommended in Behçet's uveitis, thus reducing the side effects of either drug.[101,102] Anterior segment inflammation may respond to topical steroids only.

The role of systemic corticosteroids in BD is not without controversy. Oral 1-2 mg/kg daily or as an intravenous pulse methylprednisolone, 1g daily, for three consecutive days, followed by oral steroids. The main indications for periocular steroids are severe and damaging inflammations like posterior uveitis, vitritis, macular edema, and unilateral sight threatening disease. Triamcinolone depot is preferred over prednisolone or dexamethasone due to its long lasting anti-inflammatory effect, although it may cause intractable elevation of intraocular pressure. Steroid mouth washes or pastes are available in some countries for oral ulcers.

Cytotoxic/Immunosuppressive Agents

Behçet's disease falls in the absolute category of indications for immunosuppressive chemotherapy. The most common indications of these drugs in BD are severe uveitis with retinal involvement and involvement of visceral structures. The therapeutic benefits of cytotoxic drugs in ocular Behçet's has received huge acceptance from the Middle-East and Mediterranean regions.[103,104] The most feared complications of these agents are the future development of malignancies, such as leukemia's, lymphomas, etc. Because of such serious side effects their use in the treatment of Behçet's uveitis should be restricted. International Uveitis Study Group has categorized BD as an absolute indication for the use of immunosuppressives.

Management of Ocular Complications

Common ocular complications of BD include cataract, cystoid macular edema, glaucoma, optic atrophy and posterior synechiae, while uncommon complications include retinal neovascularization, retinal tears, retinal detachment, macular hole, hypotony and phthisis bulbi. Most common causes of vision loss in BD are maculopathies and optic atrophy.

- Cataract surgery should be planned after three months of inactive uveitis. Prophylactic systemic and topical preoperative steroids are mandatory, and should be continued postoperatively. In-the-bag intraocular lens implantation has been found to reduce intraocular inflammation.[105] It should be explained to the patient that cataract surgery in an otherwise quite Behçet's eye may not yield satisfactory visual acuity postoperatively due to possible pre-existing posterior segment complications.[36,39,106] Overall cataract surgery is tolerated well in inactive BD.[17,105]
- Cystoid macular edema respond to periocular injections of steroids.[107] However, pseudophakic CME in Behçet's uveitis is difficult to treat.
- Evaluation of glaucoma in BD is not easy because it is difficult to perform and interpret visual field tests in these eyes. Glaucoma may be secondary or neovascular in type. Medical management often may not suffice to control intraocular pressure. Trabeculectomy with anti-metabolites[3,5,91,108-110] or drainage shunts are viable options. Ahmed glaucoma valve is preferable,[111] Molteno tube shunt is a reasonable option.[112] Surgery would be safer if it is insured by perioperative steroids.
- Retinal and optic disc neovascularization are major complications of recurrent and prolonged retinal vasculitis in BD. Retinal photocoagulation, theoretically an option in retinal neovascularization, has been discouraged as some investigators believe the release of retinal antigens following laser may activate the systemic sensitization, leading in exacerbation of inflammation.[113] Tugal-Tutkun and associates found that optic disc neovascularization associated with BD was more successfully treated with IFN-α than photocoagulation.[114]
- Vitreous hemorrhage is frequent in BD with severe posterior segment involvement. It may resolve spontaneously or require vitrecomy.
- Macular holes, retinal tears and retinal detachments are common in late stages of the disease. Rubeosis and phthisis bulbi follow chronic large retinal detachments. Overall vitrectomy and scleral buckling procedures are tolerated well in these patients if the disease is inactive.[17,105,115-118]
- End stage Behçet's eye disease is characterized by optic atrophy, vascular sheathing, ghost blood vessels (Refer to Fig. 19.11), diffuse atrophy, retinal

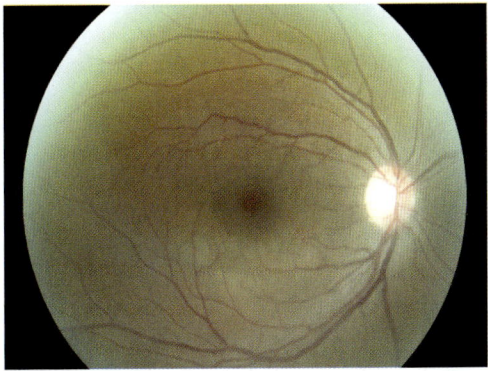

Fig. 19.12: There is marked improvement in vitritis and macular edema (same patient as in Figs 19.3 and 19.4) following treatment with infliximab. The vision at this time is 1.0

gliosis, pigmentation, chorioretinal and macular scarring (Fig. 19.12).[16] According to previous reports, 25%–45% of patients with ocular Behçet's eventually become blind despite therapeutic interventions.[119-122] Recent data suggest reduced (20%) incidence of eyes becoming blind despite treatment.

It turns out to be a confusing cocktail of drugs, their combinations, and above all, decision of which drug, or its combination, to be used where, for the best results with least complications. Different authors outline different strategies for the same indication. As a general rule, and what is followed in most parts of the world, a standard protocol says "any Behçet's patient with posterior segment involvement should be treated with azathioprine and corticosteroids, and any patient with severe (sight threatening) disease should receive additional ciclosporin or infliximab infusions. Results of treatment are encouraging (Fig. 19.12). lternately, interferon-alpha therapy can be considered.[99] Lee and Dick strongly support the evidence that time has come to embrace biologicals like anti-TNF-α drugs and use them as first line therapy for the treatment of uveoretinitis in BD. However, the editorial expresses concerns over exacerbation of CNS demyelination, compromise in innate immune control of tuberculosis and increased mortality with such therapy.[123]

PROGNOSIS FOR VISION IN BEHÇET'S DISEASE

The chronic, relapsing nature of the disease with frequent exacerbations after long periods of remissions makes it difficult to predict the visual prognosis in BD. No definitive prognostic factors for visual outcome have been identified and recurrent attacks and cumulative damage usually determine the visual outcome. Some authors link skin lesions, arthritis and posterior uveitis with loss of vision while others predict retention of vision in female gender, and anterior uveitis.[120] Another study reports age of 30 years or less, male gender, vascular thrombosis and neuro-Behçet's as risk factors for ocular involvement, associated with more severe disease and worse visual prognosis.[124] Whatever the scenario may be, prompt and aggressive treatment for severe disease with close monitoring for recurrences is the key to visual prognosis in BD. Complications like cataract, glaucoma, retinal and optic disc neovascularization, and vitreous hemorrhage, all require complex surgical interventions, and have a profound effect on the final visual outcome. The greatest mortality in BD comes from the CNS involvement.[125] Majority of these patients will loose all or part of their vision within five years. Other risk factors proposed as indicators of poor visual prognosis include more than three uveitis attacks per year, dense vitreous opacities, exudates within the retinal vascular arcades and FFA confirmed disc neovascularization and macular ischemia.[124,126]

Using immunosuppressive as first line therapy in Behçet's uveitis yields better final visual acuity.[127] Vision loss occurs an average of 3.36 years after onset of the visual symptoms in Behçet's disease.[128]

CONCLUSION

Behçet's disease is a chronic, recurrent, multisystem inflammatory disease characterized by the classic triad of recurrent oral and genital ulcers, skin lesions and ocular inflammation. The disease is most common in Turkey, Far East and Mediterranean basin. The unconfirmed etiopathogenesis involves infectious agents, immune mechanisms, and genetic factors. There is no universally approved diagnostic test for BD and the diagnosis is based on combination of clinical features. Early diagnosis and treatment has improved the prognosis but untreated cases bear the burden of very poor vision. Overall, treating BD is not an easy issue. Balancing the effects and risks of therapy largely depends on patient to patient disease and response. Although treatment of skin and mucosal lesions, and eye disease has improved considerably in the past decade, the treatment of CNS lesions and thrombophilia continue to be a challenge.

Behçet's ocular disease may remain one of the most difficult diseases to treat in an ophthalmologist's career. Its relentless and explosive nature causes severe ocular morbidity or even blindness. All agree with Lee, Dick and Yamada's evidence that it is wiser to implement biologicals as first line therapy in Behçet's uveitis.[123]

REFERENCES

1. Kaktos, ed: Hippocrates. Third book on Epidemiology. Case 7. 1993;13:209.
2. Behçet H. Uber rezidivierende apthöse durch ein virus verursachte Gxeschwüre am Mund, am Auge und am den Genitallien. Dermatol Wochen Schr. 1937;105:1152-57.
3. Keino H, Okada AA. Behçet's Disease: Global epidemiology of an old Silk Road disease. Br J Ophthalmol. 2007;91:1573-4.
4. Yazici H. Behçet's Syndrome. In: Klippel JH, Dieppe PA, (Eds). Rheumatology 6.20.1-6.20.6. London Mosby;1994.
5. Azizlerli G, Kose AA, Sarica R, Gül A, Tutkun IT, Kulaç M, et al. Prevalence of Behçet's Disease in Istanbul, Turkey. Int J Dermatol. 2003;42:803-6.
6. Shimuzu T. Clinical and Immunological studies on Behçet's Syndrome. Folia Jpn. 1971;22:801-10.
7. Stratigos AJ, Laskaris G, Stratigos JD. Behçet's Disease. Semin Neurol. 1992;12:346-57.
8. Kitaichi N, Ohno S. Behçet's Disease in children. Int Ophthalmol Clin. 2008;48:87-91.
9. Tugal-Tutkun I, Urgancloglu M. Childhood-onset uveitis in Behçet's Disease: A descriptive studies of 36 cases. Am J Ophthalmol. 2003;136:1114-9.
10. Saricaoglu H, Karadogan SK, Bayazit N, Yucel A, Dilek K, Tumal S. Clinical features late-onset Behçet's Disease: report of nine cases. Int J Dermatol. 2006;45:1284-7.
11. Mizuki N, Ohno S, Tanaka H, et al. Association of HLA B-51 and lack of association of class II alleles with Behçet's Disease. Tissue Antigens. 1992;40:22-30.
12. Vaiopoulos G, Sfikakis PP, Hatzinikolaou P, et al. Adamantiades-Behcet-Disease sisters. Clin Rheumatol. 1996;15:382-4.
13. Hamuryudan V, Yurdakul S, Ozbakir F, et al. Monozygotic twins concordant for Behçet's Syndrome. Arthritis Rhematol. 1991;34:1071-2.
14. Verity DH, Marr JE, Ohno S, Wallace GR, Stanford MR. Behçet's Disease, the silk road and HLA-B51: Historical and geographical perspectives. Tissue Antigens. 1999;54:213-20.
15. Baarsma GS. The epidemiology and genetics of endogenous uveitis; a review. Curr Res. 1992;11:1-9.
16. Tugal-Tutkun I, Onal S, Altan-Yaycioglu R, Altunbas HH, Urganciolu M. Uveitis in Behçet's Disease: an analysis of 880 patients. Am J Ophthalmol. 2004;138:373-80.
17. Mishima S, Masuda K, Izawa Y, et al. Behçet's Disease in Japan: ophthalmologic aspects Trans Am Ophthalmol Soc. 1979;76:225-79.
18. Behçet's Disease Research Committee of Japan: Behçet's Disease: guide to diagnosis of Behçet's Disease. Jpn J Ophthalmol. 1974;18:291-4.
19. International study group for Behçet's Disease: criteria for diagnosis of Behçet's Disease. Lancet. 1990;335:1078-80.

20. Yazici H, Fresko I, Yurdakul S. Behçet's syndrome: Disease manifestations, management, and advances in treatment. Nat Clin Prac Rheumatol. 2007;3:148-55.
21. Evereklioglu C. Current concepts in the etiology and diagnosis of Behçet's Disease. Surv Ophthalmol. 2005;50:297-350.
22. Yates PA, Michelson JB. Behçet's Disease. Int Ophthalmol Clin. 2006;46:209-23.
23. Akman–Demir G, Kurt BB, Serdaloglu P, et al. Seven-year follow up of neurologic involvement in Behçet's Syndrome. Arch Neurol. 1996;53:691-4.
24. Nussenblatt RB, Whitcup SM, Palestine AG. Behçet's Disease. In: Craven L, Buckwater, (Eds). Uveitis: Fundamentals and Clinical Practice, 2nd edn. St Louis, Mosby. 1996; 334-53.
25. Shimuzu T, Ehrlich GE, Inaba G, Hayashi K. Behçet's Disease (Behçet's Syndrome). Semin Arthritis Rheum. 1979;8:223-60.
26. Dilsen N, Konice M, Aral O. Our diagnostic criteria for Behçet's Disease: In: Hamza M, (Ed) Behçet's Disease. Proceedings of the third Mediterranean Congress of Rheumatology. 1986;11-15.
27. Pande I, Uppal S, Kailash S, et al. Behçet's Disease in India. A clinical, immunological, immunogenetic and outcome study. Br J Rheumatol. 1995;34:825-30.
28. Urajama A, Sakuragi S, Sakai F, et al. Angio-Behçet's Syndrome. In: Inaba GI (Ed). Proceedings of the International Conference of Behçet's Disease. Tokyo, University of Tokyo Press. 1980;171-6.
29. Bletry O, Mohattane A, Wechsler B, et al. Alleinte Cardiaque de la maladie de Behcet: Douze Observations, Press Med. 1988;17:2388-91.
30. Lakhanpal SH, Tani K, Lie JT, et al. Pathologic features of Behçet's Syndrome. A review of Japanese Autopsy registry data. Hum Pathol. 1985;16:790-5.
31. Kotake S, Higashi K, Yoshikawa K, et al. Central nervous system symptoms in patients with Behçet's Disease receiving cyclosporine therapy. Ophthalmology. 1999;106:586-9.
32. Anaba G. Clinical features of neuro- Behçet's Syndrome. In: Lehner T, Barnes CG, (Eds). Recent advances in Behçet's Disease. London, Royal Society of Medicine, Service. 1986;235-46.
33. James DG, Spiteri MA. Behçet's Disease. Ophthalmology. 1982;89:1279-84.
34. Pamir MN, Kansu T, Erbengi A, Zileli T. Papilledema in Behçet's Syndrome. Arch Neurol. 1981;38:643-5.
35. Wechsler B, Bousser MG, Du LTH, et al. Central venous sinus thrombosis in Behçet's Disease (letter). Mayo Clin Proc. 1985;60:891.
36. Scouras J, Koutroumanos J. Ischemic optic neuropathy in Behçet's syndrome. Ophthalmologica. 1976;173:11-8.
37. Kural-Seyahi E, Fresko I, Seyahi N, Ozyazgan Y, Mat C, Hamuryudan V, et al. The long-term mortality and morbidity of Behçet's syndrome; a 2-decade outcome survey of 387 patients followed at a dedicated center. Medicine (Baltimore). 2003;82:60-76.
38. Yang P, Fang W, Meng Q, Ren Y, Xing L, Kijlstra A. Clinical features of Chinese patients with Behçet's Disease. Ophthalmology. 2008;115:312-8.
39. Michelson JB, Chisari FV. Behçet's Disease. Surv Ophthalmol. 1982;26:190-203.
40. Mamo JG, Baghdassarian A. Behçet's Disease: A report of 28 cases. Arch Ophthalmol. 1964;71:4-14.
41. Zamir E, Bodhagi B, Tugal-Tutkun I, See RF, Charlotte F, Wang RC, et al. Conjunctival ulcers in Behçet's Disease. Ophthalmology. 2003;110(6):1137-41.
42. Cohen S, Kremer I, Tiqra P. Bilateral corneal immune ring opacity in Behçet's Syndrome. Arch Ophthalmol. 1991;109:324-5.
43. Tarzi MD, Lightman S, Longhurst HJ. An exacerbation of Behçet's syndrome presenting with bilateral papillitis. Rheumatology. 2005;44:953-4.

44. Hammami S, Yahia SB, Mahjoub S, Khairallah M. Orbital inflammation associated with Behçet's Disease. Clin Exp Ophthalmol. 2006;34:188-90.
45. Jabs DA, Rosenbaum JT, Foster SC, et al. Guidelines for the use of immunosuppressive drugs in patients with ocular inflammatory disorders: recommendation of an expert panel. Am J Ophthalmol. 2000;130:492-513.
46. Horiuchi T, Yoneya S, Numaga T. Vitreous involvement may be crucial in the prognosis of Behçet's Disease. In: Blodi F, Bracanto R, Cristini G, et al. eds. Acta XXV Concilium Ophthalmologicum. Rome, Kugler and Ghedini. 1986;2624-31.
47. Ehrlich GE. Vasculitis in Behçet's Disease. Int Rev Immunol. 1997;14:81-8.
48. Al-Mujaini A, Wali UK. Frosted Branch Angiitis, Neuroretinitis as initial manifestations in Behcet's Syndrome. Indian J Ophthalmol. 2010;59(3):240-1.
49. Michelson JB, Michelson PE, Chisari FV. Subretinal neovascular membrane and disciform scar in Behçet's Disease. Am J Ophthalmol. 1980;90:182-3.
50. Richards RD. Simultaneous occlusion of the central retinal artery and vein in Behçet's Disease. Trans Am Ophthalmol Soc. 1979;77:191-209.
51. Kalbian VV, Challis MT. Behçet's Disease. Report of twelve cases with three manifesting as papilleodema. Am J Med. 1970;49:823-9.
52. Fain O, Mathieu E, Lachassinne E, et al. Neonatal Behçet's disease. Am J Med. 1995;98:310-1.
53. Stark AC, Bhakta B, Chamberlain MA, et al. Life-threatening transient neonatal Behçet's Disease. Br J Rheumatol. 1997;36:700-2.
54. Sarica R, Azizlerli G, Kose A, et al. Juvenile Behçet's Disease among 1784 Turkish Behçet's patients. Int J Dermatol. 1996;35:109-11.
55. Bang D, Chun YS, Haam IB, et al. The influence of pregnancy on Behçet's Disease. Yonsei Med J. 1997;38;437-43.
56. Marsal S, Falga C, Simeon CP, et al. Behçet's Disease and pregnancy relationship study. Br J Rheumatol. 1997;36:234-8.
57. Sciuto M, Porciello G, Occhipinti G, et al. Multiple and reversible osteolytic lesions. An unusual manifestation of Behçet's disease. J Rheumatol. 1996;23:564-6.
58. Gül A. Behçet's Disease as an autoinflammatory disorder. Curr Drug Targets Inflamm Allergy. 2005;4:81-3.
59. Direskeneli H. Autoimmunity versus autoinflammation in Behçet's disease: do we oversimplify a complex disorder? Rheumatology. 2006;45:1461-5.
60. Hamza M. Foreward. In: VIIth International conference on Behçet's Disease. Rev Rhum Engl Ed. 1996;63:508.
61. Bang D, Cho YH, Choi H-J, et al. Detection of Herpes simplex virus DNA by polymerase chain reaction in genital ulcer of patients with Behçet's Disease. In: VIIth International Conference on Behçet's Disease. Rev Rhum Engl Ed. 1996;63:532.
62. Mizushima Y. Behçet's Disease. Curr Opin Rheumatol. 1991;3:32-35.
63. Hasan A, Fortune F, Wilson A, et al. Role of gamma delta T cells in pathogenesis and diagnosis of Behçet's disease. Lancet. 1996;347:789-94.
64. Mosmann TR, Sad S. The expanding universe of T cell subset: Th 1, Th2 and more. Immunol Today. 1996;17:138-46.
65. Sayinap N, Ozcebo O, Ozdeiner O, et al. Cytokines in Behçet's disease. J Rheumatol. 1996;23:321-2.
66. Kasp E, Graham EM, Stanford MR, et al. Retinal autoimmunity and circulating immune complexes in ocular Behçet's Disease. In: Lehner T, Barnes CG, eds. Recent advances in Behçet's Disease, London, Royal Society of Medicine Services. 1986;67-72.
67. Zouboulis CC, Buttner P, Tebbe B, Orfanos CE. Anticardiolipin antibodies in Adamantiades Behçet's disease. Br J Dermatol. 1993;128:281-4.

68. Ozyazgan Y, Yurdakul S, Yazici H, et al. Low dose cyclosporine A versus pulsed cyclophosphamide in Behçet's syndrome: A single masked trial. Br J Ophthalmol. 1992;76:241-3.
69. BenEzra D, Nussenblatt RB, Timonen P. Optimal Use of Sandimmum in Endogenous Uveitis. (Berlin: Springer-Verlag), 1988;7.
70. Atmaca LS, Batioglu F. The efficacy of cyclosporine in the treatment of Behçet's disease. Ophthalmic Surg. 1994;25:321-7.
71. O'Duffy JD, Taswell HF, Elveback LR. HLA antigens in Behçet's disease. J Rheumatol. 1976;3:1-3.
72. Ohno S, Oghuchi M, Hirose S, et al. Close association of HLA Bw51 with Behçet's disease. Arch Ophthalmol. 1982;100:1455-8.
73. Numaga J, Matsuki M, Mochizuki M, et al. An HLA-D region restriction fragment associated with refractory Behçet's disease. Am J Ophthalmol. 1988;105:528-33.
74. Charteris DG, Barton K, McCarteny AC, Lightman SL. CD4+ lymphocytic involvement in ocular Behçet's Disease. Autoimmunity. 1992;12:201-6.
75. Tugal-Tutkun I, Urgancloglu M, Foster CS. Immunopathologic study of the conjunctiva in patients with Behçet's disease. Ophthalmology. 1995;102:1660-8.
76. Handschumacher RE. Immunosuppressive agents. In: Gilnan AC, Rail TW, Nies AS, Taylor P, (Eds). Goodman and Gilman's The pharmacological basis of therapeutics. New York, Pergamon Press. 1990;1264-76.
77. Gül A, Esin S, Dilsen N, et al. Immunopathology of skin pathergy reaction in Behçet's disease. Br J Dermatol. 1995;132:901-7.
78. International Study Group for Behçet's Disease. Evaluation of diagnostic (Classification) criteria in Behçet's disease—towards internationally agreed criteria. Br J Rheumatol. 1992;31:299-308.
79. Mason RM, Barnes CG. Behcet's syndrome with arthritis. Ann Rheum Dis. 1969;28: 95-103.
80. O'Duffy JD. Suggested criteria for diagnosis of Behçet's disease. J Rheumatol. 1974;1:18.
81. Dilsen N, Konice M, Aral O. Our diagnostic criteria of Behcet's disease—an overview, recent advances in Behcet's Disease. London Royal Society of Medicine Services. Int Congr Sympos Series. 1986;103:177-80.
82. Atmaca LS. Fundus changes associated with Behçet's disease. Graefes Arch Clin Exp Ophthalmol. 1989;227:340-4.
83. Gass JDM. Stereoscopic Atlas of Macular diseases: Diagnosis and Treatment. St Louis, Mosby, 1997.
84. Matsuo T, Sato Y, Shiraga F, et al. Choroidal abnormalities in Behçet's disease observed in simultaneous indocyanine green and fluorescein angiography with scanning laser ophthalmoscopy. Ophthalmology. 1999;106:295-300.
85. Atmaca LS, Batioglu F. Indocyanine green videoangiography and color Doppler imaging in Behçet's disease. Acta Ophthalmol Scand. 1999;77:444-7.
86. Cruz CD, Adachi-Usami E, Kakisu Y. Flash Electroretinography and pattern visually evoked cortical potentials in Behçet's disease. Jpn J Ophthalmol. 1990;34:142-8.
87. Tugal-Tutkun I, Cingü K, Kir N, Yeniad B, Urganciolu M, Gül A. Use of laser flare cell photometry to quantify intraocular inflammation in patients with Behçet's uveitis. Graefes Arch Clin Exp Ophthalmol. 2008;246:1169-77.
88. Yang P, Fang W, Huang X, Zhou H, Wang L, Jiang B. Alterations of aqueous flare and cells detected by laser flare cell photometry in patients with Behçet's disease. Int Ophthalmol. 2010;30:485-9.
89. Gedik S, Akova YA, Yilmaz G, Bozbeyoglu S. Indocyanine green and fundus fluorescein angiography findings in patients with active ocular Behçet's disease. Ocul Immunol Inflamm. 2005;13(1):51-8.

90. Tugal-Tutkun I. Uveitis update. Middle East African Journal of Ophthalmology. 2009;16(4):219-224.
91. Kötter I, Zierhut M, Eckstein AK, Vonthein R, Ness T, Günaydin I, et al. Human recombinant interferon alfa-2a for the treatment of Behçet's disease with sight threatening posterior or panuveitis. Br J Ophthalmol. 2003;87:423-31.
92. Tugal-Tutkun I, Güney-Tefekli E, Urganciolu M. Results of interferon alfa therapy in patients with Behçet's uveitis. Graefes Arch Clin Exp Ophthalmol. 2006;244 (12):1692-5.
93. Krause L, Altenburg A, Pleyer U, Köhler AK, Zouboulis CC, Foerster MH. Long term visual prognosis of patients with ocular Adamantiades Behçet's disease treated with interferon-alfa-2a. J Rheumatol. 2008;35:896-903.
94. Sfikakis PP, Kaklamanis PH, Elezoglou A, Katsilambros N, Theodossiadis PG, Papaefthimiou S, et al. Infliximab for recurrent, sight-threatening ocular inflammation in Adamantiades Behçet's disease. Ann Intern Med. 2004;140;404-6.
95. Sfikakis PP, Markomichelakis N, Alpsoy E, Assad-Khalil S, Bodaghi B, Gül A, et al. Anti-TNF therapy in the management of Behçet's disease-review and basis for recommendations. Rheumatology (Oxford). 2007;46(5):736-41.
96. Tugal-Tutkun I, Mundun A, Urganciolu M, Kamali S, Kasapoglu E, Inanc M, et al. Efficacy of Infliximab in the treatment of uveitis resistant to the combination of azathioprine, cyclosporine and corticosteroids in Behçet's disease. An open-label trial. Arthritis Rheum. 2005;52(8):2478-84.
97. Niccoli L, Nannini C, Benucci M, Chindamo D, Cassara E, Salvarani C, et al. Long-term efficacy of infliximab in refractory posterior uveitis of Behçet's disease. A 24-month follow up study. Rheumatology (Oxford). 2007;46(7):1161-4.
98. Tabbara KF, Al-Hemidan A. Infliximab effects compared to conventional therapy in the management of retinal vasculitis in Behçet's disease. Am J Ophthalmol. 2008;146:845-60.
99. Hatemi G, Silman A, Bang D, Bodhagi B, Chamberlain AM, Gül A, et al. EULAR recommendations for the management of Behçet's disease. Ann Rheum Dis. 2008;67(12):1656-62.
100. Ben Ezra DE, Cohen E. Treatment and visual prognosis in Behçet's disease. Br J Ophthalmol. 1986;70:589-92.
101. Reed BJ, Morse LS, Schwab IR. High-dose intravenous pulse methylprednisolone hemisuccinate in acute Behçet's retinitis. Am J Ophthalmol. 1998;125:410-11.
102. Santamara J. Steroidal agents. The systemic and ocular complications. Ocul Inflamm Ther. 1988;1:19-25.
103. Mamo JG. Treatment of Behçet's disease with chlorambucil. A follow-up report. Arch Ophthalmol. 1976;94:580-3.
104. Hijikata K, Masuda K. Visual prognosis in Behçet's disease. Effects of cyclophosphamide and colchicine. Jpn J Ophthalmol. 1978;22:506-19.
105. Tabbara KF, Chavis PS. Cataract extraction in Behçet's disease. Ocul Immunol Inflamm. 1977;5:27-32.
106. Ghate JV, Jorrizo JL. Behçet's disease. In: Ruddy S, Harris ED, Sledge CB, et al. (Eds). Kelly's Textbook of Rheumatology, 6th edn. Philadelphia: Saunders: 2001:1205-9.
107. Yoshikawa K, Ichiishi A, Kotake S, et al. Posterior sub-Tenon's space injection of repository corticosteroids in uveitis patients with cystoid macular edema. Nippon Ganka Gakkai Zasshi. 1993;97:1070-4.
108. Zafirakis P, Fosters CS. Adamantiades Behçet's disease. In: Fosters CS, Vitale AT. Diagnosis and treatment of Uveitis. Philadelphia: WB Saunders: 2002;632-52.
109. Feron EJ, Rothova A, van Hagen PM, Baarsma GS, Suttorp-Schulten MS. Interferon-alpha-2b for refractive ocular Behçet's disease. Lancet. 1994;343:1428.

110. Sfikakis PP, Theodossiadis PG, Katsiari CG, Kaklamanis P, Markomichelakis NN. Effect of infliximab on sight-threatening panuveitis in Behçet's disease. Lancet. 2001;358:295-6.
111. Da Mata A, Burk SE, Netland PA, Baltatzis S, Christen W, Foster CS. Management of uveitic glaucoma with Ahmed glaucoma valve implantation. Ophthalmology. 1999;106(11):2168-72.
112. Hill RA, Nguyen QH, Baerveldt G, et al. Trabeculectomy and Molteno implantation for glaucomas associated with uveitis. Ophthalmology. 1993;100(6):903-8.
113. Atmaca LS. Experience with photocoagulation in Behçet's disease. Ophthalmic Surg. 1990;21:571-6, 107-100.
114. Tugal-Tutkun I, Onal S, Altan-Yaycioglu R, Kir N, Urganciolu M. Neovascularization of the optic disc in Behçet's disease. Jpn J Ophthalmol. 2006;50:256-65.
115. Soylu M, Demircan N, Pelit A. Pars plana vitrectomy in ocular Behçet's disease. Int Ophthalmol. 2001;24(4):219-23.
116. Ozerturk Y, Bardak Y, Durmus M. Vitreoretinal surgery in Behçet's disease with severe ocular complications. Acta Ophthalmol Scand. 2001;79(2):192-6.
117. Sullu Y, Alotaiby H, Beden U, Erkan D. Pars plana vitrectomy for ocular complications of Behçet's disease. Ophthalmic Surg Lasers Imaging. 2005;36(4):292-7.
118. Krause L, Altenburg A, Bechrakis NE, Willerding G, Zouboulis CC, Foerster MH. Intraocular surgery under systemic interferon-alpha therapy in ocular Adamantiades-Behçet's disease. Graefes Arch Clin Exp Ophthalmol. 2007;245(11):1617-21.
119. Nussenblatt RB. Uveitis in Behçet's disease. Int Rev Immunol. 1997;1467-79.
120. Sakamoto M, Akazawa K, Nishioka Y, et al. Prognostic factors of vision in patients with Behçet's disease. Ophthalmology. 1995;102:317-21.
121. Takeuchi M, Hokama H, Tsukahara R. et al. Risk and prognostic factor of poor visual outcome in Behçet's disease withocular involvement. Graefes Arch Clin Exp Ophthalmol. 2005;243:1147-52.
122. Pivetti-Pezzi P, Accorinti M, La Cava M, et al. Endogenous uveitis: an analysis of 1,417 cases. Ophthalmologica. 1996;210:234-8.
123. Lee WJR, Dick DA. Treat early and embrace the evidence in favor of anti-TNF-α therapy for Behçet's uveitis. Br J Ophthalmol. 2010;94:269-70.
124. Demiroglu H, Barista I, Dundar S. Risk factor assessment and prognosis of eye involvement in Behçet's disease in Turkey. Ophthalmology. 1997;104:701-5.
125. Chamberlain MA. Behçet's syndrome in 32 patients in Yorkshire. Ann Rheum Dis. 1977;36:491-9.
126. Yu HG, Kim MJ, Sewoong F. Fluorescein angiography and visual acuity in active uveitis with Behçet's disease. Ocul Immunol Inflamm. 2009;17(1);41-6.
127. Khairallah M, Attia S, Yahia SB, JenzeriS, Ghrissi R, Jelliti B, et al. Pattern of uveitis in Behçet's disease in a referral center in Tunisia, North Africa. Int Ophthalmol. 2009;29:135-41.
128. Yamada Y, Sugita S, Tanaka H, et al. Comparison of infliximab versus cyclosporine during the initial 6-month treatment period in Behçet's disease. Br J Ophthalmol. 2010;94:282-6.

Index

Page numbers followed by *f* refer to figure and *t* refer to table.

A

Acanthamoeba 129
Accommodation failure 244
Achromatopsia 244
Acinetobacter baumannii 113
Acne vulgaris 264
Acquired nystagmus 235
 signs in 243*t*
Acquired red-green dyschromatopsia 43
Acrylic IOLs 135
Acyclovir resistance 20
Adeno-associated virus vectors 165, 168
Adnexa lacrimal glands 125
Advanced glycation end products 139, 141*f*
Aflibercept 150, 155
Agents of phototoxicity 186
All India Ophthalmological Society 114
Amikacin 104
Amniotic membrane 28
 transplant 18
Amphotericin B 104
Amyloid-β targets 163
Ancillary investigations 39
 role of 51
Ancillary tests 277
Aneurysms 265
Angiomatous proliferation 171
Angiotensin converting enzyme 50, 147
Angle hypopyon 268
Angular vein 219*f*
Ankyrin repeat protein, designed 165, 167
Anterior chamber reaction with hypopyon 120*f*
Anterior venous drainage 219*f*
Anticoagulants 171
Anti-inflammatory therapies 161
Anti-neutrophilic cytoplasmic antibody 278
Anti-oxidative stress therapies 161, 163
Antiplatelet agents, role of 171
Anti-platelet-derived growth factor agents 165, 166
Anti-tubercular drug 43
 ocular side-effects of 43*t*
Anti-tubercular therapy 42
Anti-vascular endothelial growth factor
 agents 59,
 drugs 165, 175
 injection 128
 therapy 150
Aperiodic alternating nystagmus 238
Arcuate scotoma, inferior 88*f*, 92*f*
Argon-fluoride excimer laser 1
Arteriovenous malformations 208
Arthritis 263
Aspergillus species 129
Automated nystagmus acuity function 239, 240
Azathioprine 53
Azopt eye drops 245*f*

B

Bacillus cereus 128, 136
Bacillus species 100
Bacterial endophthalmitis 100
Bacterial endotoxin residues 118
Balanced salt solution 118
Band-shaped keratopathy 51
Behçet posterior uveitis 272*f*
Behçet's disease 261, 263, 263*t*, 270*f*, 271*f*, 237*f*, 274*t*, 278, 278*t*, 279
 in children 273
 in pregnancy 274
 prevalence of 262*t*
 sex ratio of 262*t*
Behçet's eye disease 281
Behçet's ocular disease 283
Behçet's patients 265
Behçet's uveitis 263, 275, 279, 282
Behçet's vasculitis 273*f*
Bevacizumab 150, 155
Biomechanical response, coefficient of 5
Birdshot retinochoroidopathy 51
Birefrigerant interstitial crystals in kidney, depositoin of 258*f*
Blau syndrome 51
Blind spot 211*f*
 enlarged 210*f*

Blood pressure control 147
Blue-light hazard 186
Borreliosis 36
Bronchoalveolar lavage 46, 52
Brucellosis 36
Budd-Chiari syndrome 265
Bullous keratopathy 16

C

Candida 136
   albicans 129
     chorioretinitis 136
     species 100, 129
Cardiac disease 263
Cardiac manifestations 265
Carotico-cavernous fistula 218, 219*f*
Carotid artery, internal 207, 223
Carotid cavernous fistula 208, 218
Cataract 51, 54
   surgery 14, 281
     after 15*f*
Cavernous aneurysm 217
   neck of 217*f*
Cavernous carotid artery 208
Cavernous internal carotid artery aneurysms 215
Cavernous sinus 219*f*, 222*f*
Cefazoline 104
Ceftazidime 104, 104*f*
Cell based therapies 26
Central corneal thickness 86
Central nervous system disease 263
Central scotomas 43
Cerebellar artery, superior 208
Cerebellar hemispheres 243
Cerebral angiogram 206
   findings 208, 212, 215, 223, 225
Cervicomedullary junction 243
Chalky white retinitis 270
Chemoreduction 197
Chemotherapy 197
Children's Hospital Los Angeles 194
Chorioretinal degeneration, diffuse 271*f*
Choroidal blood flow enhancing agents 161, 164
Choroidal granuloma 40, 48
Choroidal invasion 201
Choroidal neovascular membrane 160
Choroidal neovascularization 171
Choroidal polyp 171
Ciclosporin-A 280
Clindamycin, intravitreal injection of 62
Cluster infections 114
Cochrane systemic 17
Collagen cross-linking 14

Computer-assisted tomography 41
Conbercept 166
Confocal microscopy in smile 7
Confocal scanning laser ophthalmoscope 69, 82
Confusional states 263
Congenital nystagmus waveforms 235
Congenital stationary night blindness 244
Conjunctiva 125
Conjunctival granulomas 47
Conjunctival limbal autografts 26
Contact lenses 244
Control cardiovascular risk in diabetes, action to 147, 148
Convergence dampening 244
Cornea 125
   in smile, biomechanical properties of 5
Corneal abscess 107*f*
Corneal cap precision in smile 7
Corneal edema 120, 121*f*
Corneal endothelial deposits 43
Corneal perforation 16
Corneal scar 16
Corneal surface, anterior 4*f*
Corneal tensile properties 5*f*
Corneal transplant 14
Cortical vein 214*f*
   abnormal 213*f*
   reflux to 214*f*
Corticosteroids 14, 53, 280
Cultivated limbal epithelial transplantation 26
Cutaneous pathergy 263
Cyclosporin A 18
Cyclosporine 53
Cystadrops 259
Cystagon 259
Cystaran 259
Cystinosis 255, 257*f*
Cystoid edema 144*f*
Cystoid macular edema 53, 57, 281
Cytomegalovirus retinitis 62
Cytotoxic agents 280

D

Darpin 168
Demographics 170
Dendritic ulcer 17*f*
Dexamethasone 104, 154, 155
Diabetes
   complication 147
     epidemiology of 147
   control trial 147
   intervention, epidemiology of 147
   mellitus 14

Index

Diabetic eye disease 140*f*
Diabetic macular edema 57, 139, 141, 142, 145, 146, 149, 156
    classification of 142, 143
    diffuse 144*f*
    pathogenesis of 141*f*
Diabetic retinopathy 139, 156
    disease severity scale 141
    study, early treatment 139
Diacylglycerol 141
Diencephalon 243
Diet 189
Diquafosol 24, 26
Disciform keratitis 17, 19*f*
Disk edema 43
DNA
    replication 60
    synthesis 17
    viruses 12
DNA-dependent RNA polymerase 42
Drainage systems 24
Drugs 189
Dry eye 4
    advances in diagnosis of 24
    disease, management of 24*t*
    novel therapies for 25
DSA machine 206
Dural arteriovenous fistula 208, 212

E

Eales' disease 36
Eccentric gaze nystagmus 230, 231
Eccentric horizontal null position 250
Eculizumab 161, 162
Eczema, severe 14*f*
Electrophysiology 277
Embryonic organogenesis 255
Emerging therapeutic options 161, 165
Emixustat 164
Encapsulated cell technology 165, 167
Endocrine 256
Endogenous bacterial 136
Endophthalmitis 36, 107*f*, 126, 127, 135
    after intravitreal avastin 111*f*
    chronic 109
    classification of 100*t*
    epidemiology of postoperative 126
    legal issues to 115
    postoperative 99, 127
    types of 135*t*
    vitrectomy study 127
    with corneal involvement 111*f*
Endothelial keratitis 13, 19
Endothelial keratoplasty, after 16*f*
Endothelin 141

Endovascular intervention 206-208, 212, 216, 223
Endovascular therapy in neuro-ophthalmic lesions 208
End-tuberculosis strategy 32
Epiretinal membrane 272f
Epithelial keratitis 16, 19
Epstein Barr virus 46
Erythema nodosum 264
Erythrocyte sedimentation rate 206
Esotropia 195
Ethambutol 42
European league against rheumatism 279
Excited dimer 1
Exotropia 195
Extraocular muscles 125
Extrascleral extension 201
Extremely drug resistant 43
Eye 28f, 68f
    disease study, age-related 161, 163
    dressings 133
    drops 133
    infection 125
    movement
        abnormalities, classification of 230
        recording 238
    normal 76f
    pathogenesis involving 258
    perimetry, left 210f, 211f
    report
        both 71f
        single 70*f*
Eyelid 47, 125
    eversion of lower 223f

F

Facial vein 219*f*
Femtosecond laser technology 1
Femtosecond-laser in situ keratomileusis 4, 6
Fenretinide 164
Fever primes retina 186
Fibrotic sequelae 171
Fine needle aspiration cytology 40*f*
Fluocinolone 155
Fluocinolone acetonide 57
Fluorescein angiography 143, 171
Focal macular edema 143, 143*f*
Focal therapy 197, 200
Food and drug administration 57
Fovea 43
Foveal avascular zone 144
Foveation domain, longest 245
Fundus autofluorescence 39, 40*f*, 162, 173
Fundus examination 119

Fundus fluorescein angiography 39, 145, 176f
   role of 145t
Fungal endophthalmitis 108, 108f
Fusarium species 129
Fusion maldevelopment nystagmus syndrome 231, 237-239

G

Gallium 52
Ganglion cell 78
   complex 78, 78f, 86f
   layer 78
Gastrointestinal disease 266
Gene therapy 260
Genetic 180
   factors 275
Genexpert omni 43
Genital ulcers 263, 265
Genitourinary involvement 266
Gentamicin 104
Geographic atrophy 160
Ghost vessels 273f
Glaucoma probability score 73f
Glaucoma 51, 54
   diagnosis of 80
   future developments in 93
   management 65
   probability score 72, 73, 73t
   secondary 54
Glaucomatous damage, early 88f
Glucocorticoid family 57
Glycemic control 147
Gonads 257
Gonioscopy 120
Gram-negative bacteria 100
Granuloma 49f
Granulomatous uveitis, anterior 48f
Graphic recording of nystagmus 235, 237f
Growth retardation 256
Guglielmi detachable coils 207

H

Hand-washing technique 130
Head posture 244
   abnormal 237, 238f
Heerfordt's syndrome 47
Heidelberg engineering 69
Heidelberg retina tomograph 65, 69, 72
Helicobacter pylori 46
Hematoma, extradural 218
Hemorrhage 171
Hemorrhagic peds, large 174
Hemorrhagic retinopathy 48
Hepatitis C 46

Herpes simplex keratitis, classification of 13t
Herpes simplex virus 11-13, 15, 20, 46
   disease 12, 14
   infection 11
   keratitis 13, 15, 19
      prevention of recurrent 20
      risk factors for 14t
      type of 13
   vaccination 20
Herpetic endotheliitis 18
Herpetic eye disease 11
   study 11, 18
Herpetic retinochoroiditis 36
Herpetic uveitis 51
Hertle's criteria 243
Hilar lymphadenopathy
   bilateral 50, 51f
   chest X-ray-bilateral 50
HIV infection 14
Human central nervous system stem cells 165
Hyperdense serpiginous, abnormal 213f
Hyperglycemia, chronic 139
Hypertrophied feeding artery 226f
Hypopyon uveitis 43

I

Idiopathic intracranial hypertension 208, 211
Iluvien 154
Immune stressors 14
Immunity, altered 14
Immunosuppressive agents 280
Improvement in visual fields 211f
Incision lenticule extraction, small 2
Indocyanine green angiography 39, 171, 277
Induced pluripotent stem cells 165
Infantile nystagmus
   diagnostic criteria of 232t
   syndrome 231
Infection in ocular surgery, control of 125
Inflammatory cells, pearls of 270f
Inflammatory neovascular membrane 51
Inflammatory vitreous exudates 43
Intense pulsed light therapy 24
Intercellular adhesion molecule-1 5
Interdigitation zone 190
Inter-eye symmetry 68
Interferon- gamma release assays 36, 37, 41
Interferon-G 33
Interleukin 33, 275
International diagnosis of sarcoidosis 50t
Intra-arterial chemotherapy 198, 199f
Intracranial dural arteriovenous fistula 212

Intraocular
  cataract surgery, progress in 125
  fluids 118
  lenses 119, 189
  lymphoma, primary 51
  pressure 39, 40, 58, 86, 120, 121
    raised in 47
  retinoblastoma 195*t*
  tuberculosis 32, 37*t*
    classification of 41*t*
Intraretinal microvascular abnormality 142
Intravenous chemotherapy 197
Intravitreal 61
  antibiotics 103*f*
  anti-VEGFs 53
  chemotherapy 199
  clindamycin 62
  corticosteroid 154*t*
  dexamethasone 58
    implants 58
  drugs in endophthalmitis 104*t*
  fluocinolone acetonide 58
  ganciclovir 62
  immunosuppressives 60
  injections 56, 57, 151, 167
  methotrexate 60
  nonsteroidal anti-inflammatory drug 59
  steroids 151
  therapeutics in
    infectious uveitis 62
    noninfectious uveitis 56
    uveitis, advances in 56
  therapy 150
    current 155*t*
  triamcinolone acetonide 56, 57
  vancomycin 104*f*
Intravitreous triamcinolone acetonide 57, 155
Iris 47
  mass 47
Isoniazid 42

J

Joint involvement 267
Joubert syndrome 244
Juvenile rheumatoid arthritis in children 51

K

Keratitis, type of 19
Keratoconjunctivitis sicca 47
Keratolimbal allograft 26
Keratoprosthesis surgery 26, 27
Klebsiella pneumoniae 128

L

Lacrimal gland involvement 47
Lacrimal secretory 24
Lampalizumab 161
Laser flare photometry 277
Laser in situ keratomileusis 1, 2, 8, 14, 15
Laser refractive surgery of cornea 1
Laser source 93
Laser therapy 148
Latent nystagmus 237
Leber's congenital amaurosis 244
Leprosy 36
Leukocyte cystine levels 259
Lifitegrast 24
Light intensity 7
Light pollution 190
Light sensitivity 244
Light-emitting diodes 188
Limbal stem cell deficiency 26, 27, 27*f*, 28
  management of 26, 26*t*
Lipid control 147
Lipiflow 24
Lipopolysaccharide 113
Liver enzyme tests, abnormal 50
Lofgren's syndrome, acute 47
Low vision 244
Lung 46
LVP Keratoprosthesis 26
Lyme disease 51
Lymphocyte function-associated antigen 1 25
Lypoxygenase 141

M

Macular degeneration, age-related 57, 160, 170, 174, 189
Macular edema 139, 154, 281*f*
  diffuse 143
  type of 146, 146*f*
Macular ischemia 144, 144*f*, 269*f*
Macular phototoxicity 185
  acute 189
  chronic 189
  diagnosis of 189
Macular scar 273*f*
Macular swelling, causes of 145
Malignant melanoma lymphoma 36
Mantoux test 36, 37
Matrix metalloproteinase-9 24, 25
Mediastinal lymph nodes 46
Medications 119
Meibomian gland dysfunction 26
Meibomian glands 24
Meningeal artery, left middle 213*f*

Mesencephalon 243
Metaherpetic ulcer 16f
Metastatic disease 195
Metastatic tumor 36
Methotrexate 53
Microaneurysm 149
Microperimetry 146
Middle cerebral artery 225
Moderate myopia 3f
Moorfield's regression analysis 71, 73, 73t
Multicenter uveitis steroid treatment 58
Multidrug resistance TB 43
Multifocal chorioretinal lesions 48f
Multifocal choroiditis 36, 51
Multifocal placoid pigment epitheliopathy, acute posterior 36, 48
Multifocal serpiginoid choroiditis 40
Multiple lymph nodes 52f
Multiple sclerosis 51
Multi-resistant *Staphylococcus aureus* 134
Mutton fat keratic precipitates 47
MYC mutation 193
Mycobacterium tuberculosis 32, 36, 37, 46, 274
Mycophenolate mofetil 53
Myoclonic triangle 243
Myopathy 256
Myopia, changes in high 3f

N

Natural killer 275
Necrotizing keratitis 17
Needle-stick injury 130
Negative mantoux test 53
Negative tuberculin test 50
Nephropathic cystinosis 258f
Nerve fiber indicator 66, 68
Nerve fiber layer 78
Nerve growth factor 5
Neuro-Behçet's disease 263, 266
Neurology 257
Neuro-ophthalmic involvement 266
Neuroretinal rim 78
Neuroretinitis 35
Neurotrophic keratopathy 16
New anti-VEGF agents 166
New anti-VEGF drugs 165
Newer intravitreal antibiotics 113
Nitric oxide 141
Nodular periphlebitis 48
Nodule in trabecular meshwork 47
Nongranulomatous anterior uveitis 47
Non-infectious uveitis 56
Nonocular manifestations 264
Non-proliferative diabetic retinopathy 139, 142, 156
Nucleic acid amplification tests 38

Nystagmus 230, 239t, 242t, 244, 244t
    acuity function 240
        expanded 239
    classification of 239t
    interpretation of 236I
    pathophysiology of 235
    pharmacological treatment of 245
    surgical treatment of 250
    syndrome 234f
    types of 246t
        pathological 231t

O

Occipital arteriovenous malformation 224
Occipital artery 213f
Occult chroidal neovascular membrane 171
Ocular complications 51
    management of 280
Ocular conditions, abnormal 244t
Ocular disease 263
Ocular histopathology 276
Ocular HSV infection 12
Ocular hypertension treatment study 69
Ocular manifestations of Behçet's disease 267
Ocular media 188
Ocular recurrences 20
Ocular sarcoidosis 45, 47, 50
    diagnosis of 51
    prognosis of 54
Ocular surface
    disease 4
    disorders 29
        management of 24, 28
        treatment of 28t
    squamous neoplasia 28
Ocular tissues 32
Oculocutaneous albinism 234f
Ophthalmic artery 208
    infusion, selective 199
Ophthalmic disorders 206
Ophthalmic practice 132
Ophthalmic treatment 259
Ophthalmic vein
    left superior 219f
    superior 218, 219f, 221f, 222f
Ophthalmoscopic features 171
Optic atrophy 43
Optic disc 71
    edema 51
    granuloma 40
    neovascularization 51, 281
    size 71
Optic nerve 276
    head 66, 77f, 78f
        analysis 77

sarcoid granuloma 49*f*
involvement 36
Optic neuritis 43
Optic neuropathy 40
Optic OCT, adaptive 94
Optical coherence tomography 39, 65, 73, 74, 85, 145, 162, 171, 172, 239
    angiograms 95
    angiography 95, 146, 173
    role of 146*t*
Optical management of nystagmus 244, 244*t*
Optokinetic nystagmus 230
Oral
    acyclovir 18
    medication 148
    steroids 14*f*
    ulcers 263
Orbital retinoblastoma 202*f*
Organ transplant recipients 14
Oscillopsia 244
Ozurdex 154

P

Pain 120
Palsy 263
Panophthalmitis 36
Panretinal photocoagulation 156
Panuveitis 36
Pars plana vitrectomy 156
Pathergy test 267
Pazopanib 167
Periarteritis nodosa 278
Periocular Subtenon's chemotherapy 198
Periodic alternating nystagmus 238
Peripapillary atrophy 89*f*
Peripapillary nerve fiber layers 77*f*
Peripapillary splinter hemorrhages 43
Periphlebitis, acute 269
Peroxisomal disorders 244
Persistent fetal vasculature 196
Photic injury 185
Photodynamic therapy 175
Photomechanical injury 185
Photorefractive keratectomy 1, 5
Photothermal injuries 185
Phototoxic injury 185
Phototoxicity 186
Pigment epithelial
    derived factors 149
    detachments 172
Plaque brachytherapy 200
Plexiform layer, inner 78
Polarization sensitive optical coherence tomography 94
Polylactic acid-co-glycolic acid 59
Polypoidal choroidal
    neovascularisation 172
    vasculopathy 170, 174
        management of 175
Post-cataract
    acute 135
    chronic 135
    surgery 104
Posterior communicating artery 208, 224*f*
    aneurysm 223
Prednisolone acetate 122
Pre-perimetric glaucoma 87*f*
Presumed ocular sarcoidosis 50
Primitive neuroectodermal tumors 194
Probable ocular sarcoidosis 50
Proliferative diabetic retinopathy 139, 156
Prominent posterior hyaloids 270*f*
Prophylaxis 112, 129
Propionibacterium acnes 46, 109
Protein kinase C 140, 141
Pseudomonas
    aeruginosa 129
        strains 113
        endophthalmitis 114
Pulmonary function test 52
Pulmonary involvement 267
Pulmonary sarcoidosis 46
Punctate inner choroidopathy 36
Pupil 121
Pupillary nodules 47
Pyrazinamide 42

R

Radical vitrectomy with silicone oil 107*f*
Radiotherapy, external beam 200
Ranibizumab 150, 155
Rapamycin 162
RB1 gene 193
Reactive oxygen species 139
Rebamipide 24, 25
Recurrent keratitis 16
Recurrent polypoidal choroidal vasculo-pathy 180
Refractive error 244
Refractive lenticule extraction 2, 7
Refractive procedures, effect of 4*f*
Regenerative stem cell therapies 161
Relex smile 5, 7, 8
Renal 256
Renal biopsy, stain of 258*f*
Renal manifestations, extra 256
Rennin angiotensin system 141
Restore 150
Retina 276
Retinal detachment 51
Retinal disc neovascularization 51, 281

Retinal disease 189
Retinal edema pigmentary changes 43
Retinal ganglion cells 65
Retinal hemorrhages 268*f*, 269*f*
Retinal ischemia 51, 269*f*
Retinal laser therapy, selective 150
Retinal macroaneurysm 48
Retinal nerve fiber
   bundles 94
   layer 65, 67, 72, 75, 77
      analysis 75
      curvature 73
      thickness 66, 80
Retinal perivasculitis 40
Retinal pigment epithelial 94, 161, 273*f*
   changes 271*f*
Retinal pigment epithelium mottling 186
Retinal vasculitis 35
Retinitis 270
Retinoblastoma 36, 193, 196*f*, 202
   advanced 199*f*
   gene 193
   staging system for 195*t*
Retinovascular 143
Reverse staining pattern 16
Rifampicin 42
Right eye 202*f*
   perimetry 210*f*, 211*f*
Right ophthalmic segment aneurysm 217*f*
Right palpebral fissure, obliteration of 223*f*
Right transverse sinus 209*f*
Right vertebral artery 226*f*
RNA transcription 60
Rostaglandin analogs 14

S

Sarcoid nodule 49*f*
Sarcoidosis 36, 45, 47*t*, 50, 278*t*
   clinical signs of 50
   diagnosis of 51*t*
   posterior segment in 48*t*
   prevalence of 45
Scanning laser polarimetry 65, 81
Scleral buckling, posterior 209*f*
Segment invasion, anterior 201
Segmental periphlebitis 48
Serous exudation 171
Serous retinal detachment 176
Serpiginous choroiditis 36
Serpiginous-like choroiditis 34
Serum ace levels 50
Sexual transmission 262
Sigmoid sinus 209*f*
Simple limbal epithelial transplantation 26, 27
Sirolimus 161, 162

Skin
   disease 263
   lesions 264
Slit lamp
   biomicroscopy 132
   examination 119
Smile 1, 4-6, 8
   advantages of 4
   patients 4
   surgery, enhancements after 7
Snellen visual acuity 188*f*
Snowballs 48
Spasmus nutans syndrome 234, 235*f*
Spectacles 133
Spectral domain optical coherence tomography 190
Staphylococcus aureus 100, 128
Staphylococcus epidermidis 129
Staphylococcus infection, cycle of 128*f*
Stem cell therapy 165
Stereometric parameters 71
Steroids 165, 166
   intensive 102*f*
   response to 120
Stevens-Johnson syndrome 28
Stop-TB strategy 32
Strabismus 230
Streptococcus species 128
Strokes 263
Stromal keratitis 13, 17, 19
Subretinal abscess 35
Subretinal fluid 161
Subretinal haemorrhage, management of 178
Subretinal scarring 273*f*
Subthreshold micropulse laser 149
Sunlight 186
Superior petrosal sinus 221*f*
Supplements 189
Surgery, benefits of 248*t*
Surgical instruments 131*t*
Sustained drug-delivery devices 165, 167
Sustained release implants 151
Sustained release intravitreal implants 154
Sympathetic ophthalmia 36, 51
Synechiae, broad posterior 40
Syphilis 36, 51
Systemic immunosuppression 14
Systemic intravenous chemotherapy 197, 198*f*
Systemic lupus erythematosus 278
Systemic sarcoidosis 46

T

T cell ratio 46
Taut attached posterior hyaloid 145

T-cell predominance 276
Tear inflammatory mediators in smile 5
Tear meniscus height 4
Temporal arachnoid cyst 225f
Tent-shaped peripheral anterior synechiae 47
Thermal laser 175
Thiazolidinediones 141
Third generation laser refractive surgery 2
Thrombophlebitis 263
Time-domain technology 74
Tissue
 biopsy 53
 plasminogen activator 178
Tonometer prisms 132
Toxic anterior segment syndrome 100, 117
Toxic endothelial cell destruction syndrome 117
Toxocara species 129
Toxoplasma gondii 129
Toxoplasmosis 36, 51
Tractional macular edema 146f
Tractional retinal detachment 156
Traimcinolone 155
Transbronchial lung biopsy 53
Transpupillary thermotherapy 200
Transverse sinus 214f
 junction of right 209f
 left 213f
Triamcinolone acetonide 57, 151
TSNIT average 67
TSNIT standard deviation 68
TSNIT symmetry graph 67
Tubercular anterior uveitis 34f
Tubercular retinal vasculitis 35f
Tuberculin skin test 36, 37, 41
Tuberculoma 34
Tuberculosis 33, 33f, 41, 51
 diagnosis of 36t
Tumor necrosis factor alpha 5, 33, 275

U

Umbilical cord serum 29
United Kingdom Prospective Diabetes Study 147
Untreated retinoblastoma 197
Uvea 276
Uveitis 33, 56, 267, 273f
 anterior 33, 270f
 chronic posterior 273f
 compatible 50
 in immunocompetent 41
 intermediate 33, 47
 posterior 33, 271f
 severe acute anterior 43
 treatment, double-masked 61

V

Valacyclovir 20
Vancomycin 104
Vascular endothelial growth factor 58, 59, 141
 expression 56
 injections 161f
 threshold 156
Vascular network, branching 170, 172
Vascular occlusions 51, 265
Vasculitis 263, 265
Venous sinus 214f
Vermis, anterior 243
Vernal keratoconjunctivitis 28
Vertebral artery 207
 left 213f
Vestibular nucleus, superior 243
Vestibular nystagmus 230
Video nystagmography 239
Viscoelastic residues 118
Vision 120
 in Behçet's disease 282
 in left eye, blurred 34f
 loss, evaluate unexplained 145, 146
Visual acuity
 best corrected 101
 corrected distance 7
 reduction in 270f
Visual cycle modifying agents 161, 164
Visual fields 211f
Vitrectomy 155
Vitreo macular traction 146
Vitreous 120, 270f
 cytology 52
 hemorrhage 51, 281
 infiltrates 35
Vitritis 35, 269, 269f
Vogt-Koyanagi-Harada
 disease 36
 syndrome 51
Voriconazole 104

W

Wegener's granulomatosis 278
Welding arc 186
White reflex 196f

Z

Zimura 161, 162